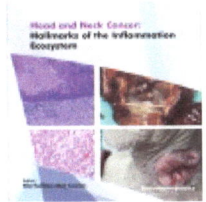

Head and Neck Cancer:
Hallmarks of the Inflammation
Ecosystem

Table of Contents

Frontiers in Inflammation

(Volume 2)

Head and Neck Cancer: Hallmarks of the Inflammation Ecosystem

Edited by

Norhafiza Mat Lazim
Department of Otorhinolaryngology-Head & Neck Surgery,
School of Medical Sciences,
Universiti Sains Malaysia,
Health Campus, Kubang Kerian,
Kelantan,
Malaysia

BENTHAM SCIENCE PUBLISHERS LTD.

End User License Agreement (for non-institutional, personal use)

This is an agreement between you and Bentham Science Publishers Ltd. Please read this License Agreement carefully before using the ebook/echapter/ejournal (**"Work"**). Your use of the Work constitutes your agreement to the terms and conditions set forth in this License Agreement. If you do not agree to these terms and conditions then you should not use the Work.

Bentham Science Publishers agrees to grant you a non-exclusive, non-transferable limited license to use the Work subject to and in accordance with the following terms and conditions. This License Agreement is for non-library, personal use only. For a library / institutional / multi user license in respect of the Work, please contact: permission@benthamscience.net.

Usage Rules:

misuse of the Work or any violation of this License Agreement, including any infringement by you of copyrights or proprietary rights.

Disclaimer:

Bentham Science Publishers does not guarantee that the information in the Work is error-free, or warrant that it will meet your requirements or that access to the Work will be uninterrupted or error-free. The Work is provided "as is" without warranty of any kind, either express or implied or statutory, including, without limitation, implied warranties of merchantability and fitness for a particular purpose. The entire risk as to the results and performance of the Work is assumed by you. No responsibility is assumed by Bentham Science Publishers, its staff, editors and/or authors for any injury and/or damage to persons or property as a matter of products liability, negligence or otherwise, or from any use or operation of any methods, products instruction, advertisements or ideas contained in the Work.

Limitation of Liability:

In no event will Bentham Science Publishers, its staff, editors and/or authors, be liable for any damages, including, without limitation, special, incidental and/or consequential damages and/or damages for lost data and/or profits arising out of (whether directly or indirectly) the use or inability to use the Work. The entire liability of Bentham Science Publishers shall be limited to the amount actually paid by you for the Work.

General:

1. Any dispute or claim arising out of or in connection with this License Agreement or the Work (including non-contractual disputes or claims) will be governed by and construed in accordance with the laws of Singapore. Each party agrees that the courts of the state of Singapore shall have exclusive jurisdiction to settle any dispute or claim arising out of or in connection with this License Agreement or the Work (including non-contractual disputes or claims).
2. Your rights under this License Agreement will automatically terminate without notice and without the need for a court order if at any point you breach any terms of this License Agreement. In no event will any delay or failure by Bentham Science Publishers in enforcing your compliance with this License Agreement constitute a waiver of any of its rights.
3. You acknowledge that you have read this License Agreement, and agree to be bound by its terms and conditions. To the extent that any other terms and conditions presented on any website of Bentham

Science Publishers conflict with, or are inconsistent with, the terms and conditions set out in this License Agreement, you acknowledge that the terms and conditions set out in this License Agreement shall prevail.

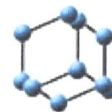

Bentham   Science   Publishers   Pte.   Ltd.
80   Robinson   Road
Singapore   #02-00
Singapore   068898
Email: subscriptions@benthamscience.net

**BENTHAM
SCIENCE**

FOREWORD

It is a privilege to foreword this research book which is unique in ways more than one. I congratulate Assoc. Prof. Norhafiza Mat Lazim for her great initiative in conceptualizing this book. This book is in the arena of uncharted territory which will, in years to come, demand more attention and work. Assoc. Prof. Norhafiza Mat Lazim has shown that path into future thinking for all of us in this book.

The book offers several chapters in a systemic way written by competent authorities in their area of work.

We are increasingly aware that there are biomarkers which almost define the biological behavior of the tumor. This biomarker is used in diagnostic workup as detailed in the book which will guide the treatment planning. The book also deals with the detection of other virological markers which will help to prevent and plan surgical/radiation therapy.

The relation between the inflammatory process and malignancy is beautifully mentioned in the chapters. Prof. Norhafiza Mat Lazim has clarified the cascade of chemical reactions in inflammation and malignancy. She has driven similarities and conclusions. In her words, she has an opened a window of opportunity to control/treat head and neck cancer by intervening biochemically at these cascades. This philosophy of drawing parallels in inflammation and malignancy reflects through this book. Author compels us to revisit and strategize our treatment policies by studying the micro-environment, a complex ecosystem.

I wish Prof. Norhafiza Mat Lazim great success not only with this book but also for her in future in this new philosophy of micro-environment and complex eco system of the cancer cells. I also acknowledge the great contribution of all other contributory authors. I am sure this book will make very interesting reading and open a window of sort.

Madan Kapre
Neeti Clinics Pvt. Ltd.
Neeti Gaurav Complex; 21
Nagpur – 440010
Maharashtra
India

Foreword by Naoki Otsuki

I am honored to write a foreword to the publication of this wonderful book. First of all, I would like to congratulate Assoc. Prof. Norhafiza Mat Lazim for making this book. I met Assoc. Prof. Lazim at the same session at the 2017 ASHNO conference in Bali, Indonesia. She presented the results of her basic research at this session. At this time, I found out that she was not only an excellent head and neck surgeon, but also an outstanding scientist in basic research on head and neck cancer. Two years later, I heard about a plan to publish a book on inflammation ecosystem in head and neck cancer, and now we have a wonderful and unique book like this.

Physiological inflammation is one of the body's initial immune defenses against infection and tissue damage. Researchers have previously identified that inflammation is frequently associated with tumor progression, but the underlying mechanisms to contribute to proinflammatory tumorigenesis are not fully understood. Much evidence has emerged regarding the infiltration of inflammatory cells into tissues and their contribution to the deleterious alterations of DNA, RNA, proteins, lipids, and metabolites in the local tissue microenvironment of chemical mediators.

In this book, based on the knowledge about the inflammatory ecosystem that has been obtained in the area of head and neck cancer, risk factors in development, diagnostic tools, biomarkers, the role of inflammation in the microenvironment associated with treatment, and tumor-related factors as therapeutic targets are also mentioned. This book brings new research into inflammatory ecosystems to significant progress in developing, diagnosing, and treating head and neck cancer.

Finally, I wish Professor Lazim a success in future, who has made a generous contribution to this book's production, and I would like to thank all other contributory authors who wrote this book.

Naoki Otsuki
Faculty of Medicine
Department of Otolaryngology
Kindai University Osaka-sayama
Japan

PREFACE

The idea for this research book 'Head and Neck Cancer and Hallmark of Inflammation ecosystem' was cultivated during an assembly with the international experts at one of Academy of Science Malaysia scientific events. This research book aims to highlight the significant roles of inflammation in head and neck malignancy. This entails the screening, diagnosis, treatment as well as follow-up schemes of head and neck cancer patients. Now, we know that the inflammation is the 7th hallmark of malignancy, and it has intimate relationship with the development and promotion of carcinogenesis, dictates the behaviour of cancer and may responsible for recurrent and metastatic disease.

Inflammation is significant, and the scope of this book is wide and encompasses all critical issues faced by clinicians, researchers, students, and other health-related personnel in managing head and neck malignancies. The book provides details on inflammation and its interaction in an ecosystem. Myriads of newly emerging inflammatory markers are interacting within a cohesive system in promoting carcinogenesis, tumour recurrent and metastases. Understanding these exquisite roles of inflammation may also serve for the development of potent therapeutic agents at the near future.

The chapters are nicely arranged with a start on a description of head and neck malignancy and its' types, followed by the risk factors where roles of inflammation in discovered and discussed in great depth. The inflammatory markers that are commonly studied which involved in the pathogenesis of head and neck malignancy are elaborated. Roles of specific inflammatory markers, especially in patient's stratification, prognosis, and survival, are pivotal, hence deserve critical attention from the scientific community.

I would like to express my deepest gratitude to Ms. Fariya Zulfiqar for her continuous commitment and dedicated work as well as to all managing team at *Bentham Science* for their relentless support. This book will be a great addition to current scientific literature on head and neck malignancy, especially in relation to the significant roles of inflammation.

Norhafiza Mat Lazim
Department of Otorhinolaryngology-Head & Neck Surgery
School of Medical Sciences, Universiti Sains Malaysia
Health Campus, 16150, Kubang Kerian
Kelantan, Malaysia

List of Contributors

Anani Aila Mat Zin	Department of Pathology, School of Medical Science, Universiti Sains Malaysia, Health Campus 16150, Kubang Kerian, Kelantan, Malaysia
Baharudin Abdullah	Department of Otorhinolaryngology-Head and Neck Surgery, School of Medical Sciences, Universiti Sains Malaysia, Health Campus 16150, Kubang Kerian, Kelantan, Malaysia
Belayat H Siddiquee	Department of Otolaryngology-Head and Neck Surgery, Bangabandhu Sheikh Mujib Medical University (BSMMU), Dhaka-1000, Bangladesh
Carlo Cavaliere	Scientific Institute for Research, Hospitalization and Healthcare - IRCCS, SDN, Naples, Italy
Gabriela Ramírez Arroyo	Otolaryngology–Head and Neck Surgery Department, Instituto Nacional de Rehabilitación, Luis Guillermo Ibarra Ibarra, Mexico City, Mexico
Giacomo Spinato	Depatment of Neurosciences, Section of Otolaryngology and Regional Centre for Head and Neck Cancer, University of Padova, Treviso, Italy Department of Surgery, Oncology and Gastroenterology, Section of Oncology and Immunology, University of Padova, Treviso, Italy
Giuseppe Azzarello	Oncology and hematology department, ULSS 3 Serenissima, Mirano Hospital, Venice, Italy
Jose Gutiérrez Jodas	Department of Otorhinolaryngology-Head and Neck Surgery, Hospital Universitario Reina Sofia, Cordoba, Spain, Avenida Menendez Pidal, Cordoba, Spain
Juan Carlos Hernaiz-Leonardo	Otolaryngology–Head and Neck Surgery Department, Instituto Nacional de Rehabilitación, Luis Guillermo Ibarra Ibarra, Mexico City, Mexico
Liberatore Tramontano	Scientific Institute for Research, Hospitalization and Healthcare - IRCCS, SDN, Naples, Italy
Marco Salvatore	Scientific Institute for Research, Hospitalization and Healthcare - IRCCS, SDN, Naples, Italy
Mario	Otolaryngology–Head and Neck Surgery Department, Instituto

Sergio Dávalos-Fuentes — Nacional de Rehabilitación, Luis Guillermo Ibarra Ibarra, Mexico City, Mexico

Maria Cristina Da Mosto — Depatment of Neurosciences, Section of Otolaryngology and Regional Centre for Head and Neck Cancer, University of Padova, Treviso, Italy

Michelle Marvin Huergo — Otolaryngology–Head and Neck Surgery Department, Instituto Nacional de Rehabilitación, Luis Guillermo Ibarra Ibarra, Mexico City, Mexico

Norhafiza Mat Lazim — Department of Otorhinolaryngology-Head and Neck Surgery, School of Medical Sciences, Universiti Sains Malaysia, Health Campus, Kubang Kerian 16150, Kelantan, Malaysia

Paolo Boscolo Rizzo — Depatment of Neurosciences, Section of Otolaryngology and Regional Centre for Head and Neck Cancer, University of Padova, Treviso, Italy

Rohaizam Japar Jaafar — Hospital Sultanah Bahiyah, Alor Setar, Kedah, Malaysia

Roman Carlos Zamora — Department of Otorhinolaryngology-Head and Neck Surgery, Hospital Universitario Reina Sofia, Cordoba, Spain, Avenida Menendez Pidal, Cordoba, Spain

Samuele Frasconi — Depatment of Neurosciences, Section of Otolaryngology and Regional Centre for Head and Neck Cancer, University of Padova, Treviso, Italy

Sharifah Emilia Tuan Sharif — Department of Pathology, School of Medical Science, Universiti Sains Malaysia, Health Campus 16150, Kubang Kerian, Kelantan, Malaysia

Simonetta Ausoni — Department of Biomedical Sciences, University of Padua, Padua, Italy

Zakinah Yahaya — Hospital Kuala Lumpur, Kuala Lumpur, Malaysia

Zulkifli Yusof — Hospital Sultanah Bahiyah, Alor Setar, Kedah, Malaysia

Introduction to Inflammation Ecosystem in Head and Neck Cancer

Norhafiza Mat Lazim*

Department of Otorhinolaryngology-Head and Neck Surgery, School of Medical Sciences, Universiti Sains Malaysia, Health Campus 16150, Kubang Kerian, Kelantan, Malaysia

Abstract

Head and neck cancer is on the rise around the globe. At present, the disease affects both the elderly and younger patient populations. This type of cancer is significant as it involves crucial anatomic regions of the head and neck, which are vital for breathing, mastication, swallowing, speech, and olfaction. The treatment options for head and neck malignancies are mainly surgery and chemoradiation, depending on the stage of the tumors. Inflammation plays an important role, and it has a strong relationship with the risk factors, assessment, and treatment of head and neck cancer. Multiple risk factors for head and neck squamous cell carcinoma like smoking, alcohol, viruses, chemicals, and foods have some elements of inflammation that play a dominant role in promoting and sustaining carcinogenesis. The inflammation cascades are complex, and multiple factors cohesively interact within the microenvironment that eventually leads to carcinogenesis, tumor recurrence, and metastasis. Recent evidence suggests that numerous anti-inflammatory biomarkers have effective therapeutic roles in the management of head and neck cancer. This chapter highlights the prominent relationship and interaction that exists between head and neck cancer and inflammation, not only in its etiopathogenesis but also in the assessment and overall management approaches. The significant focus is on the role of inflammatory agents that contribute to the process of carcinogenesis, as well as discussion on several significant inflammatory markers and molecules which may serve as a potential effective target for personalized treatment in head and neck cancer management armamentarium in the near future.

Keywords: Anti-inflammation, Carcinogenesis, Chemoradiation, Epstein Barr viruses, Head and neck cancer, Immunomodulation, Loco-regional recurrence, Malignancy, Metastases, Nasopharyngeal carcinoma, Oncogenic viruses, Oncologic surgery.

---

* **Corresponding author Norhafiza Mat Lazim:** Department of Otorhinolaryngology-Head and Neck Surgery, School of Medical Sciences, Universiti Sains Malaysia, Health Campus 16150, Kubang Kerian, Kelantan, Malaysia;
Tel: +60199442664, +6097676418, Fax: +6097676424; E-mail: norhafiza@usm.my

INTRODUCTION

At this juncture, the incidence of head and neck malignancy has shown an increasing trend, approaching similar incidence with lung and colon cancers globally. In our practice, we observed that not only the middle-aged and elderly populations are affected by the disease, but also the trend is on the rise in pediatric patients. The types of head and neck malignancy include an oral cavity carcinoma, oropharyngeal carcinoma, salivary glands carcinoma, thyroid carcinoma, sinonasal carcinoma, nasopharyngeal carcinoma, temporal bone tumors, soft tissues sarcomas, and laryngeal carcinoma. The most common histopathology of head and neck cancers is squamous cell carcinoma. Certain types of head and neck squamous cell carcinoma (HNSCC) are prevalent in specific geographic locations. For instance, nasopharyngeal carcinoma is common in China, Taiwan, Hong Kong, and South East Asia region, whereas oral and oropharyngeal carcinoma is prevalent in Europe, India, Middle East, and several other Western countries.

There are multiple identified risk factors for HNSCC, which include smoking, alcohol consumption, viral infections, dietary habits, chemicals, and other environmental pollutants. These so-called inflammation-associated molecules commonly acting in concert with the presence of other environmental and lifestyle-related co-factors promote carcinogenesis. These factors include sedentary lifestyles, stress, home environment, obesity, self-hygiene, and genetics, which together are thought to drive as much as 90% of all cancers [1]. In addition, selected endogenous and exogenous stimuli might lead to various genetic mutations and modulations, which can serve as a possible trigger for the tumor of the head and neck [2]. Certain head and neck cancer only take a short duration, *i.e.*, 5 to 10 years, to develop, whereas others appear in a case with long-standing head and neck masses of more than 20 years.

Clinical presentation of patients with head and neck cancer varies, and it depends on the patient's age, duration of symptoms, size of the mass, the location involved, presence or absence of distant metastases, and patient's comorbidities. Generally, a patient will present with a progressive mass or swelling at the head and neck region that causes constant pain or bleeding associated with reduced appetite and significant weight loss. Other associated symptoms will depend on the location of the mass. For instance, suspicious cancerous mass in the nasal cavity may cause epistaxis, mass in the nasopharynx may cause hearing complaints, mass in the oropharynx area may cause dysphagia and odynophagia, and so forth. The other symptoms such as cranial nerve involvement, pulmonary symptoms, or bony tenderness may present in aggressive and late-stage diseases.

Imperatively, the majority of patient presents at late-stage diseases, where the treatment is more challenging, and multimodality therapy is required.

The malignancy around the head and neck region deserves greater attention as it involves important anatomic regions that are crucial for breathing, speech, mastication, swallowing, hearing, olfaction, and vision. Preserving all the structures is paramount to maintain the function of all organs within the head and neck region, to ensure the patient's daily functioning and quality of life are maintained. To illustrate, for instance, facial nerve paralysis that is caused by malignant infiltrative parotid malignancy can cause significant social embarrassment and affect a patient's social interaction and integration within the community due to facial disfigurement. Thus, it is equally crucial to understand the true biology of head and neck malignancy and its sequelae in order to provide finesse care for these subsets of patients.

More than a century ago, Rudolf Virchow proposed the connection between inflammation and cancer, who found the infiltration of leukocytes in malignant tissues [3]. He noted leukocytes in the neoplastic tissue and indicated that the lymphocytic infiltrate might represent cancer origin at chronic inflammatory sites. From this evidence and documentation, there was a surge in the literature that reveals the association of inflammation in cancer formation as well as its roles in cancer therapeutics. Numerous studies have been performed to assess in-depth the relation of inflammatory cascades in the etiopathogenesis, risk factors, therapeutic and sequelae of procedures, and overall treatment in head and neck malignancy.

At this juncture, numerous studies include experimental, clinical, and epidemiological studies have revealed that chronic inflammation significantly contributes to carcinogenesis and cancer progression and predisposes to the occurrence of different types of human cancers [3]. Cancer-related inflammation is considered to be the seventh hallmark of cancer, according to Bonomi *et al.,* and numerous scientific researches have shown that the tumors develop and evolve in and from inflammatory diseases [4]. Imperatively, the steps of carcinogenesis always involve an inflammatory process as the initial step. The primary insult results in inflammation at the very beginning before other reactionary cascades coming in and subsequently promote the carcinogenesis and its sequelae.

INFLAMMATION AND CANCER

The strong relationship and interaction that exist between cancer and inflammation are evident not only in the etiopathogenesis of head and neck cancer but also in investigative procedures, assessment tools, and treatment strategies that take place during head and neck cancer management. The process of carcinogenesis and its progression are dependent on multiple important factors involving the tumor microenvironment and surrounding cells that, most of the time, are not cancerous themselves. Multiple inflammatory cascades, mediators, and inflammatory markers are interrelated and highly interactive within a cohesive inflammation ecosystem. Imperatively, these molecules and markers are able to influence, with a switch on and switch off mechanism, and *via* these, they are able to stimulate or dampen the effects of other tumor microenvironment factors, which finally will result in carcinogenesis.

Chronic inflammation induces different forms of nucleic acid, protein, and lipid damage through the production of reactive oxygen species, which has resulted in tissue damage. Tissue injury can also activate progenitor and stem cells to facilitate regeneration of the tissue. As such, stem cells are damaged by reactive oxygen species that is produced by inflammation, and the resulting mutations can accumulate over time, leading to cancerous stem cells [5]. For instance, in the case of periodontitis where significant inflammation has been shown to have a strong relationship with the development of oral cavity carcinoma. Of note, periodontitis induces a persistent inflow into the saliva of bacterial and inflammatory markers within the oral cavity and the blood to a lesser extent due to the systemic spread of the diseases [6]. Periodontal bacterial and inflammatory cytokines migrate from affected tissues to the neighbouring anatomic regions and distant sites with saliva and blood. Studies from Tezal *et al.* suggested that oral premalignant tumours, tongue carcinoma, and human papillomavirus (HPV) related tongue base and oropharyngeal tumours may be associated with chronic periodontitis [6, 7]. Additionally, another study by Rezal *et al.* reported that periodontitis as a chronic inflammatory condition could be associated with HPV positivity of HNSCC. There was a greater strength of this association among patients with oropharyngeal squamous cell carcinoma (OPSCC) than those with laryngeal and oral cavity carcinomas [7]. Currently, it is known that tongue base tumor and other oropharyngeal subsites tumor are strongly associated with HPV [8, 9]. Importantly, the HPV positivity determines the prognosis and treatment outcomes of these subsets of patients.

Another study by Murata *et al.* examined the stemness markers in human nasopharyngeal carcinoma tissues. They performed an immunohistochemical assessment of cells that were derived from the cancer tissues and revealed that in the positive cancer cells, the development of a nitroguanidine inflammation-specific DNA lesion marker was observed. Further flow cytometric analysis revealed positive cells in a human nasopharyngeal carcinoma cell line population. This highlights the importance of nitroguanidine formation, which is derived from inflammation cascade in nasopharyngeal cancer stem cells [5].

The other important role that we need to consider is immunomodulation. The role of immunomodulation is crucial in carcinogenesis and its progress and advancement. Immune cell infiltration facilitates the tumor progression through multiple factors and substances produced that mitigate carcinogenesis, and importantly it enables the tumors to escape immune response from the host. Interesting molecules like cytokines, chemokines, and growth factors all play key roles in inflammation and cancer through the promotion of proliferation, angiogenesis, and carcinogenesis [4]. Immunomodulation and inflammation are the key elements in therapeutic strategies applied to combat head and neck cancer.

Cancer initiation and growth are also closely related to angiogenesis. In clinical practice, a mass that is highly vascularized is likely to be associated with malignancy. These feeding vessels secrete and produce arrays of substances to maintain the viability of the cancer cells. Such substances include macrophages, peptides, erythrocytes, cytokines, and many more that play multiple crucial roles in the tumor microenvironment. Macrophage infiltration is a dramatic and natural characteristic of inflammation, angiogenesis, and cancer and has been recently emphasized in an effort to establish selected potent new cancer treatment strategies [10]. A reactive stroma with an excess of inflammatory mediators and leukocytes, dysregulated vessels, and proteolytic enzymes characterize the microenvironment of solid tumors [11]. With the technological advancement and refined techniques, multiple arrays of agents, biomarkers, molecules, and extracts can be further assessed and tested as effective, promising roles not only in the application of cancer therapeutics but also in cancer prophylactics. Recently, the emergence of high-quality scientific literature and research have lucidly illustrated the role of anti-inflammatory biomarkers as potential effective antitumorigenic agents.

INFLAMMATION ECOSYSTEM AND CARCINOGENESIS

Generally, as aforementioned, infectious agents, dietary patterns, and environmental factors are responsible for the global cancer burden. This is true not only for head and neck malignancy but also for other significant human malignancies like lung, breast, renal, brain, and gastrointestinal malignancies. Generally, as everybody is aware, inflammation is the major component of these infectious agents and environmental factors that form the initial insults to the mucosa and cause a subsequent chain reaction, the release of mediators and cascades that lead to carcinogenesis. The process involved is complex and requires many factors and co-factors that are derived from systemic circulation or exogenously from the environmental stimuli.

Acute inflammation usually protects against infectious agents, while chronic inflammation exaggerates the mechanism of infection. The chronic inflammation of the tissue and DNA, which includes genetic and epigenetic changes, leads to the formation of cancer, such as squamous cell carcinoma of the head and neck. This chronic infection is associated with the derangement of vital intracellular and cellular processes. Noteworthy, this persistent inflammation may trigger irreparable tissue damage and significant changes in the inflammatory cells and cytokines contained in the tumor microenvironment. For instance, Krüger *et al.* documented that oral squamous cell carcinoma (OCSCC) is promoted by chronic inflammation either due to traumatic ulceration or periodontitis [12]. Indeed, the trauma and ulceration due to sharp tooth is a well-known risk factor for OCSCC. Premalignant lesion progression to OCSCC is a multi-step process and complicated. In this case, chronic oral cavity species, the microbiota *P. gingivalis* triggers enzymatic changes that will eventually increase a complex cellular invasion and promote the formation of OCSCC. Sequentially, these changes facilitate the eventual production of tumors into a highly malignant oral cavity carcinoma phenotype.

Chronic inflammation is known to be associated with an increased incidence of human malignancy. This chronic inflammation can be induced by chemical and physical agents, autoimmune state, infectious agents, radiation, and dietary components [13]. The ties between chronic inflammation and cancer in different species can be confirmed by clinical, epidemiological and animal studies. Cervical cancer, colorectal cancer, pancreatic cancer, skin cancer, esophageal cancer, and liver cancer are some of the most significant examples where carcinogenesis is initiate by inflammation [14]. Increased production of pro-inflammatory mediators, like cytokines and chemokines, reactive oxygen intermediates, increased expression of oncogenes, cyclo-oxygenase-2 (COX-2), 5-lipoxygenase (5-LOX) and matrix metalloproteinases (MMPs) are the molecular mechanisms by which chronic inflammation drives cancer initiation and promotion. Other important factors involved include nuclear factor κB (NF-κB), activator of transcription 3 (STAT3), and hypoxia-inducible factor1α (HIF-1α) that mediate tumor formation, metastasis, and chemoradioresistance [1].

In carcinogenesis and tumor development, chronic inflammation is a significant occurrence and it has been regarded as the seventh distinctive sign of cancer. Macrophages, dendritic cells, and lymphocytes are established inflammatory cells of a tumor microenvironment. Cancer stem cells are seen as the seed of cancer. Recently, chronic inflammation has been shown to modulate the survival of cancer stem cells. Huang *et al.,* stated that the activation of inflammasome NLP3 was linked with cancer genesis and progression in many cancers, and the role of inflammasome NLRP3 was found to be specific to the tissues of different cancers. Of note, they stressed that head and neck squamous cell carcinoma is inflammation-related cancer [15]. Latest evidence has emerged that showed most tumor formation is associated with dysregulated inflammation. The molecular pathways of inflammation and cancer are uncovered by numerous recent studies. The discovery of transcription factors such as and their gene products has provided the molecular basis for the decisive role of inflammation in carcinogenesis [16]. Cancer-associated inflammation includes leukocyte infiltration and cytokine expression along with active tissue remodeling and neo-angiogenesis [3]. Reactive oxygen species damage biomacromolecules including DNA, proteins, and lipids, in the inflammatory microenvironment. Inflammatory factors recruit inflammatory cells to induce the cytokines. Superoxide is generated by NADH oxidase and inducible nitric oxide synthase (iNOS) in inflammatory and epithelial cells [5]. This superoxide possessed numerous abilities and interfere with the tissue's inflammatory activity that worsens the carcinogenesis.

The primary component of tumor infiltrates is tumor-associated macrophages (TAMs), and it is derived from circulating monocytic precursors. Chemoattracting cytokines such as chemokines direct associated macrophages into the tumor cells. TAM survivals are prolonged by colony stimulating factors. With specific activation, TAM able to kill the tumor cells or initiate destructive tissues reactions that centered on the endothelium of the involved vessels [13]. Most malignant tumors are known to contain macrophages as major tumor microenvironmental stromal cells. TAMs are modified in the tumor environment, unlike macrophages in normal tissue, with some losing the ability to phagocytize or present tumor antigens to T-cells. TAMs harbor two distinct antitumor activity phenotypes [17]. These multiple roles of macrophages are essential in the malignancy development to sustain a viable cohesive microenvironment.

INFLAMMATION AND ASSOCIATION WITH GENETIC CHANGES

Chronic inflammation promotes cancer initiation and progression. Chronic inflammation, based on recent studies, can increase mutagenic DNA lesions through the generation of ROS/RNS and can promote proliferation for tissue regeneration *via* stem cell activation. ROS and RNS are able to cause damage to different cellular components, including nucleic acids, proteins, and lipids. Multiple sources generate ROS, including inflammatory cells, carcinogenic chemicals, and their metabolites. ROS can cause formation of oxidative DNA lesion products [18]. ROS may induce the formation of mutagenic DNA oxidative lesion products [19]. This is the stepping-stone that lead to accumulated tissue damages, which persistent leads to malignancy development.

Different studies have shown that epigenetic changes might culminate in an epigenetic translation that transforms premalignant cells into tumor cells or invasive tumor cells and thus, promotes metastasis. An initiating event, which can be inflammation, is required by epigenetic switches. In addition, this switch is induced and maintained by DNA methylation and histone modifications [20]. Accumulating evidence has shown that epigenetic silencing plays an important role in carcinogenesis through the downregulation of tumor suppression genes and microRNAs. Exposure to ROS or pro-inflammatory cytokines like interleukin 6 in the inflammatory microenvironment results in increased DNA methylation of the tumor suppressor and microRNAs [5]. DNA hypermethylation has been associated with multiple head and neck malignancies including salivary glands carcinoma, laryngeal carcinoma, and OCSCC.

INTRATUMOURAL HETEROGENEITY

Significant evidence highlights that intratumoral heterogeneity between malignant and non-malignant cells and their interactions within the microenvironment of the tumor are critical to various aspects of tumor biology. Great advancement has been made in the study of intra-tumoral heterogeneity that can foster the knowledge of cancer and its carcinogenesis. Indeed, intra-tumoral heterogeneity represents a major challenge in oncology. There are various intra-tumoral heterogeneity sources that intermingle and point to its importance in the tumor microenvironment. In a micro-environment, tumor cells consist of stromal cells such as cancer-associated fibroblasts (CAFs), immune cells, and endothelial cells. Each of those cell types plays an active role in the proliferation of tumor cells. CAFs, for example, may release growth factors that are obtained in cancer cells and function to signal them. It is essential that an established malignant tumor's immune compartment is collectively immunosuppressive [21].

Besides common metabolic reprogramming routes in malignant cells, metabolism is also influenced by placement, degree of micronutrient supply, and interactions with other adjacent cells. It is vital to investigate the segment of cellular metabolism that are affected by these humoral factors. In order to identify major players to this metabolic heterogeneity in the malignant cells, many researchers have subsequently demonstrated the pivotal role of selected biomarkers in cancer-related immune response [21]. Among emerging technologies, RNA-sequencing technique has assisted in highlighting the new drug resistance programs, and specific types of immune infiltration that are highly relevant to tumor biology and management inclusive those for diagnostic and therapeutic approach [22].

MACROPHAGES AND ITS ROLES IN INFLAMMATION ECOSYSTEM

TAMs are the principal player that connect inflammation to the development of malignancy. They are the activated macrophages that are recruited to facilitate and promote carcinogenesis process in cancer related ecospheres. Numerous evidences showed that in the tumor ecospheres, TAMs have numerous functions in facilitation of the tumor growth which includes matrix proteases and growth factors expression, adaptive immunity suppression and promoting the angiogenesis [3, 23]. All of these secreted substances play dominant roles in producing desired and controlled effects by cancer cells in a complex manner. A study by Ono *et al.*, reported that macrophages invade the tissue in response to inflammation and release and yield cytokines and angiogenic factors, for instance, matrix metalloproteinases, vascular endothelial growth factor, interleukin-8, and reactive oxygen species. In addition, inflammatory markers including interleukin and cytokines able to enhance tumor proliferation and vascularization with activation and stimulation of macrophages [10].

Another dominant role of TAM is highlighted by a study by Kimura *et al.*, who investigated the roles of macrophages activation in cancer formation and neovascularization in response to interleukin production. Their results showed that recruitment of the macrophages into tumors by monocytes, activated proteins and other chemokines may play a crucial role in promoting tumor formation and neoangiogenesis, through cancer cells interactions which is mediated by inflammatory markers [24]. Angiogenesis is crucial for the restoration of cancer cell viability and survival. Other vital factors and protein also secreted by TAMs that can strongly influence the process of infiltration and metastases. TAMs, neutrophils and mast cells have been shown to produce proteases during experimental carcinogenesis. TAMs also secrete angiogenic and growth factors and enzymic proteases that denuded the extracellular matrix. Subsequently, TAMs can activate tumor cell progression, facilitate angiogenesis and promote invasion, infiltration and metastases [13]. These significant roles of TAMs can be exploited in the quest for novel therapeutic markers in the coming years.

Of note, during the inflammation process, the extracellular matrix is altered which have important sequelae. This altered extracellular matrix provides structural support for the tumor development and progression. In cancers, hypoxia is a common phenomenon and inflamed tissues can result in damage to DNA which sequentially leads to tumorigenic events. In tumor microenvironment, vascularization of tissues plays critical roles by providing nutrients, oxygen, growth factors to the active dividing cells and this serves as a mechanism for metastases [4]. The hypoxia is another promising target that can be used to alter cancer biology and its capacity to spread. In the coming years, with the advancement of the molecular work, productive research and clinical trial, it is highly possible to generate a novel agent as cancer-hypoxia targeting agent that combat cancer progression at the very early phase during its process.

Additionally, another factor such as the migration inhibitory factor (MIF), which is derived from the T-cell, has the ability to inhibit the migration of macrophages. Interestingly, the molecule was proved to be secreted by many cells which includes lymphocytes, eosinophils, and macrophages. Evidences showed that MIF belongs to proinflammatory protein group [25]. Further studies have demonstrated that MIF involves in the carcinogenesis and tumors formation including HNSCC. It has pleiotropic roles in modulating hypoxia and angiogenesis that can regulate the HNSCC cells proliferation, invasion, apoptosis, and metastases. Importantly, MIF levels are found to be higher in HNSCC patients, and the expression of MIF can be used for prediction of clinical outcomes of these selected patient's category [25]. This is another critical biomarker that can be further explore in tumor microenvironment and future studies will enable the development and expansion of effective therapeutic agents based on these unprecedented findings.

RISK FACTORS OF HEAD AND NECK MALIGNANCY AND ROLE OF INFLAMMATION

The bio-mechanism of the relationship of chronic inflammation with cancer has been extensively discussed but continues to evolve, as both inflammation and cancer are complex processes controlled by a wide range of driving forces. Inflammation is the primary insult that progress and alters the microenvironment and subsequently result in carcinogenesis. Acute inflammation does not relate to the carcinogenesis, but chronic inflammation does. As highlighted previously, many human malignancies have been closely associated with chronic inflammation such as colonic carcinoma with colitis, bronchogenic carcinoma with bronchitis, cervical carcinoma with chronic infection with human papilloma virus (HPV) and so forth. In the surrounding epithelial cells, viruses, pollutants, bacterial products, including endotoxins, enzymes and metabolic byproducts, are able to cause genetic and epigenetic changes. They also have capacity to increase carcinogenic acetaldehydes and nitrosamines. Significant cells for instance monocytes, lymphocytes, fibroblasts, and epithelial cells, produce cytokines, growth factors and prostaglandins in respond to activation by bacteria. All these factors are vital for cell proliferation, angiogenesis and migrations [14]. In addition, the epithelial cells drive the mutation accumulation which flourish under the positive microenvironment influence.

Noteworthy, it is important to understand the process that occurs between chronic inflammation and malignancy development. An association between chronic inflammation and HPV infection is important to be understand as it is critical for cancer progression. The HPV enters through a breach in the mucosa and consequently infects basal cells of the epithelium. Subsequently, basal cell proliferation occurs with the virus replicates simultaneously. These lead to mucosal damage, micro-ulcerations, and consequent epithelial proliferation mediated by inflammatory cytokines released from inflamed sites. Additionally, in this inflammatory environment, the risk of HPV transmission is high as due to increase number of virus particle produced [7]. There have been many studies that validate the association between infection and chronic inflammation that transgress into malignant cervical cancer. Vaccination against HPV has been developed based on the study directed at cervical cancer-related HPV.

Concerning this oncogenic virus, the incidence of head and neck malignancy is equally important. At present, human papillomavirus (HPV)-positive head and neck squamous cell carcinoma (HNSCC) is showing an increasing trend in several countries such as Europe, North America, India, and so forth.

Interestingly, there have been records of high variations in the HPV16 viral load and different physical viral status proportions among the HNSCC. HPV positivity was associated with the younger age group and with the oropharyngeal site. Other sites of the head and neck region are also significant in terms of relevance for HPV positivity. This is revealed by a study by Faust *et al.,* who stated that HPV was found in 73 % of tonsillar carcinoma cases, 56 % of the base of tongue cancer cases, 27 % of oral cavity cancers, 14 % of laryngeal cancers [26]. To support the role of inflammation as the etiopathogenesis of malignancy are the study focusing on periodontitis. Tezal *et al.,* stated their study provide the first evidence, of an association between chronic periodontitis and HNSCC especially for the oral cavity, oropharynx and larynx, especially in patients who never used tobacco and alcohol [6]. Imperatively, this study highlights that poorly differentiated tumor is associated with that periodontitis history, which signify role of inflammation in patient's prognosis. Generally, the poorly differentiated tumor has worse prognosis and outcomes compared to well differentiated tumors (Tables 1 and 2).

Table 1 **Specific type of head and neck malignancy and its risk factors and associated inflammatory mediators/markers.**

S. No.	Cancer Type	Inflammation Inducer/Risk Factors	Major Pathogenesis/Inflammatory Markers
1.	Oral cavity cancer	Sharp teeth Periodontitis Leukoplakia/Erythroplakia Betel nut chewing	Cytokines Interleukin TAMs T regs
2.	Oropharyngeal cancer Tonsillar carcinoma	Human Papilloma Virus (HPV) Alcohol	Chemokines Proteases
3.	Laryngeal carcinoma (Supraglottic, glottic and subglottic carcinoma)	HPV Smoking Chemicals	TAM Peptides Growth Factors
4.	Sinonasal malignancy Inverted papilloma Sinonasal undifferentiated carcinoma (SNUC)	Chemical inhalants Wood dust HPV	EGF Proteases Macrophages
5.	Nasopharyngeal	Smoked seafoods	Nitrosamines

	carcinoma	Salty fish Pickled vegetables Burnt Incest Familial inheritance	TAM Growth Factors Protease EGF
6.	Papillary thyroid carcinoma Medullary thyroid carcinoma	Radiation Familial inheritance Chemical	Macrophages Cadherin Interleukin
7.	Salivary gland tumor -Adenocystic carcinoma -Mucoepidermoid carcinoma -Pleomorphic adenoma	Chemicals Familial inheritance	Interleukin Protease TAM

Table 2 **List of cancers that are strongly related to inflammation (*Balkwill & Mantovani, 2014*).**

Malignancy	Inflammatory Stimulus/Condition
Bladder carcinoma	Schistosomiasis
Cervical carcinoma	Papillomavirus
Ovarian cancer	Pelvic inflammatory disease/talc/tissue remodeling
Gastric cancer	*H. pylori* induced gastritis
MALT lymphoma	*H. pylori*
Oesophageal carcinoma	Barrett's metaplasia
Colorectal cancer	Inflammatory bowel disease
Hepatocellular carcinoma	Hepatitis virus (B and C)
Bronchial carcinoma	Silica, asbestos, cigarette smoke
Mesothelioma	Asbestos
Kaposi's sarcoma	Human herpesvirus type 8

Reciprocal contact between cancer cells and the microenvironment of the tumor helps and allows progression of the cancer. The contribution of stromal cell-secreted factors in cancer development was recognized over the last decade, but the underlying secretory machinery remains mysterious [27]. Among these secreted molecules includes proteins, peptides, chemokines, endothelial growth factors and so forth which are the major players in the inflammatory ecosystem. These molecules are intricately interactive and tend to switch on and off of the other co-factors for different effects to take place.

For instance, Kondoh *et al.* documented that IL-10 and TGF-β have the ability to promote malignant cells immune escape since they are the representative of the immunosuppressive cytokines. IL-10 and TGF-β2 overexpression is associated with poorer prognosis of oral cancers [17].

Other factors are also important in promoting carcinogenesis in tumor microenvironment. Huang *et al.* documented that NLRP3 inflammasome is a recent critical focus in cancer development and progression, but its role is complicated in tumorigenesis and stimulating antitumor immunity. They stated that recent evidence showed that activated NLRP3 inflammasome contributed to the progression of colon cancer cells, human melanoma cells, and lung cancer cells. In addition, they stated that when gemcitabine and 5-fluorouracil were used to treat cancer cells, the activated NLRP3 inflammasome reduces antitumor efficacy and promote tumor growth [15]. Importantly, IL-10 inhibits antigen-presenting cells *i.e.*, macrophages and dendritic cells and it also confers resistance to the action of cytotoxic T cells. In addition, they documented that hypoxic stress causes immune suppressive molecules such as IL 10 and TGF-β to activate the tumor-associated macrophage division into M2 forms, thus eliminating anti-tumor immunity [17].

Growth Factors and Inflammation Ecosystem

The other major player in the inflammation systems is the growth factors. Such delicate example like transforming growth factor β1 (TGF-β1), which in many types of cancers is over-expressed and correlates with invasion of tumor. Generally, it is known that at an early stage of HNSCC development, TGF-β1 inhibits head and neck malignant cell proliferation. On the other end of the spectrum, TGF-β1 facilitate tumor invasion by its paracrine effects within the tumor microenvironment [28]. These dual effects of a specific molecule in tumor microenvironment is common and mediated by many other molecules, some are secreted by the tumor cells whereas others are secreted in response to tumor cells infiltration. In head and neck cancer tissues, the TGF-β is overexpressed. The study by Lu *et al.* showed that a transgenic oral epithelium inducible TGF-β1 expression comparable to that seen in human HNSCC patients causes inflammation, epithelial hyper-proliferation and vascularization. They suggested that TGF-β1 has significant tumor promotion role during early stages of HNSCC development [28].

Lu *et al.* stated that TGF-β1 overexpression may also involves chronic inflammation. Chronic inflammation as we know is a precursor for many human malignancies due to its pro- carcinogenesis effects. TGF-β1 is among the most active chemotactic leukocyte cytokines. Their study data suggested that over-expression of TGF-β1 in the head and neck can be an important mechanism for chronic inflammation, thereby promoting the development of

HNSCC [28]. Other supporting evidence of TGF as a major player in inflammation and carcinogenesis are highlighted by Rosenthal *et al.* They reported that in the tumor-associated stroma, TGFβ1 and IGFII overexpression were substantially over-expressed (3.4-fold) in normal and tumor-associated stromal cells with only TGFβ1. In comparison to normal mucosa, high levels of TGFß1 were identified by immunohistochemical analysis in the stromal compartment of HNSCC tumors [29].

The study reported that the lack of EGF immunological expression in the carcinomatous areas associated with pseudoepitheliomatous hyperplasias and the almost exclusive presence of EGF inflammatory conditions in the hyperplasia lesions [30]. Pseudoepitheliomatous hyperplasia is a lesion that develops as a response to a great diversity of neoplastic, infectious, inflammatory, or traumatic stimuli being associated with different pathologies. It can be grouped according to pseudoepitheliomatous hyperplasia-related etiopathogenic conditions. Infectious, neoplastic, dermatosis with chronic irritation and inflammation, and various other pathological processes are the four major categories [30].

The pseudoepitheliomatous hyperplasia-associated tumor lesions include both benign and malignant entities. The association between pseudoepitheliomatous hyperplasia and granular cell tumour is frequently observed, but lesions of pseudoepitheliomatous hyperplasia associated with spitz nevi have also been described. There are many more malignant tumors associated with pseudoepitheliomatous hyperplasia, including malignant melanoma, lymphoproliferative diseases, basocellular carcinoma, and the malignant variant of clear cell hidradenoma [31]. Other proliferative markers that have been linked to malignancy include MMP, p53, and E-Cadherin. Invasive adenocarcinomas display substantially greater stain of p53 and MMP-1 and less E-cadherin. A related panel consisting of head and neck hyperplasia has shown that p53, MMP-1 and E-cadherin have significant staining patterns of p53 and Ki67 in order to differentiate the carcinoma from reactive epithelial hyperplasia [32].

Chemokines

In spite of therapeutic progress, the survival of patients with squamous cell carcinoma in the head and the neck (HNSCC) remains stagnant. The role of the tumor microenvironment in promoting cancer progression and resistance to therapy has attracted great attention in the past decade. The predominant non-malignant type of cell in the HNSCC microenvironment is cancer-associated fibroblasts (CAFs). Studies have shown that CAFs play a critical role in mediating HNSCC progression. CAFs facilitate HNSCC development by secretion of growth factors, extracellular matrix remodeling, and modulating therapy resistance. HNSCC cells interact symbiotically with CAFs through secreted variables. Recent findings indicate that fibroblasts associated with cancer (CAF) contribute to the tumor progression. The autophagy-dependent secretion by HNSCC-associated CAFs of tumor-promoting factors may explain their role in malignant development [27]. Molecular studies have further demonstrated that inflammatory cytokines, including IL-1, IL-6, and TNF-α, modulate HPV proliferation and expression in the cervical epithelial cells of its oncogenes E6 and E7 [14].

Interaction between Mediators in the Tumor Microenvironments

In a study, the author applied the characterization strategy for primary HNSCC tumors and matched metastatic lymph node. The study analysis highlights a complex cell ecosystem with an active crosstalk between malignant and non-malignant cells. This research represents a significant move in understanding the heterogeneity of intra-tumoral expression in epithelial tumors, which involve most of solid malignancies [22].

A change in cancer cells to a mesenchymal phenotype has been established as a significant contribution to the progression and metastasis of malignant epithelial tumors, including HNSCC. This epithelial-mesenchymal transition (EMT) is a fundamental biological process for wound healing and embryonic development while it plays a role in organ fibrosis and cancer in the pathophysiological context. Growing invasiveness and migration, avoidance of apoptosis, contributions to immunosuppression and immunotherapy resistance in transformed cancer cells, have been documented for EMT. In addition, loss of cell adhesion and epithelial markers, an increase in mesenchymal markers and an alteration of the cytoskeletal structure, are among the features that can be observed in the microenvironment of the tumor [33].

An increase in invasiveness and metastases was associated with a shift toward a mesenchymal phenotype in epithelial tumors. It is assumed that this phenomenon plays a key role in the progression and the prognostication of the disease. In this study, epithelial-mesenchymal transition (EMT) was investigated in human papillomavirus negative pharyngeal squamous cell carcinoma. This study revealed the complex role of EMT in HPV-negative pharyngeal squamous cell carcinoma during the metastasis process. In comparison to lymph node metastases, primary tumor tissue showed surprisingly high stemness characteristics [33]. HNSCC-specific metabolic fingerprints were mainly defined by a staining immunohistochemistry, and serologic examination in the early years. For example, the expression of CRABP in tumor tissue was enriched with its adjacent normal tissue, while further studies have shown that external administration of retinoic acids could modulate the activity of the Epidermal Growth Factor Receptor, which is a critical key in HNSCC progression [2].

ROLE OF INFLAMMATORY MARKERS AND THEIR CRITICAL ACTION

The most important step towards the discovery of effective HNSCC prevention and treatment is to understand the interactions that exist between the risk factors. The fact that carcinogenesis is a multifactorial process is well established and the presence of a single risk factor is usually not adequate to cause cancer. However, the majority of studies focused on the independent effects of particular risk factors [14].

Therapeutics

Tumor angiogenesis and inflammatory angiogenesis can be inhibited by administering either nuclear factor-kappa B-targeting or cyclooxygenase 2 inhibitor drugs or macrophage depletion. Therefore, both inflammatory and angiogenic responses in tumor stroma are the potential targets for the development of therapeutic anticancer drugs [10]. Inflammation contributes to malignant cell survival and proliferation, tumor angiogenesis, metastasis and reduced chemotherapy response. Inflammatory pathways are attractive targets for cancer prevention and therapy given their involvement at different stages of tumor development [16].

The key players that link the inflammation and cancer is TAM. TAM has various functions which includes repression of the adaptive immunity, promoting tumor cell angiogenesis and proliferation and stimulating matrix turnover. These functions have significant effects on the tumor progression. TAM is thus an attractive target of novel biological tumor therapies, together with other myeloid-related cells present at the tumor site [11]. Literature shows that chemotherapeutic and radiation both encourage cytoprotective autophagy in tumor cells. Research into the therapeutic potential of autophagy inhibition in HNSCC is lacking, despite multiple studies in a variety of cancer cell types.

For the first time, the study results provide evidence of inhibition of autophagy that can be used as the therapeutic potential in HNSCC. High doses of drugs for instance the chloroquine, which may not achieve sufficient intra-tumoral concentrations to limit autophagy, and lack of accepted autophagy monitoring methodology in patients' tumors to confirm successful inhibition, were the major limitations of autophagy treatment in clinical trials.

A variety of anticancer therapies have been found to induce autophagy in human cancer cell lines, including radiation therapy and chemotherapy. The autophagy is a highly regulated mechanism of large-scale lysosomal degradation of long-lived proteins, macromolecules, ribosomes, and organelles [34].

Prevention of Head and Neck Malignancy with Anti-Inflammation Agents

The consumptions of natural compounds have been practices for decades due to it beneficial medicinal properties. Due to its safety, low toxicity and general acceptance as a healthy dietary supplement, the use of natural compounds for chemoprevention is highly compelling. Because of their ability to reduce the occurrence of cancer, these natural dietary agents hold great promise for chemo-preventive use and has been used consistently by selected local populations. The use of natural compounds, however, poses many difficulties. If used excessively, it can cause toxicity, potentiate resistance and due to its low bioavailability, the desired effects may take time to be produced. There have been limited scientific studies available for several substances used. On the other end of spectrum, some compounds have been investigated extensively and showed positives effects in treating ailments and cancers. Imperatively, the compound must be well tolerated and have long-lasting benefits if chemical prevention is to be feasible in premalignant populations. In addition, the different signaling pathways that contribute to HNSCC tumorigenesis require the use of compounds with multiple molecular targets [35].

For instance, lycopene has been used to treat premalignant lesions in the oral cavity such as leukoplakia. It showed positive clinical outcomes with regression of leukoplakia size and it is safe to use without significant side effects. The action of lycopene is the inhibition of selected signaling pathway which is depend on the dosage used. The study documented that lycopene has the ability to decrease the HNSCC cell growth, induced apoptosis in cells and prevention of tumor invasion. Lycopene significantly reduced multiple forms of other HNSCC including oral cavity carcinoma, laryngeal and pharyngeal carcinoma [35].

Curcumin is an active ingredient from the natural plant *Curcuma longa L.,* In certain geographic region, it is also known as turmeric. This turmeric is widely used as a coloring and flavoring agent in the food industry and formed part of traditional herbal medicine in Asian countries for thousands of years. It is used to treat many ailments including hypertension, skin eczema, vomiting, headache, diarrhea, post-partum illness *etc.* due to its many positive properties. Curcumin has been shown to have strong anti-microbial, anti-inflammatory, antioxidant, and anticancer activities in modern pharmacological studies. Numerous evidences show that curcumin can prevent carcinogenesis, sensitize cancer cells to chemotherapy, and protect normal cells from damage caused by chemotherapy [36]. In addition, curcumin has been shown to have the ability to enhance the therapeutic efficacy of chemotherapy and to protect normal cells from chemotherapy-related toxicity.

Increasing evidence shows the bioeffect of curcumin is by facilitation a series of target molecules, which includes adhesion molecules, inflammatory factors, transcription and growth factors, proteins linked to apoptosis, and certain enzymes and kinases, *etc.* Epidemiological studies indicate the reduced risk of HNSCC due to diets that are rich in the Cruciferae family vegetables such as cabbage, broccoli, and cauliflower. Importantly, cytoprotective enzymes that promote detoxification of chemical carcinogens like benzene, aldehydes and polycyclic aromatic hydrocarbons are strongly induced by broccoli extracts.

The phytochemical sulforaphane, a glucoraphanin metabolite, drives majority of inducer activity in the broccoli extract [37]. Many research studies show the chemoprevention potential of sulforaphane-rich broccoli seed preparations for oral carcinogenesis and justify further clinical research in patients at risk for HNSCC-related tobacco [36]. Other substances such as vitamin A derivative, 13-cis-retinoic acid has been consistently shown positive outcomes as chemoprevention of head and neck cancer. The EGFR targeted chemoprevention also has been extensively studied in oral cavity cancer [38].

Prognostications of Head and Neck Malignancy

Recent studies reported that external and intrinsic metabolic derangement and changes can modulate the progression of HNSCC and act as clinical treatment response. This indicates that a thorough knowledge and understanding of dynamic metabolic changes during the development and progression of HNSCC could be of great benefit to the discovery of adjuvant anti-cancer regimens [2].

TAMs reflect many tumor stroma's main inflammatory component and can impact different malignant tissue aspects. It can be derived from the bone marrow and possess high plasticity where it can differentiate into the 2 phenotypes [39]. Importantly, hypoxia is the major driver for the macrophage recruitment. Several findings indicate that TAMs represent several M2-related pro-tumor functions, such as matrix remodeling, angiogenesis promotion, and adaptive immunity suppression. Clinical studies further support the pro-tumoral role of TAM in cancer. This is in lieu of numerous evidences that showed a significant correlation between high tumor macrophage content and poor patient prognosis [37]. In future, more research on the macrophages and TAM can shed a light into head and neck cancer carcinogenesis.

The other important factor that can be used as a prognostic marker of head and neck cancer is the neutrophil lymphocyte ratio (NLR). It is a reliable and accurate indicator of systemic inflammation and has been associated with prognosis of major solid tumors such as lung prostate and colorectal cancers [40]. Studies in HPV related HNSCC showed that the NLR can be an indicator of both recurrence-free and overall survival. However, the NLR does not have independent prognostic significance in HPV positive cases.

In addition, clinical studies that show a link between HPV positivity and NLR level in determining the prognosis of the patient reported that HNSCC patients with low NLR have a better prognosis in comparison to those with high NLR [41]. HPV positive patients have lower NLR value compared to HPV negative patients. Critically, NLR is able to predict survival for both positive and negative HNSCC patients [41]. Zhang *et al.* reported in oral cavity cancer, that a high NLR is related to reduced overall and disease-free survival [42, 43]. Importantly, this reflects the significance of systemic inflammation that play critical roles in the prognostication of HNSCC [44, 45]. Rachidi *et al.* reported that higher NLR ratio is associated with reduced survival rates and the death risk is increase by 4% with the increment of I unit of NLR [46].

Subsequently, the systemic inflammatory response measurement was refined using a selective combination of albumin and C-reactive protein (called the modified Glasgow Prognostic Score, mGPS) and it has been proved to have prognostic value in renal, gastrointestinal, and lung cancers, regardless of tumor stage [47]. The prognostic value of squamous cell carcinoma antigen (SCC-Ag) in patients with HNSCC has been investigated in several studies, with contradictory findings. The study found that high levels of SCC-Ag have a major association with TNM stages but cannot be used as a predictive marker for DFS and OS in patients who have HNSCC [48].

Inflammation and immune evasion are significantly related to carcinogenesis. The Systemic Inflammation Response Index (SIRI) was suggested to be used as a pre-treatment peripheral blood biomarker for cancerous tissues. A study comprising 824 patients assessing the prognostic capacity of SIRI in HNSCC patients has been conducted. The SIRI was measured by using the monocytes, neutrophils, and lymphocytes counts. Valero *et al.,* showed that in their study, the SIRI value was significantly higher for males, patients with alcohol and cigarette smoking history, pharyngeal carcinoma, and advance tumors [49].

A significant decrease in survival rates was observed as SIRI increased. SIRI was a significant predictor of survival rates of local, regional, and distant recurrence tumor. Indeed, in HNSCC, SIRI has independent prognostic capacity. The higher the SIRI level, the lower survival the patients have [50]. This is a potential novel target that can be further developed in the head and neck cancer management research armamentarium.

Another study also emphasized that an NLR increment and numbers of monocytes and neutrophils have strong association with a reduction in disease-specific survival rates. Patients with lower lymphocytes level has reduced disease specific survival (DSS). The monocytes and peripheral neutrophil count also related to poor prognosis of HNSCC patients. Importantly, these findings which based on pretreatment neutrophil and monocyte counts enabled the identification of different prognostic profiles of HNSCC [51].

The Negative Impact of Inflammation for Future Research Consideration

Several factors related to inflammation and tumorigenesis can have negative impacts on selective head and neck management aspects. Hypoxia underlies the result of poor treatment response, recurrent tumor and progression to metastases. A rapid increase in the tumor growth resulted in inadequate blood supply, which underlies the basis of hypoxia.

Multiple inflammatory reactions and markers are involved in the genesis of hypoxia. Eventually, this will result in the development of areas of deficient of oxygen [52]. This deficient oxygen areas, are normally chemo-resistant, and are at risk of developing the residual disease and recurrent tumors despite chemoradiation treatment. The state of hypoxia is not clear-cut with the evidence of many factors that may play a role inclusive of HIFs. In tumor areas which are not significantly hypoxic, several factors have been shown to induce expression of HIF-1 alpha. Various oncogenic mechanisms, such as inactive p53 mutations, oxygen radical accumulation, and RAS mutations, have been attributed to this. In order to counteract the effects of hypoxia in interfering with the desired treatment outcomes, these factors represent specific genomic changes which can be fully investigated.

Hypoxia and inflammation occur at various stages in the cancer setting. Activation of HIF in hypoxic tumors stroma increases tumor angiogenesis. This increase in angiogenesis alters the morphological characteristics of the tumor vessels and their endothelial wall in ways that compromise the delivery of oxygen to the tissues. Inflammatory cells also contribute to vascular abnormalities in tumors by releasing the numerous associated growth factor [53]. In the presence of hypoxia, the radiation induced DNA damage is lessen which explains the reason for radio-resistance [54].

On the other spectrum, hypoxia itself causes inflammation. The idea that hypoxia can cause inflammation has been generally accepted by studies of the signaling pathways of hypoxia. For example, levels of circulating pro-inflammatory cytokines are increased in people with mountain sickness, and fluid leakage or vascular leakage results in pulmonary or cerebral edema. These changes also lead to an increased serum interleukin-6, interleukin-6 receptors, and C-reactive protein levels [44, 55]. Concentrations of oxygen are reduced in solid tumors compared with those in normal tissues. It has been shown that most solid tumors have elevated levels of HIF-1α and HIF-2α and these high levels associate with death from cancer. This discovery can be extrapolated to produce a refined treatment strategy of solid malignancy inclusive of head and neck malignancy.

Despite progress in treatment, recurrence of locoregional disease in patients with advanced disease is still a major problem. In approximately 10-30 percent of cases involving advanced tumors, local recurrences occur, even with histopathologically tumor-free surgical margins after resection. This may be attributed to the aggressive nature of the tumor with high grade and poorly differentiated features. The locoregional disease recurrences are difficult to treat as multiple patient factors and tumor factors prevail. Historically, platinum-based chemotherapy has been the standard treatment for recurrent or metastatic HNSCC, although the survival and quality of life benefits are questionable. With the current treatment paradigm, multiple newer agents and drugs have shown consistently positive results in combatting head and neck malignancy.

In HNSCC, a tyrosine kinases receptor, EGFR, is abnormally activated with more than 90% of HNSCC overexpresses EGFR. Imperatively, higher levels of EGFR expression are associated with worse prognosis. In cancer cells, EGFR expression is induced by radiation. Thus, the cancer cells can be made more sensitive to the effects of radiation by blocking EGFR signaling. EGFR signaling can be inhibited by using immunotoxin conjugates, small molecules, monoclonal antibodies directed against ligands which can increase radiosensitivity of the malignant cells [56⁻58].

FUTURE PROSPECT IN THE HEAD AND NECK MALIGNANCY MANAGEMENT

While it is well recognized that there is a clear genetic alteration for cancer development, there is growing evidence that the host inflammatory reaction is a key factor in cancer growth. Multiple inflammatory reactions and cascades have been well documented in the promotion and progression of cancers, inclusive of the occurrence of recurrence and metastases. Critically, the systemic inflammatory response plays a significant role in many solid tumor developments [39]. Arsenals of therapeutic drugs and agents are working through the action of anti-inflammations. Some of the therapeutic regimens are combined to enhance their efficiency with minimal side-effects. The evolving trends in the latest research and trials will escalate the discovery of novel markers that can be used for screening, diagnosis, treatment, follow-up, and prediction of recurrent and metastases.

Numerous important factors need to be considered when designing an effective treatment agent or regimen. The tumor factor, patient factor, and host factor need to be carefully weighed and assessed during the process of investigations for newer therapeutic agents. For instance, the radiation-induced systemic changes can interact with other antitumor treatment modalities, like immunotherapy or chemotherapy. These might influence long-term treatment outcomes such as local tumor control and distant metastases occurrences.

Other critical factors also need to be investigated in a similar fashion. Of note are the complications that are sustained by the adjacent normal tissues surrounding the irradiated areas [59]. As mentioned earlier, other significant inflammatory markers that have the potential to be used in the coming years are, for example, neutrophils, leukocytes, and lymphocytes. According to a study that was performed on 182 patients with salivary glands tumor, who were treated between 2010 and 2015, the NLR and the leukocytes levels were predictive of a benign and malignant tumor of salivary glands. The study further concluded that an NLR increment could be an inflammatory marker to differentiate a low-grade tumor from high-grade malignant parotid gland tumors [60]. This is very critical, as treatment approaches for low-grade salivary malignant tumors greatly differ from those with high-grade tumors, in terms of types of necessary surgeries and the need for adjuvant chemoradiation.

CONCLUSION

Inflammation and its ecosystem are critical in cancer progression. The reflexive relationship which exists between inflammation and cancer needs to be clearly understood as many delicate physiologic processes and molecular events in the tumor microenvironment are vital and can be effective future targets for therapeutic intervention. Additionally, numerous inciting agents and risk factors of head and neck malignancy can be identified early and utilized in screening and preventive programs in combatting head and neck malignancy at a larger scale. This momentum is needed in every clinician, physician, researcher, and scientist to gear up towards personalized cancer therapeutics.

CONSENT FOR PUBLICATION

Not applicable.

CONFLICT OF INTEREST

The authors declare no conflict of interest, financial or otherwise.

ACKNOWLEDGEMENTS

Declared none.

REFERENCES

[1]   Sethi G, Shanmugam MK, Ramachandran L, Kumar AP, Tergaonkar V. Multifaceted link between cancer and inflammation. Biosci Rep 2012; 32(1): 1-15.[http://dx.doi.org/10.1042/BSR20100136] [PMID: 21981137]

[2]   Hsieh YT, Chen YF, Lin SC, Chang KW, Li WC. Targeting cellular metabolism modulates head and neck oncogenesis. Int J Mol Sci 2019; 20(16): 3960.[http://dx.doi.org/10.3390/ijms20163960] [PMID: 31416244]

[3]   Allavena P, Sica A, Solinas G, Porta C, Mantovani A. The inflammatory micro-environment in tumor progression: the role of tumor-associated macrophages. Crit Rev Oncol Hematol 2008; 66(1): 1-9.[http://dx.doi.org/10.1016/j.critrevonc.2007.07.004] [PMID: 17913510]

[4]   Bonomi M, Patsias A, Posner M, Sikora A. The role of inflammation in head and neck cancer. In: Aggarwal B, Sung B, Gupta S, eds. Inflammation and Cancer Advances in Experimental Medicine and Biology Aggarwal B, Sung B, Gupta S. 2014; Vol. 816[http://dx.doi.org/10.1007/978-3-0348-0837-8_5]

[5]   Murata M. Inflammation and cancer. Environ Health Prev Med 2018; 23(1): 50.[http://dx.doi.org/10.1186/s12199-018-0740-1] [PMID: 30340457]

[6]   Tezal M, Sullivan MA, Hyland A, et al. Chronic periodontitis and the incidence of head and neck squamous cell carcinoma. Cancer Epidemiol Biomarkers Prev 2009; 18(9): 2406-12.[http://dx.doi.org/10.1158/1055-9965.EPI-09-0334] [PMID: 19745222]

[7]   Tezal M, Scannapieco FA, Wactawski-Wende J, et al. Local inflammation and human papillomavirus status of head and neck cancers. Arch Otolaryngol Head Neck Surg 2012; 138(7): 669-75.[http://dx.doi.org/10.1001/archoto.2012.873] [PMID: 22710409]

[8]   Haeggblom L, Ramqvist T, Tommasino M, Dalianis T, Näsman A. Time to change perspectives on HPV in oropharyngeal cancer. A systematic review of HPV prevalence per oropharyngeal sub-site the last 3 years. Papillomavirus Res 2017; 4: 1-11.[http://dx.doi.org/10.1016/j.pvr.2017.05.002] [PMID: 29179862]

[9]   Craig SG, Anderson LA, Schache AG, et al. Recommendations for determining HPV status in patients with oropharyngeal cancers under TNM8 guidelines: a two-tier approach. Br J Cancer 2019; 120(8): 827-33.[http://dx.doi.org/10.1038/s41416-019-0414-9] [PMID: 30890775]

[10]   Ono M. Molecular links between tunour angiogenesis and inflammation: inflammatory stimuli of macrophages and cancer cells as targets for therapeutic strategy. Cancer Sci 2008; 99(8): 1501-6.[http://dx.doi.org/10.1111/j.1349-7006.2008.00853 x]

[11]   Solinas G, Germano G, Mantovani A, Allavena P. Tumor-associated macrophages (TAM) as major players

of the cancer-related inflammation. J Leukoc Biol 2009; 86(5): 1065-73.[http://dx.doi.org/10.1189/jlb.0609385] [PMID: 19741157]

[12] Krüger M, Hansen T, Kasaj A, Moergel M. The correlation between chronic periodontitis and oral cancer. Case Rep Dent 2013; 2013: 262410.[http://dx.doi.org/10.1155/2013/262410] [PMID: 23936684]

[13] Balkwill F, Mantovani A. Inflammation and cancer: back to Virchow? Lancet 2001; 17;357(9255): 539-45.[http://dx.doi.org/10.1016/S0140-6736(00)04046-0]

[14] Tezal M. Interaction between chronic inflammation and oral HPV infection in the etiology of head and neck cancers. Int J Otolaryngol 2012; 2012: 575242.[http://dx.doi.org/10.1155/2012/575242] [PMID: 22518158]

[15] Huang CF, Chen L, Li YC, et al. NLRP3 inflammasome activation promotes inflammation-induced carcinogenesis in head and neck squamous cell carcinoma. J Exp Clin Cancer Res 2017; 36(1): 116.[http://dx.doi.org/10.1186/s13046-017-0589-y] [PMID: 28865486]

[16] Zhu Z, Zhong S, Shen Z. Targeting the inflammatory pathways to enhance chemotherapy of cancer. Cancer Biol Ther 2011; 12(2): 95-105.[http://dx.doi.org/10.4161/cbt.12.2.15952] [PMID: 21623164]

[17] Kondoh N, Mizuno-Kamiya M, Umemura N, et al. Immunomodulatory aspects in the progression and treatment of oral malignancy. Jpn Dent Sci Rev 2019; 55(1): 113-20.[http://dx.doi.org/10.1016/j.jdsr.2019.09.001] [PMID: 31660091]

[18] Ohnishi S, Ma N, Thanan R. DNA damage in inflammation-related carcinogenesis and cancer stem cells. Oxid Med Cell Longev 2013; 387014. [http://dx.doi.org/10.1155/2013/387014]

[19] Kawanishi S, Ohnishi S, Ma N, Hiraku Y, Oikawa S, Murata M. Nitrative and oxidative DNA damage in infection-related carcinogenesis in relation to cancer stem cells. Genes Environ 2017; 38: 26.[http://dx.doi.org/10.1186/s41021-016-0055-7] [PMID: 28050219]

[20] Rokavec M, Öner MG, Hermeking H. Inflammation-induced epigenetic switches in cancer. Cell Mol Life Sci 2016; 73(1): 23-39.[http://dx.doi.org/10.1007/s00018-015-2045-5] [PMID: 26394635]

[21] Xiao Z, Dai Z, Locasale JW. Metabolic landscape of the tumor microenvironment at single cell resolution. Nat Commun 2019; 10(1): 3763.[http://dx.doi.org/10.1038/s41467-019-11738-0] [PMID: 31434891]

[22] Puram SV, Tirosh I, Parikh AS, et al. Single-cell transcriptomic analysis of primary and metastatic tumor ecosystems in head and neck cancer. Cell 2017; 171(7): 1611-1624.e24.[http://dx.doi.org/10.1016/j.cell.2017.10.044] [PMID: 29198524]

[23] Sica A, Allavena P, Mantovani A. Cancer related inflammation: the macrophage connection. Cancer Lett 2008; 267(2): 204-15.[http://dx.doi.org/10.1016/j.canlet.2008.03.028] [PMID: 18448242]

[24] Kimura YN, Watari K, Fotovati A, et al. Inflammatory stimuli from macrophages and cancer cells synergistically promote tumor growth and angiogenesis. Cancer Sci 2007; 98(12): 2009-18.[http://dx.doi.org/10.1111/j.1349-7006.2007.00633.x] [PMID: 17924976]

[25] Wang SS, Cen X, Liang XH, Tang YL. Macrophage migration inhibitory factor: a potential driver and biomarker for head and neck squamous cell carcinoma. Oncotarget 2017; 8(6): 10650-61.[http://dx.doi.org/10.18632/oncotarget.12890] [PMID: 27788497]

[26] Faust H, Eldenhed Alwan E, Roslin A, Wennerberg J, Forslund O. Prevalence of human papillomavirus types, viral load and physical status of HPV16 in head and neck squamous cell carcinoma from the South Swedish Health Care Region. J Gen Virol 2016; 97(11): 2949-56.[http://dx.doi.org/10.1099/jgv.0.000611] [PMID: 27667722]

[27] New J, Arnold L, Ananth M, et al. Secretory autophagy in cancer-associated fibroblasts promotes head and neck cancer progression and offers a novel therapeutic target. Cancer Res 2017; 77(23): 6679-91.[http://dx.doi.org/10.1158/0008-5472.CAN-17-1077] [PMID: 28972076]

[28] Lu SL, Reh D, Li AG, et al. Overexpression of transforming growth factor beta1 in head and neck epithelia results in inflammation, angiogenesis, and epithelial hyperproliferation. Cancer Res 2004; 64(13): 4405-10.[http://dx.doi.org/10.1158/0008-5472.CAN-04-1032] [PMID: 15231647]

[29] Rosenthal E, McCrory A, Talbert M, Young G, Murphy-Ullrich J, Gladson C. Elevated expression of TGF-beta1 in head and neck cancer-associated fibroblasts. Mol Carcinog 2004; 40(2): 116-21.[http://dx.doi.org/10.1002/mc.20024] [PMID: 15170816]

[30] Pascu RM, Crăiţoiu Ş, Crăiţoiu MM, et al. The role played by growth factors TGF-β1, EGF and FGF7 in the pathogeny of oral pseudoepitheliomatous hyperplasia. Curr Health Sci J 2017; 43(3): 246-52.[http://dx.doi.org/10.12865/CHSJ.43.03.11] [PMID: 30595884]

[31] Pascu RM, Crăiţoiu Ş, Florescu AM, et al. Histopathological study of oral pseudoepitheliomatous hyperplasia. Curr Health Sci J 2017; 43(4): 361-6.[http://dx.doi.org/10.12865/CHSJ.43.04.13] [PMID: 30595904]

[32] Klieb HB, Raphael SJ. Comparative study of the expression of p53, Ki67, E-cadherin and MMP-1 in verrucous hyperplasia and verrucous carcinoma of the oral cavity. Head Neck Pathol 2007; 1(2): 118-22.[http://dx.doi.org/10.1007/s12105-007-0029-y] [PMID: 20614262]

[33] Ihler F, Gratz R, Wolff HA, et al. Epithelial-mesenchymal transition during metastasis of HPV-negative pharyngeal squamous cell carcinoma. BioMed Res Int 2018; 2018: 7929104.[http://dx.doi.org/10.1155/2018/7929104] [PMID: 29693014]

[34] Rikiishi H. Autophagic action of new targeting agents in head and neck oncology. Cancer Biol Ther 2012; 13(11): 978-91.[http://dx.doi.org/10.4161/cbt.21079] [PMID: 22825332]

[35] Crooker K, Aliani R, Ananth M, Arnold L, Anant S, Thomas SM. A review of promising natural chemopreventive agents for head and neck cancer. Cancer Prev Res (Phila) 2018; 11(8): 441-50.[http://dx.doi.org/10.1158/1940-6207.CAPR-17-0419] [PMID: 29602908]

[36] Liu Z, Huang P, Law S, Tian H, Leung W, Xu C. Preventive effect of curcumin against chemotherapy-induced side-effects. Front Pharmacol 2018; 9: 1374.[http://dx.doi.org/10.3389/fphar.2018.01374] [PMID: 30538634]

[37] Bauman JE, Zang Y, Sen M. Prevention of carcinogen-induced oral cancer by sulforaphane. Cancer Prev Res (Phila) 2016; 9(7): 547-57.[http://dx.doi.org/10.1158/1940-6207.CAPR-15-0290]

[38] Mak MP, William WN, Jr. Targeting the epidermal growth factor receptor for head and neck cancer chemoprevention. Oral Oncol 2014; 50(10): 918-23.[http://dx.doi.org/10.1016/j.oraloncology.2013.12.024] [PMID: 24412287]

[39] Davis RJ, Van Waes C, Allen CT. Overcoming barriers to effective immunotherapy: MDSCs, TAMs, and Tregs as mediators of the immunosuppressive microenvironment in head and neck cancer. Oral Oncol 2016; 58: 59-70.[http://dx.doi.org/10.1016/j.oraloncology.2016.05.002] [PMID: 27215705]

[40] Yu Y, Wang H, Yan A, et al. Pretreatment neutrophil to lymphocyte ratio in determining the prognosis of head and neck cancer: a meta-analysis. BMC Cancer 2018; 18(1): 383.[http://dx.doi.org/10.1186/s12885-018-4230-z] [PMID: 29618336]

[41] Xu C, Yuan J, Du W, et al. Significance of the neutrophil-to-lymphocyte ratio in p16-negative squamous cell carcinoma of unknown primary in head and neck. Front Oncol 2020; 10: 39.[http://dx.doi.org/10.3389/fonc.2020.00039] [PMID: 32083001]

[42] Zhang B, Du W, Gan K, Fang Q, Zhang X. Significance of the neutrophil-to-lymphocyte ratio in young patients with oral squamous cell carcinoma. Cancer Manag Res 2019; 11: 7597-603.[http://dx.doi.org/10.2147/CMAR.S211847] [PMID: 31496814]

[43] Lee S, Kim DW, Kwon S, Kim HJ, Cha IH, Nam W. 2020.

[44] Sica A, Schioppa T, Mantovani A, Allavena P. Tumour-associated macrophages are a distinct M2 polarised population promoting tumour progression: potential targets of anti-cancer therapy. Eur J Cancer 2006; 42(6): 717-27.[http://dx.doi.org/10.1016/j.ejca.2006.01.003] [PMID: 16520032]

[45] Ambatipudi S, Langdon R, Richmond RC, et al. DNA methylation derived systemic inflammation indices are associated with head and neck cancer development and survival. Oral Oncol 2018; 85: 87-94.[http://dx.doi.org/10.1016/j.oraloncology.2018.08.021] [PMID: 30220325]

[46] Rachidi S, Wallace K, Wrangle JM, Day TA, Alberg AJ, Li Z. Neutrophil-to-lymphocyte ratio and overall survival in all sites of head and neck squamous cell carcinoma. Head Neck 2016; 38(Suppl 1): E1068-74.[http://dx.doi.org/10.1002/hed.24159]

[47] Rosculet N, Zhou XC, Ha P, et al. Neutrophil-to-lymphocyte ratio: Prognostic indicator for head and neck squamous cell carcinoma. Head Neck 2017; 39(4): 662-7.[http://dx.doi.org/10.1002/hed.24658] [PMID: 28075517]

[48] Proctor MJ, Morrison DS, Talwar D, et al. An inflammation-based prognostic score (mGPS) predicts cancer survival independent of tumour site: a Glasgow Inflammation Outcome Study. Br J Cancer 2011; 104(4): 726-34.[http://dx.doi.org/10.1038/sj.bjc.6606087] [PMID: 21266974]

[49] Travassos DC, Fernandes D, Massucato EMS, Navarro CM, Bufalino A. Squamous cell carcinoma antigen as a prognostic marker andits correlation with clinicopathological features in head and neck squamous cell carcinoma: Systematic review and meta-analysis. J Oral Pathol Med 2018; 47(1): 3-10.[http://dx.doi.org/10.1111/jop.12600] [PMID: 28600896]

[50] Valero C, Pardo L, Sansa A. Prognostic capacity of systemic inflammation response index (SIRI) in patients with head and neck squamous cell carcinoma. Head Neck 2019; 42(2): 336-43.[http://dx.doi.org/10.1002/hed.26010] [PMID: 31750591]

[51] Valero C, Pardo L, López M, et al. Pretreatment count of peripheral neutrophils, monocytes, and lymphocytes as independent prognostic factor in patients with head and neck cancer. Head Neck 2017; 39(2):

219-26.[http://dx.doi.org/10.1002/hed.24561] [PMID: 27534525]

[52]   Alsahafi E, Begg K, Amelio I, *et al.* Clinical update on head and neck cancer: molecular biology and ongoing challenges. Cell Death Dis 2019; 10(8): 540.[http://dx.doi.org/10.1038/s41419-019-1769-9] [PMID: 31308358]

[53]   Eltzschig HK, Carmeliet P. Hypoxia and inflammation. N Engl J Med 2011; 364(7): 656-65.[http://dx.doi.org/10.1056/NEJMra0910283] [PMID: 21323543]

[54]   Göttgens EL, Ostheimer C, Span PN, Bussink J, Hammond EM. HPV, hypoxia and radiation response in head and neck cancer. Br J Radiol 2019; 92(1093): 20180047.[http://dx.doi.org/10.1259/bjr.20180047] [PMID: 29493265]

[55]   Cripps C, Winquist E, Devries MC, Stys-Norman D, Gilbert R. Head and Neck Cancer Disease Site GroupEpidermal growth factor receptor targeted therapy in stages III and IV head and neck cancer. Curr Oncol 2010; 17(3): 37-48.[http://dx.doi.org/10.3747/co.v17i3.520]

[56]   Santuray RT, Johnson DE, Grandis JR. New therapies in head and neck cancer. Trends Cancer 2018; 4(5): 385-96.[http://dx.doi.org/10.1016/j.trecan.2018.03.006] [PMID: 29709262]

[57]   Horn D, Hess J, Freier K, Hoffmann J, Freudlsperger C. Targeting EGFR-PI3K-AKT-mTOR signaling enhances radiosensitivity in head and neck squamous cell carcinoma. Expert Opin Ther Targets 2015; 19(6): 795-805.[http://dx.doi.org/10.1517/14728222.2015.1012157] [PMID: 25652792]

[58]   Balázs K, Kis E, Badie C, *et al.* Radiotherapy-induced changes in the systemic immune and inflammation parameters of head and neck cancer patients. Cancers (Basel) 2019; 11(9): 1324.[http://dx.doi.org/10.3390/cancers11091324] [PMID: 31500214]

[59]   Damar M, Dinç AE, Erdem D, *et al.* Pretreatment neutrophil- lymphocyte ratio in salivary glands tumours is associated with malignancy. Otolaryngol Head Neck Surg 2016; 155(6): 988-96.[http://dx.doi.org/10.1177/0194599816659257] [PMID: 27436419]

[60]   Armstrong WB, Meyskens FL, Jr. Chemoprevention of head and neck cancer. Otolaryngol Head Neck Surg 2000; 122(5): 728-35.[http://dx.doi.org/10.1016/S0194-5998(00)70205-1] [PMID: 10793355]

Types of Head and Neck Malignancy

Gabriela Ramírez-Arroyo[1], [*], Juan Carlos Hernaiz-Leonardo[1], Michelle Marvin-Huergo[1], Mario Sergio Dávalos-Fuentes[1]

[1] Department of Otolaryngology–Head and Neck Surgery, Instituto Nacional de Rehabilitación "Luis Guillermo Ibarra Ibarra", Mexico City, Mexico

Abstract

Head and neck cancer (HNC) is a heterogeneous group of malignant neoplasms, and its classification is a challenge. Based on the primary site, most literature comprehends five types of HNCs: laryngeal, pharyngeal, oral cavity, nasal cavity, and salivary gland cancer. More than 90% of HCNs are of epithelial origin, making squamous cell carcinoma the most common histological type. The prototypic HNC is a moderately differentiated squamous cell carcinoma associated with tobacco and alcohol consumption that affects older men more frequently. They are usually treated in a similar fashion. Currently, the human papillomavirus epidemic and a shift in tobacco consumption patterns are changing this trend. HNCs have a high rate of genetic heterogeneity, and molecular profiling has gained importance in the classification and future treatment of HNCs.

Keywords: HPV-positive, Laryngeal cancer, Molecular profile, Nasal cavity cancer, Oral cavity cancer, Pharyngeal cancer, Salivary gland cancer, Squamous cell carcinoma, Unknown primary.

---

[*] **Corresponding author Gabriela Ramírez-Arroyo:** Department of Otolaryngology–Head and Neck Surgery, Instituto Nacional de Rehabilitación "Luis Guillermo Ibarra Ibarra", Mexico City, Mexico; Tel: +525534882547; E-mail: gabyra18@hotmail.com

INTRODUCTION

To talk about HNC is a complex task, as the term itself is ambiguous. In oncologic terms, the type of cancer in any region of the body is determined by its primary site and histology. Following this train of thought, the term HNC could comprise all tumors arising between the thoracic inlet and the skull base. Some textbooks on HNC follow this approach and include most cancers occurring in these primary sites in their discussion, but most publications concerning HNCs do not consider skin, thyroid, parathyroid, cervical esophagus, and other primaries of this anatomical region a part of HNCs.

Based on a definition proposed by the American Joint Committee on Cancer [1], most cancer societies reserve the term HNC for malignant neoplasms that arise in salivary glands or in the squamous cells that line mucosal surfaces within the head and neck [2]. These tumors are aggressive, mostly develop from squamous cells [3], are classically associated with tobacco and alcohol consumption [4], and their diagnosis and treatment are similar [5]. HNCs deeply affect the quality of life, interfering with the patients' daily life activities such as speech, swallowing, breathing, and even social interaction [6]. Hence, tumors held under the umbrella term HNC are classified into 5 main groups, each named according to the anatomic region of the head and neck where they develop:

1. Laryngeal cancer
2. Pharyngeal cancer
3. Oral cavity cancer
4. Nasal cavity and paranasal sinus cancer
5. Salivary glands cancer

Laryngeal, pharyngeal, oral cavity and salivary gland neoplasms are further classified according to the anatomic subsite or the affected salivary gland.

The metastatic carcinoma of unknown primary (MCUP) of the head and neck is another type of HNC. MCUP refers to the state in which cervical adenopathy is identified, but the primary tumor cannot be diagnosed even after an aggressive evaluation [7]. As the diagnostic workup has become more thorough, it must include a surgical search, taking biopsies of suspected primary sites and detection of Human Papillomavirus and Epstein-Bar Virus, the true incidence of MCUP is close to 1-2%. Up to 90% of the MCUPs are primaries of the oropharynx [8].

Besides the site of origin, histology is the other criteria used to classify malignant neoplasms (Table 1). More than 90% of HCNs are of epithelial origin, making squamous cell carcinoma the most common histological type.

Salivary gland tumors represent the biggest exception to this rule, as the most common histologic type is mucoepidermoid carcinoma [9]. Certain clinical guidelines on HNC management refer only to squamous cell carcinomas, coining the term head and neck squamous cell carcinoma (HNSCC). HNSCC represents the prototype of HNC that arises from the mucosal lining of upper aerodigestive tracts, is associated with tobacco and alcohol consumption, affects older males, and thus, is treated similarly. This prototypic HNSCC is a moderately differentiated squamous cell carcinoma. Other histologic subtypes or variants of HNSCC are described: spindle cell variant, papillary variant, basaloid squamous variant, and verrucous carcinoma, all of which exhibit different biologic behaviors [10].

Table 1 **Main subtypes of HNC according to the primary site and histological type.**

HNC Type	Subtypes	Histological Types
Laryngeal cancer	• Supraglottic carcinoma Includes the epiglottis, false vocal cords, ventricles, aryepiglottic folds, and arytenoids • Glottic carcinoma Includes the true vocal cords and the anterior and posterior commissures • Subglottic carcinoma 1 cm below the true vocal cords and extends to the lower border of the cricoid cartilage	Squamous cell carcinoma* Variants of SCC Includes verrucous, spindle cell and basaloid SCC Adenocarcinoma Lymphoma Includes Hodgkin's lymphoma and non-Hodgkin's lymphoma ** Sarcomas Includes chondrosarcoma, and leiomyosarcoma Miscellaneous Includes minor salivary gland tumors, malignant melanoma, neuroendocrine carcinoma, among others
Pharyngeal cancer	• Nasopharynx	Nasopharyngeal carcinoma Keratinizing squamous Non-keratinizing squamous Basaloid squamous Extranodal natural killer/T cell lymphoma***
	• Oropharynx Includes soft palate, tonsil, tonsillar pillars, base of tongue, vallecula and posterior oropharyngeal wall	Squamous cell carcinoma, HPV-positive Includes basaloid and papillary SCC, adenosquamous, undifferentiated, spindle cell, and ciliated adenosquamous carcinoma.

		Squamous cell carcinoma, HPV-negative Squamous cell carcinoma, HPV not tested, morphology highly suggestive of HPV association Small cell carcinoma Lymphoma Sarcomas Minor salivary gland tumors
	• Hypopharynx Includes pyriform sinus, postcricoid region, posterior pharyngeal wall	Squamous cell carcinoma* Variants of SCC Includes verrucous, spindle cell and basaloid SCC Adenocarcinoma Lymphoma Includes Hodgkin's lymphoma and non-Hodgkin's lymphoma ** Sarcomas Includes chondrosarcoma, leiomyosarcoma, and others Miscellaneous Includes minor salivary gland tumors, neuroendocrine carcinoma, among others
Oral cavity cancer	• Lip • Oral tongue • Alveolar ridge • Retromolar trigone • Floor of the mouth • Buccal mucosa	Squamous cell carcinoma* Minor salivary gland tumors (adenoid cystic carcinoma, mucoepidermoid carcinoma, adenocarcinoma) Mucosal melanomas Osteosarcomas
Nasal cavity and paranasal sinus cancer	Rarely classified according to the sinus of origin.	Squamous cell carcinoma* Adenocarcinoma Neuroendocrine carcinoma Esthesioneuroblastoma Sinonasal undifferentiated carcinoma Small cell carcinoma Mucosal melanoma Rhabdomyosarcoma Extranodal NK/T-cell lymphoma, sinonasal type Sinonasal teratocarcinosarcoma
Salivary gland	• Parotid • Submandibular gland	Mucoepidermoid carcinoma Adenoid cystic carcinoma

cancer	• Sublingual gland • Minor salivary glands	Secretory carcinoma Polymorphous adenocarcinoma Intraductal carcinoma Acinic cell carcinoma Carcinoma ex pleomorphic adenoma Carcinosarcoma Sialoblastoma Lymphomas Other adenocarcinomas**** Other carcinomas*****
Thyroid carcinoma	-	Papillary carcinoma Follicular carcinoma Hürthle (oncocytic) cell carcinoma Poorly differentiated thyroid cancer Anaplastic thyroid cancer Medullary carcinoma Others Mucoepidermoid carcinoma, SCC, mucinous carcinoma, lymphoma, angiosarcoma

Note: This table does not pretend to be a comprehensive list of histopathological types of HNC. For further information, we suggest to the reader to refer to the WHO Classification of Head and Neck Tumors. Fourth edition.

SCC squamous cell carcinoma
"" Despite their rarity, salivary gland neoplasms show a histological diversity that is arguably unparalleled in comparison by any other organ, which reflexes in its complex taxonomy
* SCC is further classified into keratinizing and nonkeratinizing types and graded as well, moderately or poorly differentiated
** Lymphomas are further classified according to specific features
*** Type of NHL typical of the nasopharynx
**** Including basal cell adenocarcinoma, mucinous adenocarcinoma, sebaceous lymphadenocarcinoma, cystadenocarcinoma, not otherwise specified
***** Including epithelial-myoepithelial carcinoma, sebaceous carcinoma, squamous cell carcinoma, clear cell carcinoma, myoepithelial carcinoma, small cell carcinoma, large cell carcinoma.

Even if they are not strictly considered a type of HNSCC, second primary malignancies (SPM) occurring in the head and neck region do have a worse prognosis and could be considered a unique group of HNCs. About 9% of patients with HNSCCs treated with radiotherapy develop an SPM mainly in the head and neck; tumours can also occur in the lungs. SPMs are relevant because they represent the leading long-term cause of mortality in HNSCCs patients, causing one-third of the deaths [11]. The median time to develop an SPM is 72 months, the risk of presenting an SPM increases through time with a 15-year risk of developing an SPM of 25 to 42%, according to smoking habits [12]. SPM illustrates the concept of "field cancerization" described by Slaughter [13], in which a carcinogen like tobacco leads to local inflammation, which drives a change that will eventually favor the development of a new malignancy. At the time this phenomenon was described, it was unlikely to determine a molecular profile and the genetic damage in cells could not be established. Nowadays, controversy remains and it is still unclear if the primary HNSCC and the SPM are genetically related or not [14].

It must be kept in mind that HNSCCs subtypes are clinically, histologically, and molecularly distinct [15], despite their generic management. Considering the complexity to define HNC types, a homogenous classification system is still lacking. The 11th revision of the International Classification of Diseases (ICD-11) was last updated in April 2019 and is available online at https://icd.who.int/browse11/l-m/en. ICD-11 includes 22 primary sites among HNCs. The ICD-11 should be used with caution, as some elements are not mutually exclusive nor a subset of each other, especially regarding oropharynx and oral cavity cancers, leading to an unappropriated registration of these HNC types and their respective subtypes.

The third edition of the International Classification of Diseases for Oncology (ICD- O-3), whose second version is currently pending since July 2019 due to decommissioning from the http://codes.iarc.fr website, includes topographic, morphologic, and HPV/p16 status codes providing a more extensive and specific classification system [16]. Despite these efforts, the use of several definitions for classifying types of HNCs still hampers communication amongst the oncologic community of clinicians and researchers; hence, a more standardized approach is encouraged when registering data of HNC patients.

From a clinical point of view, it is our opinion that when faced with a patient with symptoms associated with a head and neck malignancy, the differential diagnosis should not only consider neoplasms included under the term HNSSC but should also include "the other" neoplasms that might occur in this complex and fascinating anatomical region.

EPIDEMIOLOGY OF HEAD & NECK CANCER

According to data published by GLOBOCAN 2018, HNC is the sixth commonest cancer. It accounts for 4% of all cancers. In 2018, 887 659 new cases, and 453 307 deaths were reported worldwide [17]. This data does not consider paranasal sinus cancer nor MCUP. Lip and oral cavity cancers are the most common subtypes of the HNCs, with more than 50% of cases reported in Asia [18]. In the United States HNCs represent 3% of all cancers and the trend is declining. Since 2002, the incidence in men decreased by 0.29% per year *(p = .0357)* and the incidence in women decreased by 0.38% per year *(p = .0074)*, mainly due to a decline in the number of laryngeal carcinomas, parallel to a reduction of smoked tobacco [19]. Still, approximately 75% of HNSCCs are related to tobacco and alcohol use [20], which are known to have a synergistic effect. Damage caused by alcohol and tobacco is dose-dependent, as shown in a meta-analysis including 13,830 patients with HNC. In patients with alcohol consumption, the pooled odds ratio (OR) was 1.29(95% CI 1.06-1.57) for light drinkers which were defined by daily consumption of $\leq$ 12.5g, 2.67(2.05-3.48) when consumption was deemed moderate, and 6.63(5.02-8.74) for heavy drinkers which were defined by daily consumption of $\geq$50g/day. In patients with tobacco consumption the risk was stronger, the pooled OR were 2.33(95% CI 1.84- 2.95), 4.97(95% CI 3.67-6.71), and 6.77(95% CI 4.81-9.53) for light smokers consuming a maximum of 19 cigarettes/day, moderate smokers consuming 20–39 cigarettes/day, and heavy smokers consuming 40 cigarettes/day, respectively [21]. In the developing world, the incidence of HNC is higher, and it is considered the most common cancer in Southeast Asia [22]. This has been related to the use of betel quid which generally contains betel leaf, areca nut, and slaked lime, and may contain tobacco. Chewing of either betel leaf, tobacco, or areca nut by itself is also carcinogenic.

Since cigarette smoking has declined in many areas of the world, HPV-16 infection is becoming a prominent risk factor and is shifting the demographics of HNSCC towards white, male, younger patients who do not smoke nor drink. HPV-related HNC has a higher burden in developed countries, opposite to what happens with cervical cancer, another HPV-related cancer with a higher burden in less developed countries. The distribution of HNC predominates in the male population, 73% of the HNC patients are men [23], and the percentage is even higher for HPV-positive HNC. The median age of diagnosis is 60-years old but it is lower among HPV-positive HNCs [24].

Overall, 5-year survival for HNSCCs is close to 65%. In stage I, the 5-year survival is at least 80% and in advanced stages (III-IV) it is close to 40% [25]. 5-year survival varies amongst HNC subtypes, it is best for lip and oral cavity cancer with an 89.5% and 75% survival rate respectively [23, 24], and it is worst for nasal cavity and paranasal sinus cancer with a 5-year survival rate of 60.3%.

TYPES OF HEAD AND NECK CANCER

The following section briefly describes the main characteristics of each subtype of head and neck cancer according to its presentation site, emphasizing the role inflammation plays in oncogenesis:

Laryngeal and Hypopharyngeal Cancer

Laryngeal Cancer

Laryngeal cancer is one of the most important HNCs worldwide. In 2018, 177,422 cases and 94,771 related deaths were reported [26]. The incidence is higher in eastern and southeast Asia. The most common malignancy is squamous cell carcinoma, comprising 85-95% of cases. The World Health Organization (WHO) classifies premalignant laryngeal lesions as hyperplasia, keratosis, and mild, moderate, and severe dysplasia based on cellular atypia and dysplasia. Clinically, the lesions might present like leukoplakia (Fig. 1).

A comprehensive meta-analysis of laryngeal leukoplakia by Isenberg *et al.* [27], revealed no dysplasia in 53.6% biopsies, mild to moderate dysplasia in 33.5% biopsies, and severe dysplasia to carcinoma *in situ* in 15.2% biopsies analyzed. Premalignant lesions progress in 0-57% of cases into carcinoma *in situ* and eventually to invasive carcinoma (Fig. 2) [28]. Accumulation of genetic alterations favors progression. The most frequent mutations affect cell growth regulation molecules, such as epidermal growth factor receptor (EGFR), fibroblast growth factor receptor-3 (FGFR3), the catalytic subunit of phosphatidylinositol 3-kinase (PIK3CA), KRAS, and tumor suppressor genes such as PTEN, CDKN2A, and TP53. Identifying these genetic alterations in premalignant lesions may be useful to determine their risk of progression [29].

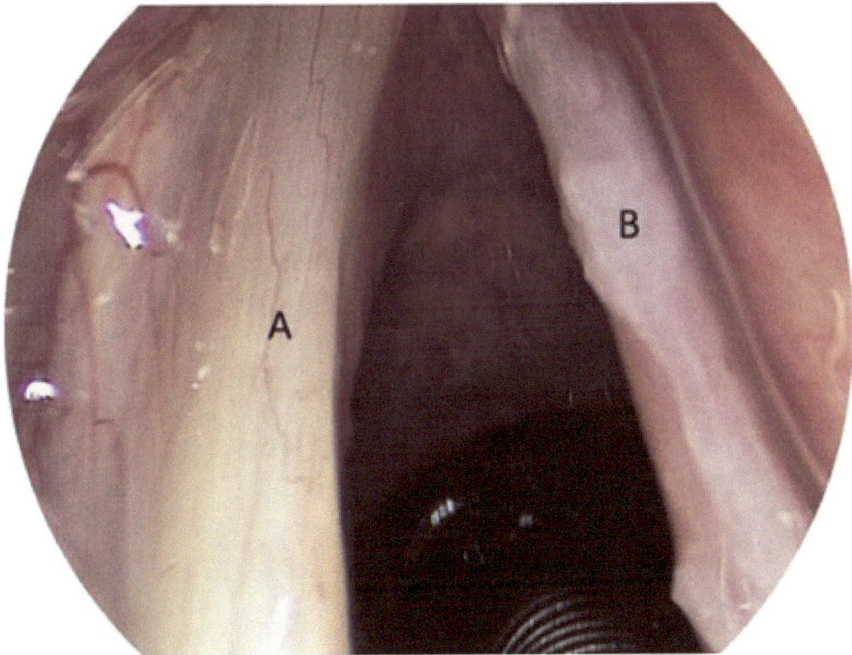

Fig. **(1))**
Endoscopic view of a larynx with leukoplakia. **A** = Left vocal cord, **B**= Leukoplakia overlying right vocal cord.

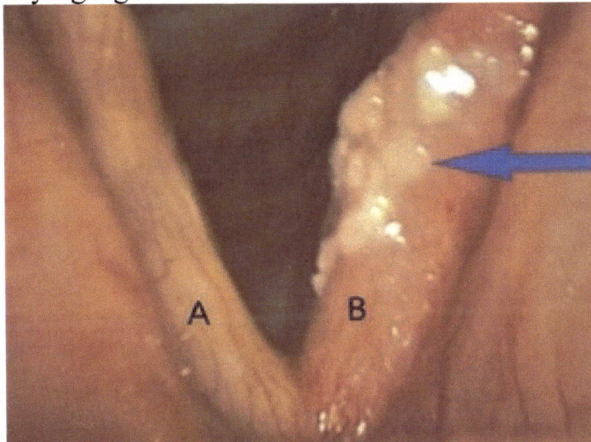

Fig. **(2))**
Endoscopic view showing left vocal cord carcinoma. Arrow indicates whitish cancerous mass. **A**=Right vocal cord, **B**=Left vocal cord.

Risk factors associated with laryngeal cancer include alcohol and tobacco exposure with an OR of 2.46 and 9.38 respectively, when used together the risk is multiplied [30, 31]. The exact mechanism through which tobacco leads to cancer is unknown, efforts to understand the molecular pathways have been made with animal models. In a pilot study using mice, Ha *et al.* described the elevation of IL-4 in the larynx of mice exposed to tobacco and vape smoke. IL-4 is a key inflammatory marker of TH2 cells [32]. On a genetic basis, TP53 mutations in HNSCCs occur more frequently in patients who smoke than in patients who do not smoke [10].

Gastroesophageal and laryngopharyngeal reflux can lead to chronic mucosal inflammation and leukoplakia, yet their role in the development of carcinoma is controversial. A systematic review and meta-analysis found that reflux disease was an independent risk factor for laryngeal malignancy after controlling for smoking and drinking covariates, with an OR 2.07 (95% CI, 1.26–3.41; p=.004) [33]. Environmental factors such as asbestos, polycyclic aromatic hydrocarbons, and textile dust have been associated [34]. Human papillomavirus (HPV) is found in approximately 20% of laryngeal tumors and has been associated with a better prognosis. HPV-positive tumors are associated with better local control and fewer recurrence and less metastasic disease, although this is still controversial [35, 36].

Anatomically, laryngeal cancer is divided into glottic, supraglottic, and subglottic tumors. Glottic cancers represent two-thirds of laryngeal tumors and most commonly occur on the anterior two-thirds of the vocal folds. Persistent hoarseness is usually the first complaint and present at an initial stage of the disease. Therefore, glottic cancer tends to be discovered early, improving prognosis. Supraglottic cancers represent one-third of laryngeal tumors and are more aggressive than glottic tumors. They usually remain asymptomatic until later stages, when they typically present with airway obstruction and cervical lymph nodes [34, 37]. Subglottic cancers are very rare and represent only 2% of laryngeal cancer cases. Patients usually remain asymptomatic until the locally advanced disease causes hoarseness, stridor, or dyspnea [38], and thus, the prognosis is poor.

Initial workup includes direct visualization with flexible endoscopy, followed by direct laryngoscopy and biopsy. Imaging techniques include computed tomography and/or magnetic resonance to evaluate local tumor extension and neck disease. Positron emission tomography has proven useful in the detection of metastatic disease [39, 40].

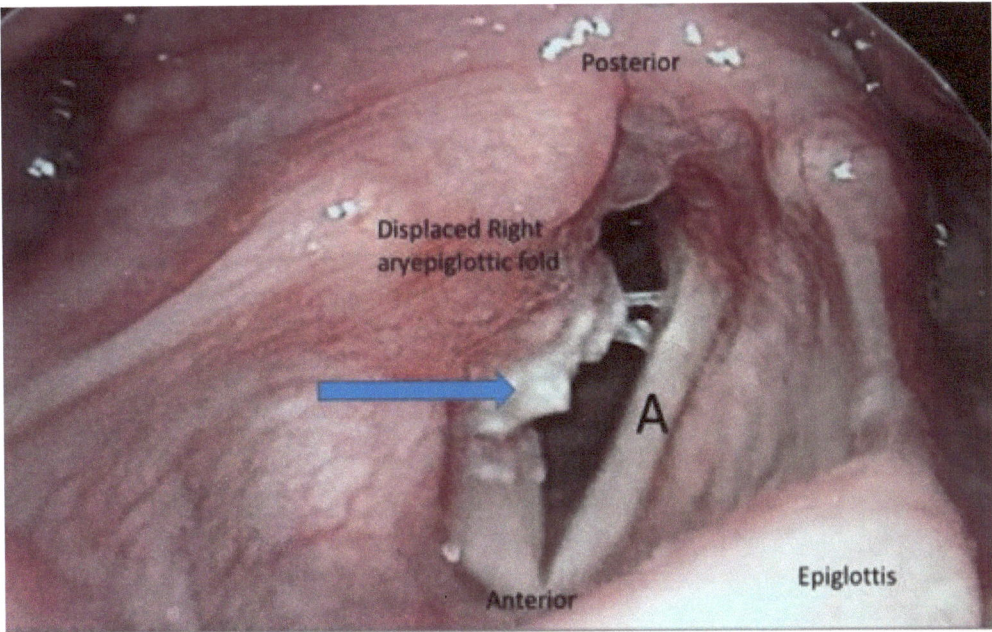

Fig. (3))

T3 supraglottic SCC right arytenoid cartilage. Arrow indicates the tumor. **A** = left vocal cord.

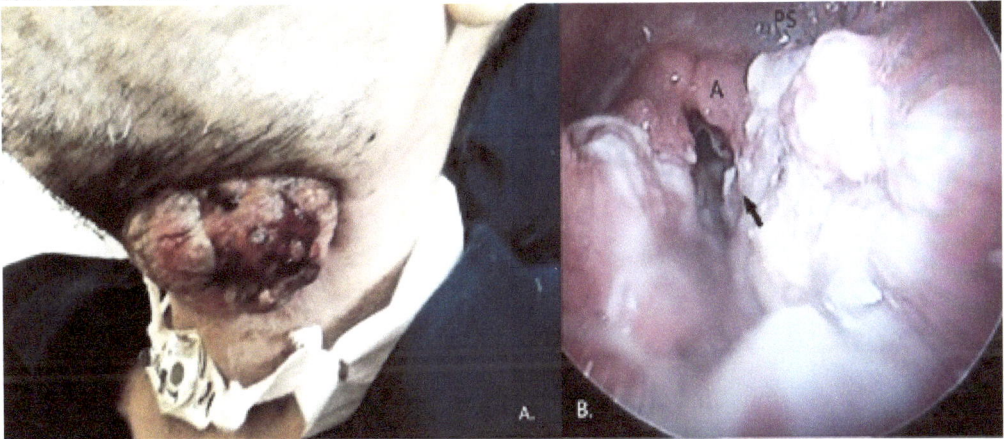

Fig. (4))

T4b laryngeal carcinoma with concomitant laryngeal tuberculosis. **A)** Soft tissue invasion of the left neck. **B)** Endoscopic view. **PS** = Pyriform sinus, **A** = Arytenoid cartilage, **arrow** = vestibular fold, **(*)** = left vocal fold.

To determine treatment laryngeal cancer is divided into early-stage laryngeal cancer (stage I and II) and advanced-stage laryngeal cancer (stage III and IV) (Figs. 3 and 4). For early stages, both radiation therapy (RT) and larynx preserving surgical techniques have a high curative rate, with a 5-year survival rate of 90% in stage I and 80% in stage II, with either treatment. Results in voice quality are also similar [34, 41, 42]. Limited RT affecting a smaller volume is being studied, and it includes carotid sparing radiation therapy and image-guided intensity-modulated hypofractionated RT. In stage I glottic cancer, this limited approach has similar locoregional control rates than classic intensity-modulated RT [43, 44]. Larynx preserving surgical techniques include partial open laryngectomy, transoral laser microsurgery, and transoral robotic surgery. Transoral laser surgery is often preferred to partial open laryngectomy due to its comparable efficacy with decreased morbidity, improved preservation of laryngeal function, lower costs, and shorter hospital stays [42].

Advanced-stage laryngeal cancer (stage III or IV) comprehends T3 and T4 tumors or any cancer that has lymph node involvement, regardless of tumor size. These patients can be treated with radical surgery or chemo-radiotherapy (CRT). There is a survival benefit for patients treated with total laryngectomy with adjuvant radiotherapy compared to those treated with chemo-radiotherapy, but the latter is superior in terms of organ preservation. Laryngeal cancer has an aggressive nature, characterized by a high recurrence and a poor prognosis. The 5-year overall survival rate is approximately 53% in late stages [33]. As of today, no molecular prognostic biomarkers have been identified for treatment stratification still, efforts are being made.

Hypopharyngeal Cancer

The prevalence of hypopharyngeal cancer varies greatly geographically. It is relatively frequent in Asia with 55,591 cases per year (69%) and extremely infrequent in North America with 3,125 (3.9%) cases per year. The most common type of hypopharyngeal cancer is squamous cell carcinoma (95%). Similar to laryngeal squamous cell carcinoma, smoking and alcohol are the main risk factors [45]. Other risk factors include tobacco chewing, vitamin C and iron deficiencies, gastric reflux, exposure to asbestos, coal dust, steel dust, iron compound fumes, and air pollution from solid fuels such as wood or crop residue [46, 47]. Exposure of hypopharyngeal epithelial cells to acidic reflux has been shown to induce nuclear factor-kB, leading to deregulation of oncogenic microRNAs, as seen in laryngeal carcinoma [33].

Hypopharynx is divided into three anatomical subsites, and the prevalence of cancer varies in each subsite. Cancer arises more often in the pyriform sinus (65-85%), followed by the posterior pharyngeal wall (10-20%), and it is uncommon in the postcricoid space (5-15%) (Fig. 5). Patients with these tumors usually remain asymptomatic until later stages of the disease, when they present with dysphagia, odynophagia, otalgia, weight loss, hemoptysis, dysphonia, dyspnea, or a painless neck mass [48].

Initial tumor assessment includes direct visualization with flexible fiberoptic endoscopy, looking for the obliteration of pyriform fossa, ulceration of the mucosa, edema of the arytenoids, and fixation of the vocal folds or the cricoarytenoid joint. Extension studies include contrast-enhanced CT to identify cartilage invasion. MRI is useful to assess soft tissue invasion, carotid involvement, and nodal extracapsular spread. Combined positron emission tomography (PET) and CT help evaluate the primary site, occult nodal involvement, and distant metastasis or synchronous primary tumors, and it is recommended in stage III/IV tumors [40]. Recently saliva microbiome studies have reported a significant difference in bacterial cultures between hypopharyngeal cancer patients and healthy controls. These changes are attributed to tobacco, betel nut, and alcohol use, which cause activation of toll-like receptors leading to a chronic pro-inflammatory state. Saliva based microbiome testing may be useful in early detection, which would lead to a better prognosis [49].

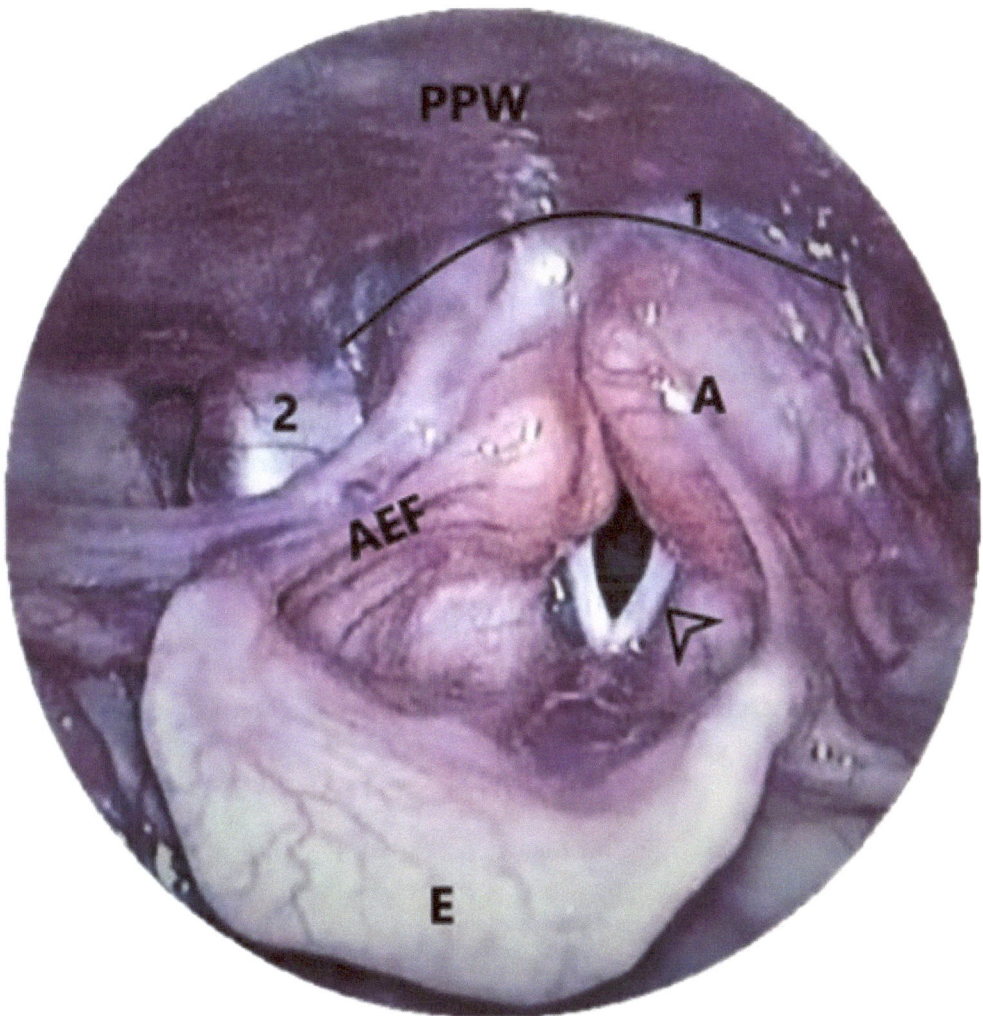

Fig. (5))
Hypopharyngeal cancer - Adenoid cystic carcinoma in the postcricoid area

invading both arytenoid cartilages. Arrowhead points to the left vocal cord. **PPW** = Posterior pharyngeal wall, **AEF** = Aryepiglottic fold, **A**= left arytenoid cartilage, **E** =epiglottis, **1**= postcricoid area, **2**= pyriform sinus.

Treatment of hypopharyngeal cancer is frequently challenging because patients usually present with advanced disease, also their health status is poor due to chronic malnutrition. At diagnosis, only 15% of tumors are confined to the hypopharynx, while 65% have local lymph node metastasis and 20% distant metastasis.

Total laryngectomy with partial pharyngectomy has been the standard of care for many years, but this paradigm is changing. Minimally invasive surgery with laser or robot-assisted has a 5-year control comparable to radical surgery with significantly less morbidity [50]. Radiotherapy combined with systemic chemotherapy has acceptable results in late stages, and most patients prefer it due to its lower morbidity [51]; nevertheless, surgery with adjuvant chemo-radiotherapy has longer disease-specific survival and overall survival in early and advanced stages [48]. Homologous recombination, specifically FaDu-R cells, has been associated with radio-resistance in hypopharyngeal cancer, indicating this protein could serve as a biomarker to predict response to radiotherapy [52].

Multimodal treatment with surgery, radiotherapy, and systemic treatment which includes biological and immunological agents is starting to gain popularity; however, immunotherapy still plays a small role in hypopharyngeal cancer. Recently an animal study by Cho *et al.*, demonstrated that colchicine can suppress cell invasion, migration, and adhesion in hypopharyngeal tumors by reducing the expression of metalloproteinase-9 (MMP9), the urokinase-type plasminogen activator (uPA) system, and the FAK/SRC complex, then colchicine might play a role as an adjuvant treatment in these tumors [55].

Unlike other HNCs, only a very small proportion of hypopharyngeal tumors have been linked to HPV with no significant overall survival differences. Specific treatment decisions for HPV-related tumors have not been established [53, 54].

Hypopharyngeal cancer has one the worst prognosis of HNC, primarily related to lymph node disease and distant metastasis. A study by Jing P *et al.* found that 3- phosphoinositide-dependent protein kinase 1 (PDK1) was overexpressed in squamous cell hypopharyngeal carcinoma. This overexpression correlated with regional lymph node and distant metastasis. PDK1 induced epithelial-mesenchymal transition and metastasis by activating the Notch 1 pathway, this pathway could be a future therapeutic target [56, 57].

Oral Cavity and Oropharyngeal Cancer

Oral Cavity Cancer

Oral cavity cancer is the 15th most frequent cancer. In 2018, there were 354,864 new cases reported worldwide and 177,384 associated deaths. Alcohol, tobacco, and betel nut use are the most important risk factors. Ethanol causes damage through its metabolite acetaldehyde (ADD), which is produced by oral and microbial alcohol dehydrogenase. Elevated levels of ADD promote DNA mutations. Alcohol also increases the permeability of oral mucosa, enhancing the absorption of alcohol and tobacco chemicals [31, 58].

Tobacco fumes and nicotine impair the saliva's antioxidant system and bring about oxidative stress, inducing genomic mutations, and the expression of pro-inflammatory genes. Mitochondrial defects acquired with age are aggravated by smoking, increasing the production of reactive oxygen species that promote the accumulation of DNA damage. Some signaling routs activated by free radicals include NF-KB, STAT3, MAPKs, PKC, Nrf2/Keap, and PAPR-a, caspase 3, NADPH oxidase 4, JNK mitogen-activated protein kinase. Tobacco also alters the cell cycle by elevating nitric oxide concentration, a regulator of the cell cycle, cell signaling, and apoptosis. Smoking promotes the expression of Ki67, a cell proliferation marker in oral keratinocytes, which overexpression results in precancerous and cancerous lesions.

Smoking weakens the innate immune function of the oral mucosa by modulating the expression of genes like hBD-1, hBD-2, NF-kB, NOD1, and RIP2. Changes in gene expression reduce the density of mature dendritic cells, elevate the expression of IL-8, inhibit phagocytosis, and promote macrophage conversion to the M2 subtype, which has anti-inflammatory, pro-tumor, and immune-suppressive characteristics. Tobacco smoke favors a pro-inflammatory environment by disturbing cellular-mediated immunity, it increases helper T cells and reduces regulatory T cells. Finally, tobacco smoke alters the mouth's microbiome, favoring a population of *Streptococci* and *Selenomonad*s, which also promotes a pro-inflammatory state [58].

Betel quid chewing plays an important role in oral cavity carcinogenesis. In a meta-analysis published by Guha *et al.*, the overall relative risk in betel nut chewing alone was 2.56, and 7.74 if associated with tobacco. About 50% of oral and oropharyngeal cancer in China, Taiwan, and India could be prevented if betel nut was no longer chewed [59].

Arecoline is the most important carcinogen in betel nut. Arecoline undergoes a nitrosation reaction with saliva, producing a variety of nitrosamines (BSNAs). These nitrosamines induce oxidative stress and subsequent carcinogenesis. The pathways involved in the production of reactive oxygen species (ROS) are NADPH, NOX-1, and cytochrome P450. These ROS are involved in epithelial aging by inhibiting auto-renewal abilities, which is associated with chemo-radiotherapy resistance and worse prognosis. Arecoline also induces chromatin relaxation by inhibiting PARP (poly ADP ribose polymerase), which constitutes a family of proteins involved in DNA repair and maintenance of genomic stability. The relaxation of the chromatin structure allows nitrosamines to interact with DNA, resulting in epigenetic silencing of tumor suppressor genes. The areca nut also contributes to malignancy by promoting cell motility through elicitation of matrix metalloproteases 1, 2, 8, 9, and suppression of tissue inhibitors of the metalloproteinase (TIMP) functions.

Other local factors have been linked with carcinogenesis. Chronic use of alcohol-based mouthwash has an increased risk of oral cavity and oropharyngeal cancer (OR 1.11). The damage mechanism is through the elevation of ADD, as with alcohol consumption [60]. Poor oral hygiene and periodontal disease have been linked to oral cavity carcinoma, through modification of the oral microbiome. Abnormal microbiome interacts with NOD-like receptors, Toll-like receptors, and RIG-I-like receptors resulting in chronic inflammation, and subsequent epigenetic mutations [61]. Recent studies have associated *Porphyromonas gingivalis* with increased risk of squamous cell carcinoma, through 3 different mechanisms: epithelial-mesenchymal transition of malignant cells, neoplastic proliferation, and tumor invasion. Proper control of this bacteria may serve as primary prevention in oral cancer [63]. Mucosal trauma secondary to sharp teeth, dentures, faulty restorations, and implants has been associated with carcinogenesis. Proposed mechanisms include DNA damage associated with increased activity of poly-ADP-ribose in mucosa with chronic trauma. The second mechanism proposes that chronic trauma promotes a pro-inflammatory state and oxidative stress [62].

SCC constitutes more than 90% of oral cancers. Other tumors arise from connective tissue, minor salivary glands (5%), lymphoid tissue, and melanocytes. Premalignant lesions include leukoplakia, erythroplakia, lichen planus, and submucous fibrosis. Each, with a varying risk of malignancy according to the degree of dysplasia. In general, leukoplakia has a very low risk of malignant transformation (1%), but erythroplakia is commonly associated with dysplasia and carcinoma *in situ*, therefore excision is recommended [64]. Mucosal and submucosal fibrosis are associated with betel nut chewing due to an increase in collagen production, reduction in degradation by proteinase, and activation of the TGF-B pathway. This increase in TGF-B raises the ratio of regulatory T cells to cytotoxic T cells in oral dysplasia, a crucial step for progression to SCC [58]. Patients usually present with advanced disease and with symptoms like mouth pain, non-healing mouth ulcers, loosening of teeth, dysphagia, odynophagia, weight loss, bleeding, otalgia, or difficulty in fitting dentures. Tongue cancer can grow as an infiltrative or as an exophytic lesion (Fig. 6), from a longstanding leukoplakia or erythroplakia.

Tongue cancer presents with symptoms such as pain, dysarthria (which indicates muscle involvement), and up to 66% of patients have cervical lymph node involvement at diagnosis. Lip cancer usually presents as an exophytic or an ulcerative lesion of the lower lip. It can be associated with bleeding, pain, and numbness of the skin innervated by the mental nerve [64]. Since most patients present with advanced disease, efforts are being made to clinically validate the detection of molecular biomarkers in saliva for early detection of oral cavity cancer. In genomics, HOX A9, NID2, and EGFR have shown promising results for the detection of oral cancer. A salivary transcriptome including 7 mRNA biomarkers has a sensitivity and specificity of 91% [65, 66].

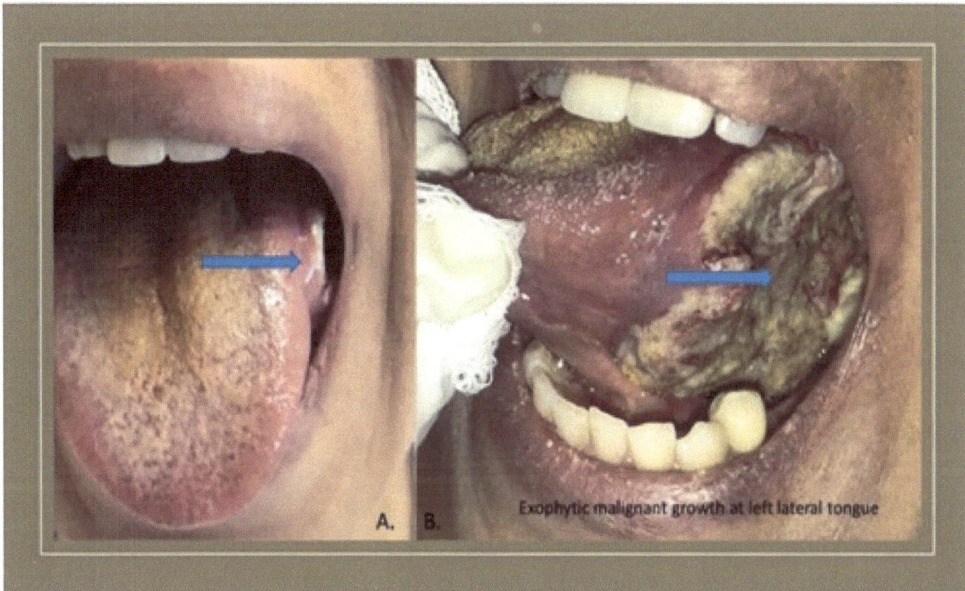

Fig. (6))
Tongue SCC. **A)** Frontal view **B)** Lateral view showing exophytic malignant growth at left lateral tongue.

The treatment of oral cancer includes surgery, radiotherapy, and chemotherapy alone or in combination according to disease extent. Surgical excision remains the primary modality of treatment in locally advanced tumors. Outcomes of treatment have improved over the last 30 years; this is associated with the ability to resect large tumors and reconstruct large defects. Technology such as intraoperative ultrasound and navigation have made surgical resection more precise [64, 67]. Molecular-based therapies approved for the treatment of oral

SCC are cetuximab (anti-EGFR), pembrolizumab, and nivolumab (anti-PD1), all with suboptimal results. Genetic biomarkers associated with good response to cisplatin include members of the Fanconi anemia/ BRCA pathway (BRCA1, BRCA2, SHFM1) [68].

Approximately 1.5% of patients with oral cancer will have a synchronous primary in the oral cavity, the larynx, the esophagus, or the lungs. Metachronous tumors develop in 10-40% of patients in the first ten years after the treatment of the primary tumor. Regular post-therapy surveillance and control of risk factors are important for secondary prevention [64].

Oropharyngeal Cancer

Cases of oropharyngeal cancer decreased in the 1980s parallel to a decrease in tobacco use, however, there was a new rise in the 1990s linked to HPV-associated cases [69]. Currently, unlike the rest of the HNCs, oropharyngeal cancer has an increasing trend per the HPV epidemic. Statistics on the association of HPV and oropharynx cancers are highly variable, with some authors reporting that 30% of oropharyngeal cancers are caused by HPV [70], and the American series reporting an HPV-positive prevalence as high as 70-80% [71, 72]. In 2018, 92,887 cases were reported worldwide with 51,005 associated deaths. Incidence is greater in Europe (30.1%) and Asia (41.7%) [73]. SCC represents 95% of oropharyngeal tumors, Waldeyer ring lymphomas, and minor salivary gland tumors represent the remaining 5% [74].

HPV, specifically type 16, has been widely associated with SCC of the oropharynx. Types 18, 32, and 33 are also related but less common. HPV-negative SCCs are associated with p53 mutations, decreased levels of p16 and increased levels of pRb. HPV-positive SCCs are associated with wild-type p53, down-regulation of pRb, and upregulation of p16 [69]. The gold standard for the diagnosis of HPV is polymerase chain reaction (PCR) to detect DNA. However, p16 serves as a useful biomarker [75]. In a meta-analysis conducted by Ndiaye *et al.* in 2014, the prevalence of HPV in oropharyngeal cancer was 46% and the prevalence of p16 was 41% [76]. The presence of HPV-16 in saliva samples has been associated with subsequent development of oropharyngeal cancer and could serve as a minimally invasive screening test in the at-risk population [77].

Oropharyngeal tumors (Fig. **7**) are more frequent in the tonsils and the base of the tongue, thus, the clinical presentation includes dysphagia, odynophagia, referred otalgia, snoring, sleep apnea, or a neck mass.

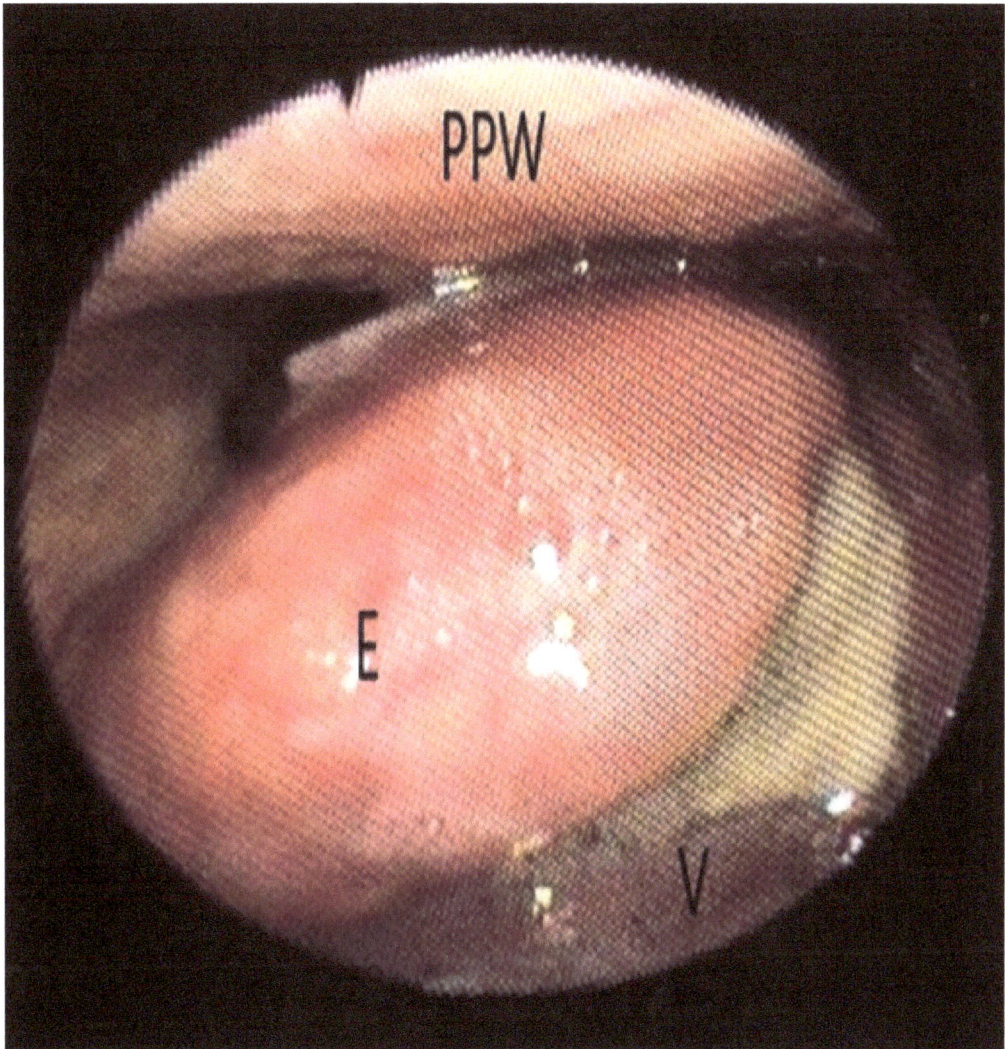

Fig. (7))
Oropharyngeal SCC of the vallecula invading epiglottis. **PPW** = posterior pharyngeal wall, **E** = Epiglottis, **V** = vallecula.

HPV-positive cancers often occur in younger patients, who present in early stages (T1 or T2) with an extensive nodal disease (N2 or N3). Patients with HPV-driven tumors have a better prognosis than those with HPV-negative tumors. The prevalence of SPM is also less frequent in HPV-positive patients. For these reasons, oropharyngeal cancer associated with HPV is staged differently to HPV-negative oropharyngeal cancer in the 2017 TNM system (AJC Staging guidelines, 8th edition [69, 78]. Younger age of presentation and the lack of association with alcohol and tobacco abuse partially explains the improved prognosis of HPV-positive tumors, but the molecular changes related to HPV *per se* also seem to play a role. In a study by Chung *et al.*, HPV tumors with a high p16 expression had a better prognosis than those with a lower expression [79]. Differences in clinical features of HPV-positive and HPV-negative cancers are summarized in Table 2.

Table 2 Clinical features of HPV-related oropharyngeal cancer *vs* non-HPV oropharyngeal cancer.

-	HPV Positive	HPV Negative
Oropharyngeal SCC cases	70-80%	20-30%
Epidemiology	Age: 33-50 Not associated with tobacco or alcohol	Age: over 50 Main risk factors tobacco and alcohol
Clinical features	Neck masses Greater risk of local metastasis	Dysphagia, odynophagia referred otalgia, snoring, sleep apnea
Biomarkers	Wild type P53 mutation Upregulation of p16 Downregulation of pRb	P53 mutation Decreased levels of p16 Increased pRb
Treatment	Surgery + deintensification chemoradiotherapy	Surgery + regular chemoradiotherapy
Prognosis 5-year OS	80%	40%
HPV: Human papillomavirus, SCC: squamous cell carcinoma, OS: overall survival.		

Regardless of HPV-status multimodal treatment for oropharyngeal cancer with radiation, chemotherapy, and/or surgery was frequent. Surgical outcomes have improved especially with the use of robotic surgery [50], and surgery as monotherapy is becoming a possibility. Due to the more favorable prognosis in HPV associated oropharyngeal cancer (80 *vs*. 40% 5-year survival), deintensification chemo-radiotherapy has been proposed, phase II non-randomized trials have reported encouraging results. In 2017, Marur *et al*. reported 80-94% 2-year progression-free survival (PFS) in T1-T3/N0-N2b treated with induction chemotherapy (cisplatin, paclitaxel, and cetuximab) and 95% 2-year PFS in those treated with adjuvant low dose radiotherapy with improved swallowing and nutritional status. Recently, Chera *et al*. reported favorable results at 2 years (95% local-regional control, 91% metastasis-free survival, 86% PFS, and 95% overall survival) with intensity-modulated radiotherapy (60 Gy) and low dose cisplatin [80]. Nevertheless, deintensification should only be performed in the context of clinical trials.

Salivary Gland Malignancy

Salivary gland malignancies are a group of rare, histologically diverse, and complex tumors with a world incidence of 0.59 cases/100,000 inhabitants [81], which represents about 3- 5% of all HNCs [82, 83]. The morphologic classification is extensive and keeps evolving. The 4th edition of the WHO Classification of Salivary Gland Tumors suffered relevant changes when compared to previous versions and currently includes 22 types of malignant tumors of epithelial origin and a borderline lesion. This last version emphasizes the importance of identifying genomic alterations to discern amongst lesions. Translocations and gene fusions are expected to be useful biomarkers [84].

Mucoepidermoid carcinoma, adenoid cystic carcinoma (ACC), and adenocarcinoma are the most common types of salivary gland neoplasms, with a prevalence of 34%, 22%, and 18%, respectively [9].

Mutations in p53 are the most common genetic alterations in mucoepidermoid carcinomas but are associated with moderate and high-grade tumors only. Mucoepidermoid carcinoma is associated with a specific genetic translocation between chromosomes 11 and 19, where exon1 from chromosome 19 interacts with exons of a gene on chromosome 11 associated with the Notch signaling pathway, called mastermind-like 2 (MAML2), resulting in the protein product CRTC1-MAML2. This protein product can activate an EGFR ligand to induce tumor growth. Overexpression of EGFR is present in 73% of high-grade tumors and is associated with a poorer prognosis. AAC also has a specific translocation, involving chromosomes 6 and 9, this translocation creates a fusion product between the myeloblastosis (MYB) oncogene and the transcription factor gene Nuclear Factor1B (NFIB). The effect of MYB-NFIB status on prognosis is controversial [85]. Overexpression of C-kit is another relevant genomic feature of ACCs.

From a clinical point of view, mucoepidermoid carcinoma is the most prevalent malignant neoplasm affecting major salivary glands. It is more common in men and tends to present as a solitary mass. A rapid growth rate, pain, facial palsy, trismus, local soft tissue invasion, bone invasion, and enlarged cervical lymph nodes should raise the suspicion for malignancy and prompt a thorough clinical workup. ACC affects minor salivary glands more frequently, has a slight gender predisposition toward women, it is indolent, and has a propensity for neural invasion. ACC also tends to produce late metastasis, a process regulated by c-kit and TGF-B [85].

Based on the primary site salivary neoplasms are divided into two groups, the first includes major salivary glands and the second comprises the minor salivary glands lining the oral cavity, the pharynx, the larynx, the nasal cavity, and the paranasal sinuses. Approximately, 70% of salivary gland tumors arise on the parotid gland, followed by submandibular tumors with a prevalence of 5-15% [86].

Possible risk factors associated with salivary gland malignancies are high consumption of processed meat, obesity, alcohol consumption, and radiation exposure [87]. Due to the rarity of salivary gland malignancies and distinctive clinical features of each histologic type, their pathophysiology remains understudied, resulting in fewer evidence-based therapies compared to other cancers. In general, surgical resection with negative margins is the mainstay in all types of salivary gland malignancies. Adjuvant radiotherapy is suggested for tumors with high-risk features and chemotherapy is reserved for a palliative setting.

Nasal and Paranasal Sinus Cancer

Nasal and paranasal sinus cancer is a very rare entity, it represents less than 3% of upper aerodigestive tumors and < 0.5% of all cancers [88]. The most common malignant neoplasms in this area are squamous cell carcinoma (Fig. 8) and adenocarcinoma. Neuroendocrine tumors and mucosal melanoma are infrequent [89]. Maxillary and ethmoid sinuses are more commonly affected, while sphenoid and frontal malignancies are rare. They are more common in the sixth decade of life and present a male predominance 1.8:1 [88].

Tobacco smoke is the most important risk factor for the development of SCC, the pathogenesis is similar to other HNSCC [90]. Chronic exposure to inhaled wood dust, glues, and adhesives is associated with adenocarcinoma [91]. Large particles of wood dust (10-20 mm), deposit on the walls of the nose and paranasal sinuses. These particles are cyto-genotoxic and induce oxidative DNA damage with a delay in DNA repair activity. Exposed cells show extensive autophagy, reduced DNA repair associated with reduced OGG1, and DNA base accumulation through phosphorylation of the EGFR/AKT/mTOR pathway [93].

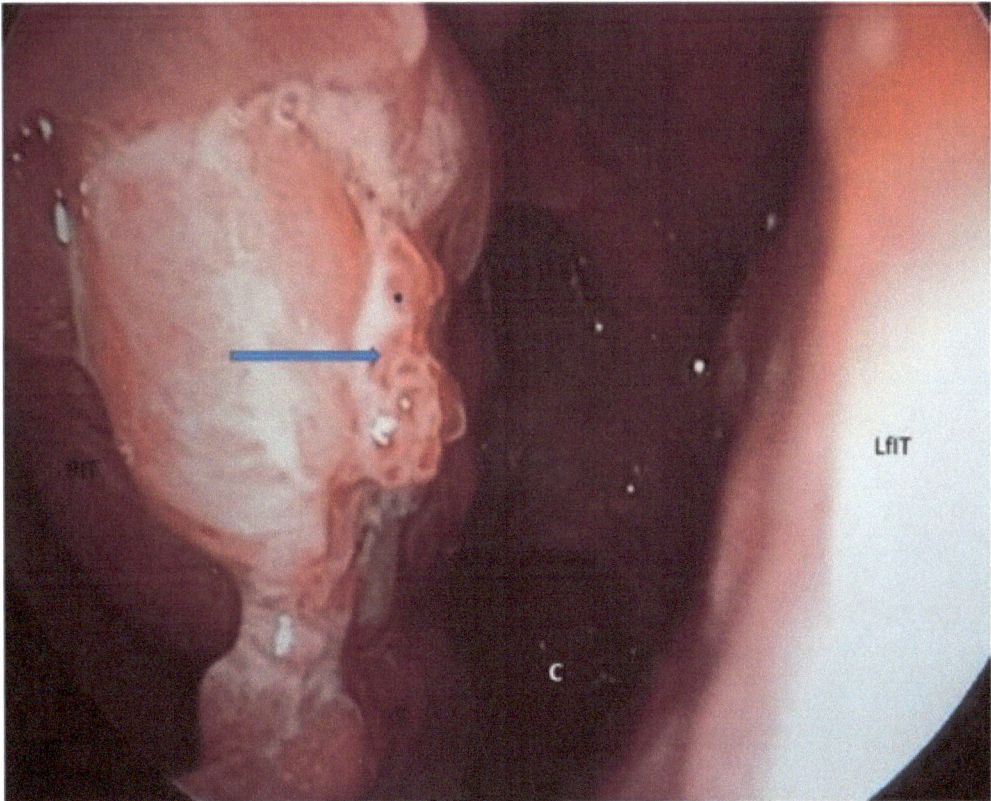

Fig.   **(8))**
Sinonasal Squamous cell carcinoma, arrow points at the tumor. **RIT** = Right inferior turbinate, **S** = perforated septum, **(*)** = tumor, **C** = choana, **LfIT** = Left inferior turbinate.

HPV infection has been associated with cases of sinonasal inverted papilloma (Fig. **9**), a benign tumor with malignant capability (Fig. **10**). Cases related to HPV-infection have a better prognosis [92]. Paranasal tumors have some correlation with the Epstein-Barr virus [89].

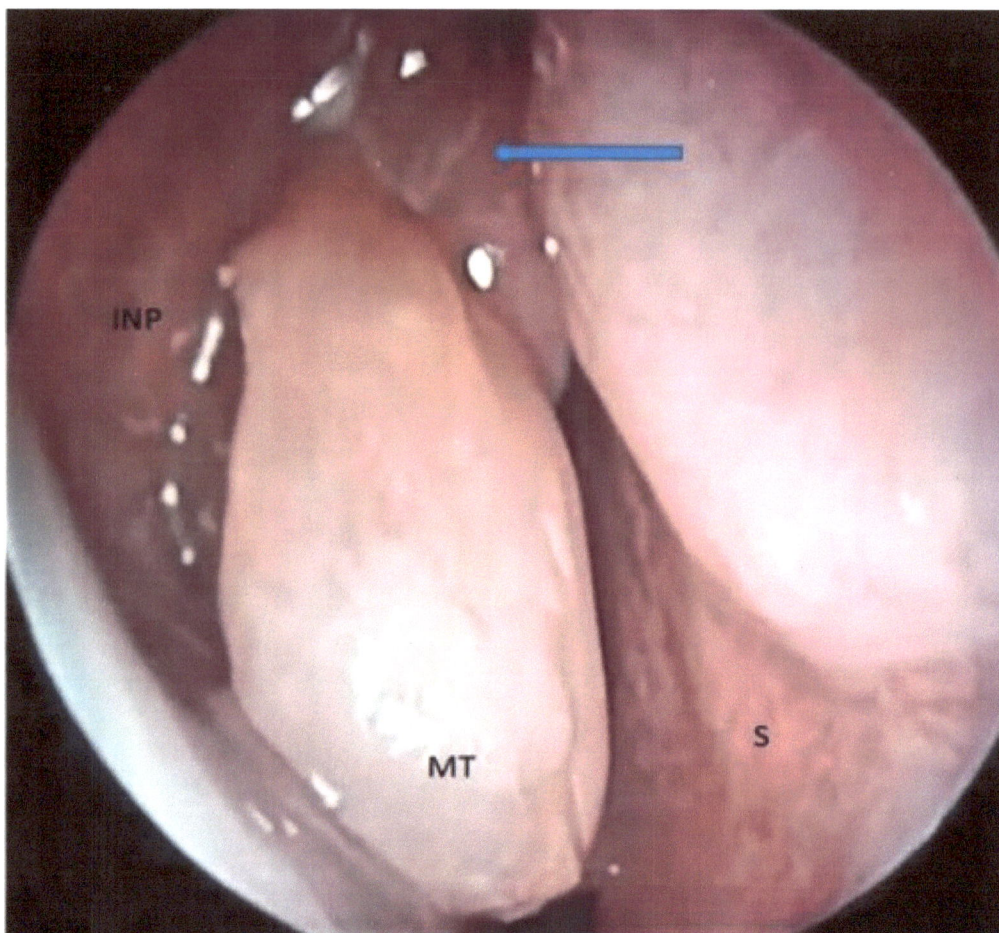

Fig. (9))
Sinonasal inverted nasal papilloma (arrow), **MT** = middle turbinate, **INP** = Sinonasal inverted nasal papilloma, **S** = septum.

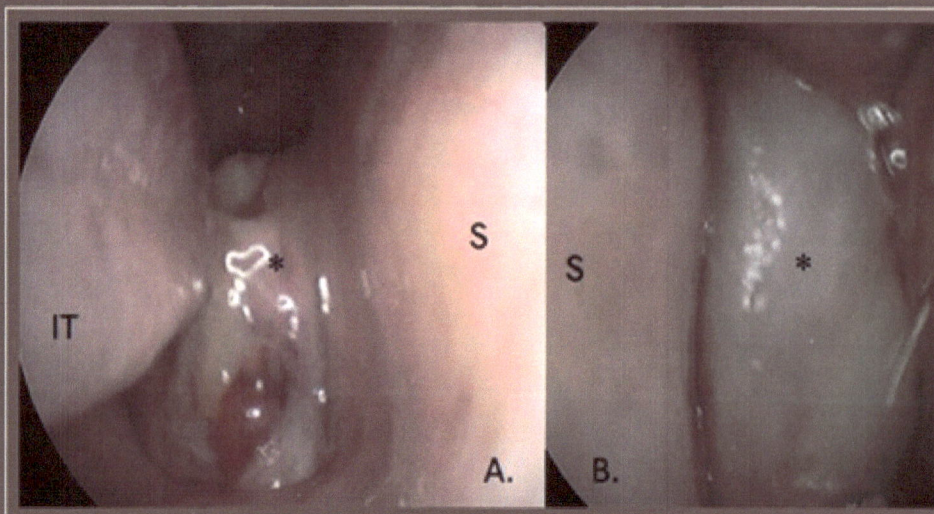

Fig. **(10))**

Malignant transformation of an inverted papilloma into sinonasal undifferentiated Carcinoma. **A)** Right nasal cavity, IT = Inferior turbinate, **S** = septum, **(*)** tumor in choana. **B)** Left nasal cavity, **S** = Septum, **(*)** tumor in the vestibular area.

Most patients with nasal cavity and paranasal sinus carcinoma present with symptoms of advanced disease such as nasal obstruction (71%) and epistaxis (42%). Facial swelling or pain, trismus, proptosis, diplopia, cranial nerve dysfunction, seizures, and other neurologic symptoms suggest invasion of adjacent structures. In the ethmoid sinus locally advanced lesions may extend to the anterior cranial fossa or the orbit and may present with anosmia or displacement of the ocular globe (Fig. 11). Sphenoid sinus tumors may extend directly into the cavernous sinus and affect cranial nerves III, IV, VI, V1, and V2. They may also invade the middle cranial fossa [89].

Initial evaluation includes a thorough physical examination with nasal endoscopy, assessment of cranial nerves, ophthalmologic function, and otoscopy. Computed tomography is the best modality to evaluate bone changes and bone destruction suggests malignancy. Neck disease must be purposefully evaluated, with emphasis on retropharyngeal lymph nodes and IB-IIA cervical levels. Magnetic resonance imaging is useful in evaluating orbital, intracranial, and perineural invasion [94]. A biopsy is required for definitive diagnosis. Treatment consists primarily of surgical resection (Fig. 12), with adjuvant radiotherapy in all tumor stages except T1N0. In irresectable tumors, chemo-radiotherapy is the treatment of choice. In recent years surgical treatment has shifted from open approaches (subfrontal, lateral rhinotomies, or degloving among others) to endonasal endoscopic resection. Improved instruments, image guidance technology, and better reconstructive techniques now allow resection of larger tumors [94].

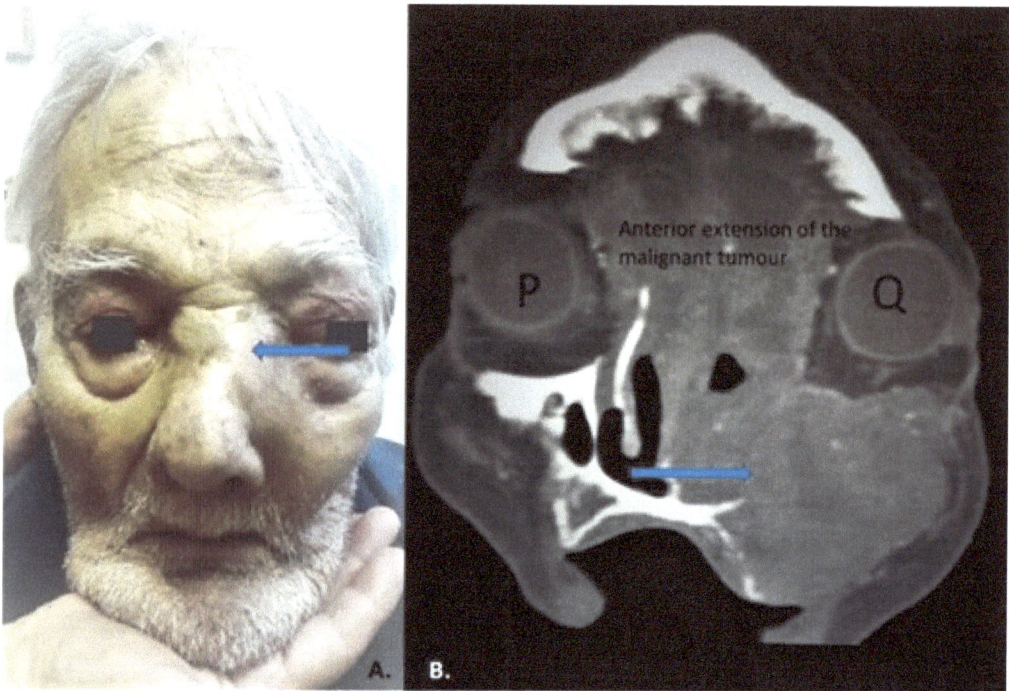

Fig. **(11))**
Extensive sinonasal carcinoma **(A)** with anterior extension **(B)** and causing deviation of nasal bridge externally. **P** = Right orbital cavity, **Q** =Left orbital cavity.

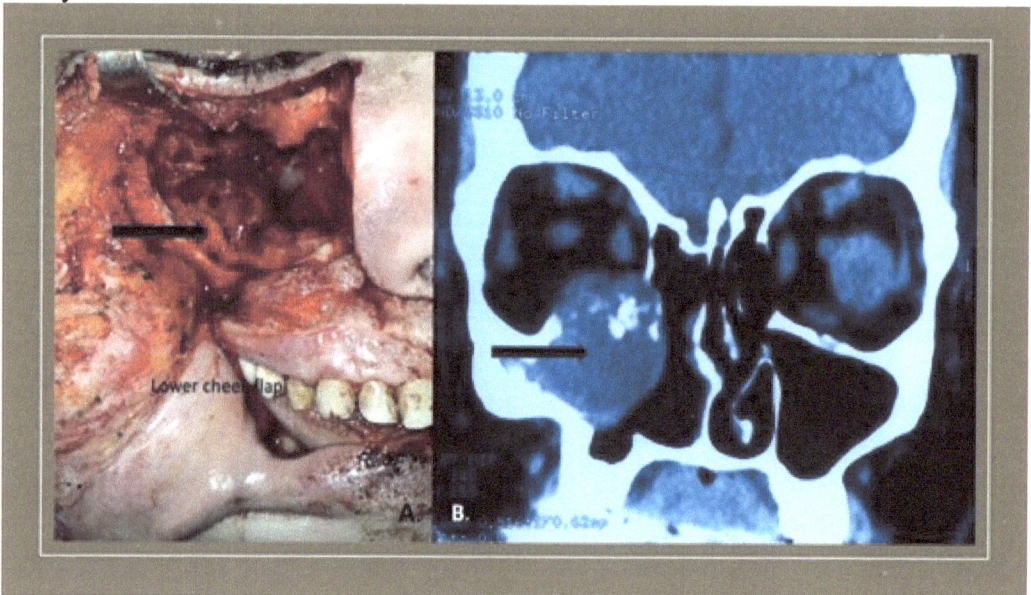

Fig. **(12))**
Subtotal maxillectomy for recurrent maxillary sinus carcinoma **A)** Intraoperative picture **B)** CT scan.

Nasopharyngeal Cancer

Nasopharyngeal cancer is an epithelial carcinoma that arises from the nasopharyngeal mucosal lining. Its incidence has gradually decreased in the last two decades [95]. In 2018, there were 129,079 reported cases with 72,987 associated deaths. The incidence of nasopharyngeal cancer varies greatly geographically. It is extremely rare in the US (1.9%) and Europe (3.9%) and frequent in Asia (85.4%). It is one of the most common cancers in Southern China, with 25 cases per 100,000 inhabitants per year. It is more prevalent in men 2-5:1, with a peak age of onset at 50- 59 years [96].

The WHO classifies 3 pathological subtypes keratinizing squamous, non-keratinizing squamous, and basaloid squamous. Nonkeratinizing is the most frequent subtype (95%) and has a close relation to the Ebstein-Barr Virus (EBV) infection [97].

There are genetic and environmental risk factors. Genetic susceptibility genes include HLA genes at the MHC region on chromosome 6p21, TNFRSF19 on 13q12, MECOM on 3q26, CDKN2A/CDKN2B on 9p21, and CLPTM1L/TERT on 5p15. Heterozygous germline variants of Macrophage stimulating 1 cell surface receptor (MST1R) is strongly associated with early age of onset and may be useful for population screening [97, 98]. Other associated genomic changes include loss of function mutations in NF-kB negative regulators, CCND1 amplification, TP53 mutations, and P13K/MAPK pathway mutations.

EBV is the primary etiologic agent in nasopharyngeal cancer. EBV-DNA and EBV gene expression has been detected in both precursor lesions and tumor cells. Mutations in NF-kB signaling promote chronic inflammation which contributes to persistent EBV infection, immune evasion of EBV infected cells, metabolic reprogramming, and cancer cell formation [99]. Nasopharyngeal carcinoma cells express a specific subgroup of EBV-latent proteins (EBNA-a, LMP-1, LMP-2) and a BamHI-A fragment of the EBV genome [97]. Due to its great association with EBV, population screening in endemic regions of Asia is becoming more and more frequent. Anti-EBV-IgA antibody (EA-IgA), anti-EBV capsid antigen (VCA-IgA), and anti-EBV nuclear antigen 1 (EBNA1-IgA) have low sensitivity and specificity. In a recent cohort study, EBV-DNA detection in plasma was reported useful in 20,000 participants with a sensitivity and specificity of 97.1% and 98.6% respectively [100].

Other risk factors include family history, tobacco smoking, consumption of salted dried fish, alcohol, and poor oral hygiene [101]. During the processing of salted dried fish, N-nitrose compounds undergo metabolic conversion into reactive nitrates that induce DNA damage [102]. An association between the inflammatory disease of the nasopharynx and nasopharyngeal carcinomas has been described in a recent systematic review by Riley *et al.* [103]. The evidence that supports this association is based on small retrospective studies, and therefore should be accepted with caution.

Patients with nasopharyngeal cancer usually present with headache, diplopia, facial numbness, otitis media with effusion, and neck mass. Unilateral otitis media with effusion in adults should always raise suspicion of nasopharyngeal cancer and endoscopic evaluation is obliged. Since the most common site of origin is the fossa of Rosenmüller, patients may be asymptomatic for a long time and present with advanced disease. Cranial nerves III, IV, V, and VI are frequently affected due to paracavernous tumor invasion. Nasopharyngeal cancer exhibits early metastatic disease, with 75-90% of patients having neck disease, and 5-11% distant metastasis (bone, lung liver) at the time of diagnosis [98, 104].

Laboratory blood count, serum biochemistry, liver function test, and alkaline phosphatase should be requested. Imaging studies should include chest X-ray, computed tomography, and magnetic resonance of the nasopharynx [104]. Definitive diagnosis is made through an endoscopically guided biopsy of the primary. An incisional neck biopsy is not appropriate for histopathological diagnosis.

Baseline plasma EVB-DNA is useful as a prognostic biomarker and as an indicator of recurrence after radical treatment [105]. Other biomarkers are programmed death 1, programmed death-ligand 1 (PD-1/PD-L1), and stromal tumor-infiltrating lymphocytes (TILs) the latter have been associated with better outcomes [97]. Recently Zhang *et al.*, published a 7- microRNA biomarker (let-7b-5p, miR-144-3p, miR-17-5p, miR-20a-5p, miR-20b- 5p and miR-205-5p) in plasma with good diagnostic results but no relation to prognosis [106].

The treatment of nasopharyngeal carcinoma consists of surgical excision, radiotherapy, and chemotherapy. Radiotherapy is effective in early-stage tumors without local or distant metastasis, with a 5-year survival of 80-90% [98]. Classical open surgical approaches (maxillary swing, midface degloving, transpalatal, transmaxillary, and transinfratemporal fossa) are being replaced with minimally invasive techniques (endoscopic nasopharyngectomy or robotic surgery). These minimally invasive surgical techniques have better overall survival than radiotherapy [107]. Tumors are considered irresectable when they have an extensive intracranial extension, cavernous sinus invasion, or encasement of the petrosal internal carotid artery. Treatment for advanced disease is a combination of chemo and radiotherapy [98].

Nasopharyngeal cancer immunotherapy has shown promising results with bevacizumab (anti-VEGF). EBV-specific cytotoxic T-lymphocytes (EBV-CTLs) combined with gemcitabine and carboplatin in advanced EBV-positive nasopharyngeal cancer had encouraging results with overall survival of 71%. Nivolumab (anti-Pd-1) was recently evaluated for heavily pretreated recurrent metastatic disease with an overall response of 20%. Currently, nivolumab and ipilimumab (CTLA-4 inhibitor) are being evaluated in patients with locally advanced tumors [97, 98, 108].

Thyroid Malignancy

Thyroid cancer is one of the most common malignant neoplasms encountered. In the US alone, 52,000 cases were reported during 2019, representing about 3.0% of all new cancer cases that year. Its incidence has been on the rise worldwide, owing in part to better imaging techniques that allow an earlier diagnosis of smaller nodules. This trend, however, is only seen in papillary subtypes and has not been reflected in lower mortality indexes, which support a true increase in frequency [109]. Risk factors associated with thyroid cancer include ionizing radiation, radioiodine administration, nitrate consumption, obesity, and insulin resistance [110, 111].

Thyroid cancers can be broadly divided into follicular derived neoplasms and neuroendocrine C-cell derived cancers. Follicular derived neoplasms represent 94% of all subtypes, being the papillary carcinoma the most common one [112]. Follicular cancer, Hurthle cell thyroid cancer, and poorly differentiated thyroid cancer can also be found in this category, all of them carrying a poorer prognosis. Anaplastic thyroid cancer accounts for <1% and is the most aggressive of the group. Medullary thyroid cancers, on the other hand, derive from parafollicular cells. This neoplasm usually arises from *de novo* mutations in the *RET* proto-oncogene, although it can present as familial syndromes like multiple endocrine neoplasia (MEN) 2A, MEN 2B, and familial medullary thyroid carcinoma (FMTC) [113].

Most thyroid cancers present mutations in the mitogen-activated protein kinase (*MAPK*) pathway. In papillary subtypes, the most frequent mutation is the *BRAFT^{1799A}* mutation. Follicular cancers and the follicular variant of papillary cancers commonly harbor mutations in the *RAS* family. These initial mutational events are thought to be responsible for cancer initiation, while mutations in phosphatidylinositol-3-kinase and p53 tumor suppressor pathway promote tumor progression [114, 115]. Chromosomal translocations are also encountered and some of them can carry prognostic significance. *ALK* rearrangements, for example, are associated with aggressive variants and its identification might have therapeutic ramifications [114]. The *STRN-ALK* fusion leads to constituent *ALK* pathway activation and TSH independent thyroid cell proliferation [116]. Inhibition of the *ALK* pathway in these patients might lead to better therapeutic outcomes.

Thyroid cancers usually present as asymptomatic thyroid nodules. With the growing use of head and neck imaging, silent nodules are being increasingly encountered in clinical practice. Correct identification of benign and malignant nodules is of uttermost importance since it can result in the avoidance of unnecessary surgery and distress. The initial evaluation of any thyroid nodule should include TSH measurements and thyroid sonography with a survey of the cervical lymph nodes [117]. According to the most recent ATA guidelines, nodules measuring >1 cm with high or intermediate suspicion sonographic pattern and nodules measuring > 1.5 cm with low suspicion sonographic pattern should routinely undergo diagnostic thyroid fine-needle aspiration (FNA). For nodules measuring > 2 cm with very low suspicion sonographic pattern, either observation of diagnostic FNA is appropriate. Purely cystic nodules should not undergo FNA [117]. Once diagnostic FNA is done, the results should be classified according to the Bethesda system. Non-diagnostic results should undergo a second FNA, while benign results should avoid surgery. If cytology results in thyroid malignancy, surgery is warranted. Intermediate results are more challenging to manage.

Galectin-3 immunohistochemistry has also been described for intermediate FNA results, although it is not as widely used as the previous methods. Galectin-3 is a β- galactosyl-binding molecule in the lectin group that is not normally present in healthy thyroid tissue. Its presence usually reflects thyroid cancer, since it is one of the targets of P53 activity [118]. Reported sensitivity and specificity for FNA cytology were 78 and 93% respectively. Though, a systematic review and meta-analysis published in 2017 found significant heterogeneity and publication bias comparing galectin-3 use in histological samples as well as FNA cytology, with a lower performance utility for FNA cytology [119]. Even though these results confirm the overexpression of galectin-3 in thyroid cancer, they question the real performance rate for FNA cytology compared to other techniques.

Once a cancer diagnosis is made, the main treatment for thyroid cancer is surgical. Depending on the stage, surgery can range from a simple lobectomy to a total thyroidectomy plus neck dissection [114, 117]. Radioiodine treatment can be used as adjuvant treatment depending on the postoperative findings and risk stratification. The overall 5-year survival rate surpasses 98% for early stages [112]. A small fraction of cases, however, are not cured by standard therapy and may require systemic treatment. Novel strategies based on the molecular pathways involved are in development at the moment, including *ALK* translocation inhibitors, *mTOR* inhibitors, *ERBB-HER2/3* inhibitors, amongst others [120].

Metastatic Carcinoma of Unknown Primary (MCUP)

MCUP account for 4-5% of all cancer diagnosis [121]. They can broadly be categorized as SCC, adenocarcinomas, neuroendocrine tumors, and poorly differentiated tumors. In the head and neck region, however, most CUPs correspond to SCCs. They usually present as solitary neck masses without any other accompanying symptoms. These patients require extensive workup to identify the primary site, including a complete physical examination, panendoscopy, CT, MRI, and FDG-PET [122]. If the primary site is identified, treatment is tailored to the appropriate staging and type of cancer. When there is no identifiable primary site on examination and imaging, bilateral tonsillectomy and lingual tonsillectomy can help in the identification of occult primaries, since most MCUPs arise in the oropharynx [123].

Specific biomarkers in FNA samples can also help narrow the possible sites. P16 positivity, for example, usually indicates an oropharyngeal origin, although this is not always the case [124]. These patients have a better prognosis compared to non-HPV associated cancer [125]. For EBV-positive cases, nasopharyngeal SCC should be suspected. Excisional lymph node biopsies should be avoided when possible, opting for a more comprehensive treatment.

If no primary site is identified, treatment should aim to control the disease in the neck while lowering the odds of growth in possible primary sites. Both surgery and radiotherapy are valid options as primary therapy in early nodal stages. Advance nodal stages usually need combined approaches. For definitive radiotherapy, the radiation field needs to be tailored to the possible primary site. The low prevalence of MCUP in the head and neck region prevents the completion of randomized trials, and its treatment remains controversial. The usual approach is to target both necks and the oropharynx. Depending on the risk factors and prevalence of nasopharyngeal cancer, the nasopharynx can be included in the radiation field. The larynx and hypopharynx are rarely involved, so avoiding treatment of these areas should be carefully considered [126, 127]. There is no clear consensus on the treatment of these types of cancers and therapy should be tailored for each case.

Lymphoma

Lymphomas are a heterogeneous group of lymphoid derived neoplasms. They are classified according to the cell of origin, morphology, immunophenotype, and genetic profile [128]. They can broadly be divided into Hodgkin's lymphoma (HL) and non-Hodgkin's lymphoma (NHL), with subsequent classifications according to specific features. NHL represents the majority of cases, with HL accounting for 12% of cases in one study [129]. Diffuse large B-cell lymphoma (DLBCL) is the most common type of NHL in the head and neck, found in one-third of the cases [129‑131].

The frequency of the different subtypes of lymphoma varies by geographical region. Places where the human T-cell lymphotropic virus 1 and Epstein-Barr virus are common, tend to have a disproportionate amount of T-cell and NK-cell lymphomas compared to the rest of the world [132, 133]. The most important risk factor described for NHL is immunodeficiency [132]. However, many risk factors are still unknown. This fact gave way to the creation of the International Lymphoma Epidemiology Consortium (InterLymph) in 2001. This interdisciplinary group is made up of epidemiologists, pathologists, clinicians, geneticists, immunologists, and biostatisticians whose goal is to facilitate the pooled analysis of individual-level data from different studies around the world, hoping to increase statistical power for rare exposures and subtypes of NHL. One of the studies published by this group was the InterLymph Non-Hodgkin Lymphoma Subtypes Project. It included studies from North America, Europe, and Australia and reported a combined dataset of 17,471 NHL cases and 23,096 controls [134]. Risk factors evaluated include a family history of malignancy, autoimmune disease, Hepatitic C virus (HCV) seropositivity, atopy, reproductive history, physical activity, alcohol and tobacco consumption, sun exposure, and occupation, among others. For DLBCL, B-cell activating autoimmune diseases, HCV seropositivity, family history of NHL, and higher young adult BMI were associated with increased DLBCL risk, whereas higher socioeconomic status, any atopic disorder, and greater recreational sun exposure were associated with decreased risk [135]. It is interesting to note that the history of B-cell activating autoimmune disease had the highest adjusted OR, 2.22 (95% CI 1.36 - 3.61) for men, and 2.42 (95% CI 1.73 - 3.38) for women. These entities included Hashimoto thyroiditis, hemolytic anemia, myasthenia gravis, pernicious anemia, rheumatoid arthritis, Sjögren's syndrome, and systemic lupus erythematosus. A detailed description of the different risk factors is beyond the focus of this chapter and the reader should consult the complete InterLymph report for further information.

The pathogenesis of NHL involves DNA damage during the maturation process that results in chromosomal aberrations and subsequent proto-oncogene activation [132]. The different subtypes depend on the degree of maturation and genetic alterations encountered. Neoplasms that do not have IgV mutations correspond to pre-germinal center-derived NHL, like mantle-cell lymphoma, since these cells

have not undergone somatic hypermutation. Diffuse large B-cell lymphomas, in contrast, derive from post-germinal center B-cells and have IgV mutations.

Clinical features vary depending on the site of origin and include cervical mass, odynophagia, dysphagia, and globus pharyngeus. B-symptoms are relatively rare and do not distinguish between aggressive and indolent subtypes [129]. Cervical lymph nodes are the most frequent site involved for both HL and NHL. For NHL, 65% of cases are found in cervical lymph nodes, while extranodal sites are involved in 25- 30% of cases [130]. The Waldeyer ring constitutes the most frequent extranodal site for head and neck NHL. They can also arise in the ocular adnexa, paranasal sinuses, salivary glands (Fig. 13), oral cavity, larynx, and the thyroid gland [131].

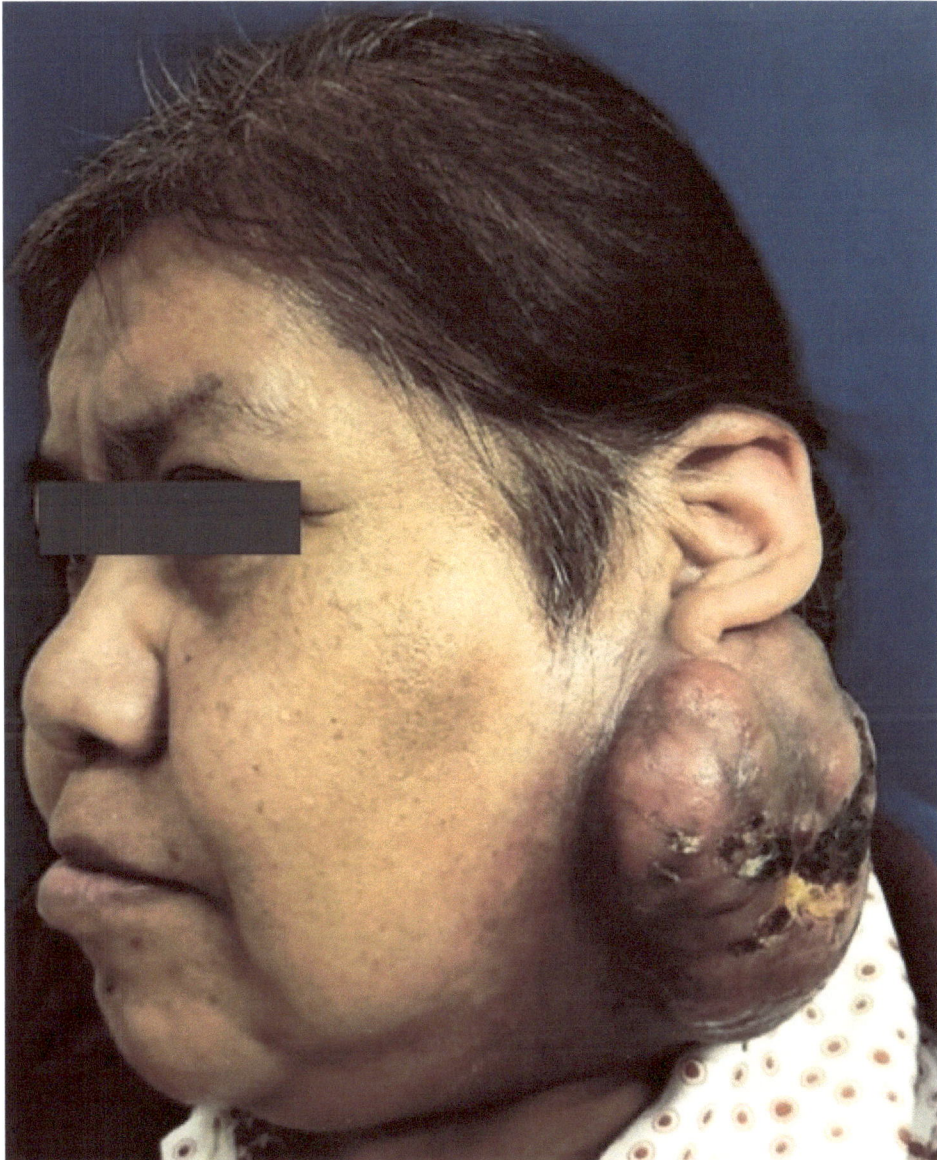

Fig. (13))
Primary lymphoma of the left parotid gland.

Adult patients presenting with an unexplained neck mass should undergo a complete evaluation to rule out lymphoma. Most lymphadenopathies in young people are due to infectious etiologies and should be evaluated as such. With increasing age, however, the probability of neoplastic disease increases. Risk factors should be investigated to help narrow the differential diagnosis. As we mentioned previously, immunodeficiency is the main risk factor for head and neck lymphoma and should raise suspicion if present. Most cases present as an indolent neck mass which can wax and wane. Obstructive symptoms develop when there is a bulky disease or extranodal extension [129].

Most cases do not develop B-symptoms at the time of diagnosis and, when present, should raise suspicion of disseminated disease. HL is usually found in younger patients compared with NHL. Mediastinal tumors are common in HL and need to be ruled out [129]. Otherwise, there are no clinical or laboratory findings that can help the clinicians distinguish between the two.

Most head and neck malignancies can present with neck masses at some point, making the clinical diagnosis of lymphoma challenging, and histology is mandatory. Nodes larger than 2 cm in diameter have a good diagnostic yield and should be evaluated when possible [136]. Although FNA is used as an initial screening test in many centers around the world, a core needle or an excisional biopsy is usually necessary for adequate diagnosis [137-139]. To make the diagnosis, the pathologist needs to evaluate histology, immunophenotyping, and genetics in the specific context of the case [128].

Contrast-enhanced CT is the imaging of choice for the initial evaluation since it permits adequate evaluation of the neck, mediastinal, abdominal, and pelvic lymph nodes. All patients should undergo a marrow biopsy from the posterior iliac crest to evaluate bone marrow involvement [130]. Clinical staging is done using the Ann Arbor system. Although originally developed for HL, this staging system can be used for NHL as well.

Treatment involves a combination of chemotherapy and radiotherapy. Since the 1980s, DLBCL was treated using a combination of radiation plus cyclophosphamide, vincristine, and prednisolone or CHOP. The MabThera International Trial, published in 2006, proved that the addition of rituximab, a monoclonal antibody targeting CD-20, improved 3-year survival compared with CHOP alone [140]. Since then, R-CHOP has been the standard regime for DLBCL. With the increasing precision of molecular methods, new therapies will arise that target specific pathways depending on the gene expression profiling (GEP).

Miscellaneous: Esophageal, Cutaneous, Temporal Bone Cancer

Carcinoma of the Cervical Esophagus

Carcinoma of the cervical esophagus (CEC) is rare in western countries. East Asia has higher rates probably due to dietary habits. Most cases correspond to SCCs. Consequently, risk factors include tobacco and alcohol use [141]. It is estimated that 75% of esophageal cancers are due to high alcohol consumption. They are frequently found during endoscopic evaluation indicated for aerodigestive symptoms. CECs are usually locally advanced at the time of diagnosis, which limits the surgical options due to the high morbidity associated with them. Treatment includes a combination of chemotherapy and radiotherapy [142], and the 5-year survival rate is less than 10% [31].

Skin Cancer

Non-melanoma skin cancer (NMSC) is the most common type of human cancer. Over 80% of these tumors arise in the head and neck [143], making it the most common type of HNC. NMSC consists of basal cell carcinomas (BCC) and SCC. The main risk factor associated with skin cancer is sun exposure. UV rays, particularly intermittent intense UVB exposure, can damage DNA [144]. The most commonly mutated gene in NMSC is the *TP53* tumor suppressor gene, and it usually involves C -> T single-base transition mutations at dipyrimidine sites. This mutation allows cells to escape apoptosis after DNA damage, which progresses to full-blown cancer. Other mutations encountered, especially in SCCs are mutations in *CDKN2A* and *Ras* [145]. This last gene is involved in the MAPK pathway. Therapies that target the epidermal growth factor receptor (EGFR) decrease signaling through the Raf-Ras-MAPK pathway, effectively control platinum-resistant SCCs [146]. The high mutational rate caused by UV light exposure results in multiple neoantigen expression. This event can promote priming and infiltration by neoantigen reactive T cells rich in PD-1. Patients with a high burden of neoantigen expression and intratumor heterogeneity could, in turn, respond favorably to anti-PD-1 therapy [147].

Most NMSCs are treated surgically with good outcomes. Advanced cases may require the addition of chemotherapy and radiotherapy for local and systemic control. Target therapy and immunotherapy have an important place in the treatment of advanced cancers, particularly in platinum-resistant cases.

Temporal Bone Carcinoma

Temporal bone carcinoma usually refers to skin cancers involving the external auditory canal (EAC). They are rare neoplasms, estimated around one to six per million inhabitants, but behave aggressively [148]. The most frequent histological subtype is SCC. Surgical excision with adjuvant radiotherapy constitutes the usual treatment. Parotidectomy and neck dissection should be considered in every case [149]. Surgical procedures vary and are usually mutilating. Some authors argue that, due to the aggressive nature of the tumor, the minimal approach should include a lateral temporal bone resection [149, 150]. Total temporal bone resections are rarely performed due to the high morbidity and mortality associated with the procedure. Prognosis is usually poor if not detected early. As with other types of SCCs, both kinase inhibitors and immunotherapy could potentially improve patient outcomes in the future.

MOLECULAR AND GENOMIC LANDSCAPE OF HEAD AND NECK MALIGNANCY

HNSCCs have a high rate of genetic heterogeneity. Mutations can lead to loss-of-function of tumor suppressor genes such as p53, retinoblastoma tumor suppressor (RB), and p16INK4a, or overexpression of oncogenes such as the epidermal growth factor receptor (EGFR)4 and PIK3CA. EGFR4 is overexpressed in 80% of HNSCCs and correlates with poor prognosis, the latter is part of the PI3K/Akt/mTOR pathway, which is the most affected pathway in HNSCCs [15].

Current research is focused on understanding the molecular, biochemical, genetic, and immunological properties of HNSCC that lead to rapid cell growth, tumor proliferation, and metastatic invasion, a task made possible with the use of cell lines derived from different primary sites [151]. A more detailed molecular profile allows a better classification of HNSCC subtypes and will enable tailored diagnosis and treatment strategies.

According to the concept of field cancerization, cells are not the only ones mutating in cancer; but genetic and epigenetic changes also take place in surrounding epithelial, stromal, and immune cells, leading to dynamic cancer-prone surrounding extracellular matrix, a concept known as tumor microenvironment [152, 153]. A well-known example of the role of the environment is hypoxia, hypoxic tumors have a worse response to treatment than none-hypoxic tumors, which is partially explained by an upregulation of Vascular Endothelial Growth Factor (VEGF) *via* Jun N terminal kinase (JNK-1) and p38 kinase. VEGF is a key player in the development of tumor vascularization, and its production by tumor cells is associated with poor prognosis, nodal metastasis, a more advanced clinical stage, and low survival in HNSCC [154]. Measuring biomarkers revealing the tumor microenvironment is another way of classifying HNSCCs. Inflammation is a hallmark of cancer, and shares pathways with diverse inflammatory processes like Alzheimer's disease and cardiovascular thrombosis, one of these pathways is modulated by the anti-inflammatory mediator Annexin A1 (ANAX1) [155, 156]. ANAX1 is an anti-inflammatory mediator that acts regulating leukocyte extravasation, macrophage phagocytosis, and glucocorticoid action interacting with the receptor FPR2.

Molecular and genomic profiling is changing the way cancers are been diagnosed and managed:

Laryngeal Cancer

From a molecular point of view, the cell's immortalization in laryngeal squamous cell carcinoma (LSCC) is associated with a downregulation of the caspase complex, which promotes cellular apoptosis [157].

As stated earlier, laryngeal carcinoma can have devastating consequences for patients, and research is looking for new and less invasive forms of diagnosis, novel therapies, and more accurate prognosis tools. Genetic silencing by DNA methylation of cell-cell adhesion molecules favors cancer progression, thus protocadherin17 (PCDH17) has a role as a tumor suppressor gene in LSCC, and testing for PCDH17 promoter DNA methylation in peripheral blood is a potential biomarker [158].

Novel therapies search to target molecular pathways, *e.g.* bleomycin-A2, demonstrated an antitumoral role by increasing caspase-dependent apoptotic rates *in vitro* in Hep-2 laryngeal carcinoma cells [157] and ANAX1. A study by Gastardelo *et al*. has shown that activated mast cells and neutrophils by the tumor microenvironment, demonstrate up-regulation of ANXA1/FPR2 as an anti-inflammatory response mechanism to resolve inflammation and proliferation in laryngeal cancer [159]. There is much research pending, but ANAX1 is a promising target for future treatment.

Based on mRNA profiling, the Cancer Genome Atlas identified laryngeal cancer subclasses, which are classic, basal, and mesenchymal subclasses; however, these do not correlate with prognostic differences. Recently, damaging mutations of methyltransferases NSD1 and NSD2 have been associated with a better prognosis [160]. NSD mutations are associated with widespread genome hypomethylation in tumors with a better response to cisplatin.

A study by Enhong *et al.* detected lung adenocarcinoma metastasis-associated transcript -1 (MALAT-1) in laryngeal squamous cell carcinoma cells and proved its role in the development of these tumors by developing a MALAT-1 silencing model in human laryngeal and hypopharyngeal tumor cells. Since this biomarker is more frequent in advanced tumor cells it is a decisive gene for regulating metastasis, and it may play a role as a biomarker indicating tumor progression [161].

Oropharyngeal Cancer

Perhaps, of the information gathered through molecular analyses, the determination of the Human Papilloma Virus (HPV) status is the most clinically relevant in current practice. Oncogenic HPV (90% of cases type 16) is associated with oropharyngeal cancer through the inactivation of p53 and pRB by viral proteins E6 and E7, respectively. Other HNCs have also been associated with HPV infection but to a much weaker extent.

HPV-related HNCs have a better prognosis, which might be explained due to genetic differences. HPV-positive HNSCCs are much less likely to harbor a TP53 mutation than HPV-16-negative HNSCCs. The risk of progression is 73% lower and the risk of death that is 64% lower in patients with HPV-positive tumors [10] compared to HPV-negative tumors. Deintensification of treatment in HPV-positive OSCC is under investigation. The importance of sorting HNC cancer into HPV-positive and HPV-negative types cannot be overstated. Efforts have been made to determine useful molecular biomarkers linked to HPV-status to establish specific treatment targets. Downregulation of caspase-8 in HPV-positive SCCs leads to decreased apoptotic rates affecting negatively cisplatin-based treatment [157], hence caspase-8 expression could be used to tailor therapy. Patients with NOTCH-1 mutations in HPV positive tumors have poorer overall survival, no difference has been found in HPV-negative tumors. This could be explained by previously reports NOTCH-1 associated chemoresistance in other tumors. SOX2 amplification has been reported in TP53 mutated cases of HPV-negative tumors and is associated with worse overall survival. Identifying these mutations may serve as a prognostic indicator and a future target therapy line [162, 163].

Thyroid Cancer

In recent years, molecular markers became a valuable tool to "rule-out" or "rule-in" thyroid malignancy. Three strategies emerged for intermediate FNA results; a seven-gene panel of genetic mutations and rearrangements, a gene expression classifier (167 GEC; mRNA expression of 167 genes), and galectin-3 immunohistochemistry [117].

The seven-gene panel tests for the most common mutations, including *BRAF V600E, NRAS* codon 61, *HRAS* codon 61, and *KRAS* codons 12/13point mutations and *RET/PTC1, RET/PTC3*, and *PAX8/PPARγ* rearrangements. A study by Nikiforov *et al.* evaluated 1056 consecutive thyroid FNA samples with indeterminate cytology, finding that molecular testing had a positive predictive value of 87 – 95% for predicting thyroid cancer [164]. It is important to note that *RAS* mutations were associated with malignancy in 85% of the cases, compared to 100% of *BRAF, RET/PCT,* and *PAX8/PPARγ* mutations. It is then safe to assume that a positive gene panel "rules-in" malignancy and should prompt surgery. Mutation negative nodules, on the other hand, had a 14 and 28% risk of malignancy for FN/SFN and SMC diagnoses, thus making it unable to "rule-out" thyroid cancer.

The gene expression classifier by comparison has better sensitivity and negative predictive value, making it a valuable tool to "rule-out" malignancy. This tool was originally developed by Veracyte and is currently marketed as Afirma GSC. It combines RNA sequencing information with machine learning algorithms to provide the clinicians with one of two results: suspicious or benign. The reported sensitivity exceeds 90%, while specificity was found to be 52% [165]. A newer supplement, called Afirma XA, is now available and can be used in Afirma GSC positive FNA samples and Bethesda V/VI nodules to detect gene variants or fusions [166]. Although no long-term data are available, the genomic classification of thyroid neoplasms will likely improve patient care in the future.

In recent years, immunotherapy has shown promising results for a wide range of malignant neoplasms. In advanced cases, poorly differentiated and anaplastic variants, targeting the immune system can be of great value. There are several potential targets for therapy in thyroid cancers. Anaplastic thyroid cancers, for example, have a dense population of tumor-associated macrophages (TAM), composing nearly 50% of their volume [120]. *BRAF* mutations found in most thyroid cancers upregulate *CSF-1* and *CCL-2* expression which in turn attracts TAMs. These macrophages are of the M2 phenotype and promote tumor growth. Selective inhibition of these chemokines can reduce tumor volume and repolarize macrophages into an M1 antitumor phenotype [167].

Treg cells play a significant role in the equilibrium and escape phases of the cancer immunoediting process. This subpopulation is increased in recurrent cases of papillary thyroid cancer and recurrent metastatic lymph node disease [168]. The expression of inhibitory molecules, particularly *CTLA-4* and *PD-1,* is also upregulated and is associated with a worse prognosis. Under normal circumstances, both pathways prevent autoreactivity; *CTLA*-4 inhibits T cells before they are activated in lymph nodes, while *PD-1* regulates previously activated T cells at a later stage. However, they allow cancer cells to escape destruction when found in tumor-infiltrating T cells [169]. Several drugs have been developed that target these pathways, including ipilimumab (anti-CTLA-4), pembrolizumab (anti-PD-1), and nivolumab (anti-PD-1). At the moment several ongoing trials are evaluating the efficacy and safety of these drugs in advanced thyroid cancer as a single treatment or in combination with multiple kinase inhibitors [120, 170].

Lymphoma

Advances in molecular profiling have led to a more precise classification of lymphomas in general. For DLBCL, GEP identified three "subgroups"; germinal center B-cell-like DLBCL (GCB), activated B-cell- like DLBCL (ABC), and DLBCL that could not be classified [128, 171]. These subgroups represented neoplasms that originated at different moments of B-cell maturation and have significant differences in the associated gene expression. Notably, the t(14;18) translocation involving the BCL-2 gene and the amplification of the c-rel locus on chromosome 2p are exclusively found in GCB. This subgroup also has the highest 5-year survival [172]. One of the theories that explain the better survival outcome for GBC involves decreased activation of the nuclear factor kappa beta pathway since it interferes with the apoptosis generated by chemotherapy [173]. Since GEP is still not widely available as a diagnostic tool, for the time being, immunohistochemistry profiles are used to classify DLBCL. The most commonly used antibodies are CD10, BCL-6, and IRF4/MUM1; however, these do not correlate perfectly with GEP. Quantification of RNA transcripts could circumvent this problem in the future [128].

CONCLUSION

Head and neck cancers arise in a complex anatomic region. Due to the heterogeneity of the area, a comprehensive classification that is broadly accepted is lacking. We encourage our readers to keep in mind that "Types of Head and Neck Malignancies", might mean different things for different authors. The most simplistic approach is based on the site of origin, yet for some, this definition contemplates every tumor arising from the thoracic inlet to the skull base; while most consider only tumors arising in salivary glands and cells that line mucosa surfaces. For others, the histological type is the most important trait to define the type of cancer. With increasing knowledge of cancer pathogenesis, molecular characteristics are gaining popularity for classification purposes. In the near future, gene expression profiling of malignant neoplasms promises better diagnosis, treatment, and prognosis of these tumors. Until a clearer definition of the types of head and neck malignancy arises, researchers and clinicians must be thorough and cautious when reporting data on head and neck cancer.

CONSENT FOR PUBLICATION

Not applicable.

CONFLICT OF INTEREST

The authors confirm that the content of this chapter has no conflict of interest.

ACKNOWLEDGEMENTS

Declared none.

REFERENCES

[1]   Lydiatt WM, Patel SG, O'Sullivan B. Head and neck cancers-major changes in the American Joint Committee on cancer. CA Cancer J Clin 2017; 67(2): 122-37.

[2]   Cohen N, Fedewa S, Chen AY. Epidemiology and demographics of the head and neck cancer population. Oral Maxillofac Surg Clin North Am 2018; 30(4): 381-95.[http://dx.doi.org/10.1016/j.coms.2018.06.001]

[3]   Alfouzan AF. Head and neck cancer pathology: Old world versus new world disease. Niger J Clin Pract 2019; 22(1): 1-8.[PMID: 30666013]

[4]   Maasland DHE, van den Brandt PA, Kremer B, Goldbohm RAS, Schouten LJ. Alcohol consumption, cigarette smoking and the risk of subtypes of head-neck cancer: results from the Netherlands Cohort Study. BMC Cancer 2014; 14: 187.[http://dx.doi.org/10.1186/1471-2407-14-187] [PMID: 24629046]

[5]   Fulcher CD, Haigentz M, Jr, Ow TJ. Education Committee of the American Head and Neck Society (AHNS)AHNS Series: Do you know your guidelines? Principles of treatment for locally advanced or unresectable head and neck squamous cell carcinoma. Head Neck 2018; 40(4): 676-86.[http://dx.doi.org/10.1002/hed.25025] [PMID: 29171929]

[6]   Cohen EEW, LaMonte SJ, Erb NL, et al. American Cancer Society Head and Neck Cancer Survivorship Care Guideline. CA Cancer J Clin 2016; 66(3): 203-39.[http://dx.doi.org/10.3322/caac.21343] [PMID: 27002678]

[7]   Hung YH, Liu SA, Wang CC, Wang CP, Jiang RS, Wu SH. Treatment outcomes of unknown primary squamous cell carcinoma of the head and neck. PLoS One 2018; 13(10): e0205365.[http://dx.doi.org/10.1371/journal.pone.0205365] [PMID: 30335795]

[8]   Chernock RD, Lewis JS. Approach to metastatic carcinoma of unknown primary in the head and neck: squamous cell carcinoma and beyond. Head Neck Pathol 2015; 9(1): 6-15.[http://dx.doi.org/10.1007/s12105-015-0616-2] [PMID: 25804376]

[9]   Adelstein DJ, Koyfman SA, El-Naggar AK, Hanna EY. Biology and management of salivary gland cancers. Semin Radiat Oncol 2012; 22(3): 245-53.[http://dx.doi.org/10.1016/j.semradonc.2012.03.009] [PMID: 22687949]

[10]   Pai SI, Westra WH. Molecular pathology of head and neck cancer: implications for diagnosis, prognosis, and treatment. Annu Rev Pathol 2009; 4(4): 49-70.[http://dx.doi.org/10.1146/annurev.pathol.4.110807.092158] [PMID: 18729723]

[11]   Morris LGT, Sikora AG, Patel SG, Hayes RB, Ganly I. Second primary cancers after an index head and neck cancer: subsite-specific trends in the era of human papillomavirus-associated oropharyngeal cancer. J Clin

Oncol 2011; 29(6): 739-46.[http://dx.doi.org/10.1200/JCO.2010.31.8311] [PMID: 21189382]

[12] Ng SP, Pollard C, III, Kamal M, *et al.* Risk of second primary malignancies in head and neck cancer patients treated with definitive radiotherapy. NPJ Precis Oncol 2019; 3: 22.[http://dx.doi.org/10.1038/s41698-019-0097-y] [PMID: 31583278]

[13] Slaughter D, Southwick H, Smejkal W. Field cancerization in oral stratified squamous epithelium; clinical implications of multicentric origin. Cancer 1953; 6(5): 963–8.

[14] Ha PK, Califano JA. The molecular biology of mucosal field cancerization of the head and neck. Crit Rev Oral Biol Med 2003; 14(5): 363-9.[http://dx.doi.org/10.1177/154411130301400506] [PMID: 14530304]

[15] Alsahafi E, Begg K, Amelio I, *et al.* Clinical update on head and neck cancer: molecular biology and ongoing challenges. Cell Death Dis 2019; 10(8): 540.[http://dx.doi.org/10.1038/s41419-019-1769-9] [PMID: 31308358]

[16] World Health OrganizationInternational classification of diseases for oncology (3rd edition, 1st revision.), 3rd edition, 1st revision.2013.

[17] Globocan WHO. 2019.https://gco.iarc.fr/today/data/factsheets/cancers/1-Lip-oral-cavity-fact-sheet.pdf

[18] Cheong SC, Vatanasapt P, Yang YH, Rosnah BZ, Ross Kerr A, Johnson NW. Oral cancer in South East Asia: Current status and future directions. Translational Research in Oral Oncology 2017; 2: 1-9.[http://dx.doi.org/10.1177/2057178X17702921]

[19] Mourad M, Jetmore T, Jategaonkar AA, Moubayed S, Moshier E, Urken ML. Epidemiological trends of head and neck cancer in the United States: A SEER population study. J Oral Maxillofac Surg 2017; 75(12): 2562-72.[http://dx.doi.org/10.1016/j.joms.2017.05.008] [PMID: 28618252]

[20] Cramer JD, Burtness B, Le QT, Ferris RL. The changing therapeutic landscape of head and neck cancer. Nat Rev Clin Oncol 2019; 16(11): 669-83.[http://dx.doi.org/10.1038/s41571-019-0227-z] [PMID: 31189965]

[21] Zhang Y, Wang R, Miao L, Zhu L, Jiang H, Yuan H. Different levels in alcohol and tobacco consumption in head and neck cancer patients from 1957 to 2013. PLoS One 2015; 10(4): e0124045.[http://dx.doi.org/10.1371/journal.pone.0124045] [PMID: 25875934]

[22] Joshi P, Dutta S, Chaturvedi P, Nair S. Head and neck cancers in developing countries. Rambam Maimonides Med J 2014; 5(2): e0009.[http://dx.doi.org/10.5041/RMMJ.10143] [PMID: 24808947]

[23] Australian Institute of Health and WelfareHead and neck cancers in Australia Cancer series no 83 Cat no CAN 80 2014.

[24] Rettig EM, D'Souza G. Epidemiology of head and neck cancer. Surg Oncol Clin N Am 2015; 24(3): 379-96.[http://dx.doi.org/10.1016/j.soc.2015.03.001] [PMID: 25979389]

[25] Cárcamo M. Epidemiología y generalidades del tumor de cabeza y cuello Epidemiology and generalities of the head and neck tumor. Rev Med Clin Las Condes 2018; 29(4): 388-96.[http://dx.doi.org/10.1016/j.rmclc.2018.06.009]

[26] Globocan WHO. 2019.https://gco.iarc.fr/today/data/factsheets/cancers/14-Larynx-fact-sheet.pdf

[27] Isenberg JS, Crozier DL, Dailey SH. Institutional and comprehensive review of laryngeal leukoplakia. Ann Otol Rhinol Laryngol 2008; 117(1): 74-9.[http://dx.doi.org/10.1177/000348940811700114] [PMID: 18254375]

[28] Gale N, Poljak M, Zidar N. Update from the 4th edition of the World Health Organization classification of head and neck tumours: What is new in the 2017 WHO Blue Book for tumours of the hypopharynx, larynx, trachea and parapharyngeal space. Head Neck Pathol 2017; 11(1): 23-32.

[29] Manterola L, Aguirre P, Larrea E, *et al.* Mutational profiling can identify laryngeal dysplasia at risk of progression to invasive carcinoma. Sci Rep 2018; 8(1): 6613.[http://dx.doi.org/10.1038/s41598-018-24780-7] [PMID: 29700339]

[30] Bosetti C, Gallus S, Franceschi S, *et al.* Cancer of the larynx in non-smoking alcohol drinkers and in non-drinking tobacco smokers. Br J Cancer 2002; 87(5): 516-8.[http://dx.doi.org/10.1038/sj.bjc.6600469] [PMID: 12189548]

[31] The LancetAlcohol and cancer. Lancet 2017; 390(10109): 2215.[http://dx.doi.org/10.1016/S0140-6736(17)32868-4] [PMID: 29165257]

[32] Ha TN, Madison MC, Kheradmand F, Altman KW. Laryngeal inflammatory response to smoke and vape in a murine model. Am J Otolaryngol 2019; 40(1): 89-92.[http://dx.doi.org/10.1016/j.amjoto.2018.10.001] [PMID: 30472132]

[33] Parsel SM, Wu EL, Riley CA, McCoul ED. Gastroesophageal and laryngopharyngeal reflux associated with laryngeal malignancy : A systematic review and meta-analysis. Clin Gastroenterol Hepatol 2019; 17(7):

1253-64.[http://dx.doi.org/10.1016/j.cgh.2018.10.028] [PMID: 30366155]

[34] Steuer CE, El-Deiry M, Parks JR, Higgins KA, Saba NF. An update on larynx cancer. CA Cancer J Clin 2017; 67(1): 31-50.[http://dx.doi.org/10.3322/caac.21386] [PMID: 27898173]

[35] Yang D, Shi Y, Tang Y, *et al.* Effect of HPV infection on the occurrence and development of laryngeal cancer: A review. J Cancer 2019; 10(19): 4455-62.[http://dx.doi.org/10.7150/jca.34016] [PMID: 31528209]

[36] Tumban E. A Current update on human papillomavirus-associated head and neck cancers. Viruses 2019; 11(10): 922.[http://dx.doi.org/10.3390/v11100922] [PMID: 31600915]

[37] Raitiola H, Pukander J, Laippala P. Glottic and supraglottic laryngeal carcinoma: differences in epidemiology, clinical characteristics and prognosis. Acta Otolaryngol 1999; 119(7): 847-51.[http://dx.doi.org/10.1080/00016489950180531] [PMID: 10687946]

[38] Garas J, McGuirt WF, Sr. Squamous cell carcinoma of the subglottis. Am J Otolaryngol 2006; 27(1): 1-4.[http://dx.doi.org/10.1016/j.amjoto.2005.05.004] [PMID: 16360814]

[39] Atula TS, Varpula MJ, Kurki TJ, Klemi PJ, Grénman R. Assessment of cervical lymph node status in head and neck cancer patients: palpation, computed tomography and low field magnetic resonance imaging compared with ultrasound-guided fine-needle aspiration cytology. Eur J Radiol 1997; 25(2): 152-61.[http://dx.doi.org/10.1016/S0720-048X(96)01071-6] [PMID: 9283844]

[40] Kuno H, Onaya H, Fujii S, Ojiri H, Otani K, Satake M. Primary staging of laryngeal and hypopharyngeal cancer: CT, MR imaging and dual-energy CT. Eur J Radiol 2014; 83(1): e23-35.[http://dx.doi.org/10.1016/j.ejrad.2013.10.022] [PMID: 24239239]

[41] Aaltonen LM, Rautiainen N, Sellman J, *et al.* Voice quality after treatment of early vocal cord cancer: a randomized trial comparing laser surgery with radiation therapy. Int J Radiat Oncol Biol Phys 2014; 90(2): 255-60.[http://dx.doi.org/10.1016/j.ijrobp.2014.06.032] [PMID: 25304787]

[42] Warner L, Chudasama J, Kelly CG, *et al.* Radiotherapy versus open surgery versus endolaryngeal surgery (with or without laser) for early laryngeal squamous cell cancer. Cochrane Database Syst Rev 2014; (12)CD002027.[http://dx.doi.org/10.1002/14651858.CD002027.pub2] [PMID: 25503538]

[43] Trotti A, III, Zhang Q, Bentzen SM, *et al.* Randomized trial of hyperfractionation versus conventional fractionation in T2 squamous cell carcinoma of the vocal cord (RTOG 9512). Int J Radiat Oncol Biol Phys 2014; 89(5): 958-63.[http://dx.doi.org/10.1016/j.ijrobp.2014.04.041] [PMID: 25035199]

[44] Al-Mamgani A, Kwa SLS, Tans L, *et al.* Single vocal cord irradiation: Image guided intensity modulated hypofractionated radiation therapy for T1a glottic cancer: Early clinical results. Int J Radiat Oncol Biol Phys 2015; 93(2): 337-43.[http://dx.doi.org/10.1016/j.ijrobp.2015.06.016] [PMID: 26264629]

[45] Hashibe M, Brennan P, Benhamou S, *et al.* Alcohol drinking in never users of tobacco, cigarette smoking in never drinkers, and the risk of head and neck cancer: pooled analysis in the International Head and Neck Cancer Epidemiology Consortium. J Natl Cancer Inst 2007; 99(10): 777-89.[http://dx.doi.org/10.1093/jnci/djk179] [PMID: 17505073]

[46] Sapkota A, Gajalakshmi V, Jetly DH, *et al.* Indoor air pollution from solid fuels and risk of hypopharyngeal/laryngeal and lung cancers: a multicentric case-control study from India. Int J Epidemiol 2008; 37(2): 321-8.[http://dx.doi.org/10.1093/ije/dym261] [PMID: 18234740]

[47] Shangina O, Brennan P, Szeszenia-Dabrowska N, *et al.* Occupational exposure and laryngeal and hypopharyngeal cancer risk in central and eastern Europe. Am J Epidemiol 2006; 164(4): 367-75.[http://dx.doi.org/10.1093/aje/kwj208] [PMID: 16801374]

[48] Hochfelder CG, McGinn AP, Mehta V, Castelluci E, Kabarriti R. OW TJ. Treatment sequence and survival in locoregionally advanced hypopharyngeal cancer: A surveillance, epidemiology, and end results – based study. Laryngoscope 2019; 00: 1-11.[PMID: 31821572]

[49] Panda M, Rai AK, Rahman T, *et al.* Alterations of salivary microbial community associated with oropharyngeal and hypopharyngeal squamous cell carcinoma patients. Arch Microbiol 2020; 202(4): 785-805.[http://dx.doi.org/10.1007/s00203-019-01790-1] [PMID: 31832691]

[50] Tamaki A, Rocco JW, Ozer E. The future of robotic surgery in otolaryngology – head and neck surgery. Oral Oncol 2020; 101: 104510.[http://dx.doi.org/10.1016/j.oraloncology.2019.104510]

[51] Eckel HE, Bradley PJ. Treatment Options for Hypopharyngeal Cancer. Adv Otorhinolaryngol 2019; 83: 47-53.[http://dx.doi.org/10.1159/000492308] [PMID: 30943512]

[52] Liu C, Liao K, Gross N, Wang Z, Li G, Zuo W. Homologous recombination enhances radioresistance in hypopharyngeal cancer cell line by targeting DNA damage response. Oral Oncol [Internet]. Elsevier; 2020; 100 (October 2019): 104469. [http://dx.doi.org/10.1016/j.oraloncology.2019.104469]

[53] Cho JH, Joo YH, Shin EY, Park EJ, Kim MS. Anticancer effects of colchicine on hypopharyngeal cancer. Anticancer Res 2017; 37(11): 6269-80.[PMID: 29061810]

[54] Dalianis T, Grün N, Koch J, *et al.* Human papillomavirus DNA and p16(INK4a) expression in hypopharyngeal cancer and in relation to clinical outcome, in Stockholm, Sweden. Oral Oncol 2015; 51(9): 857-61.[http://dx.doi.org/10.1016/j.oraloncology.2015.06.002] [PMID: 26120094]

[55] Shaughnessy JN, Farghaly H, Wilson L, *et al.* HPV: a factor in organ preservation for locally advanced larynx and hypopharynx cancer? Am J Otolaryngol 2014; 35(1): 19-24.[http://dx.doi.org/10.1016/j.amjoto.2013.08.006] [PMID: 24119488]

[56] Cho KJ, Park EJ, Kim MS, Joo YH. Characterization of FaDu-R, a radioresistant head and neck cancer cell line, and cancer stem cells. Auris Nasus Larynx 2018; 45(3): 566-73.[http://dx.doi.org/10.1016/j.anl.2017.07.011] [PMID: 28844650]

[57] Jing P, Zhou S, Xu P, *et al.* PDK1 promotes metastasis by inducing epithelial-mesenchymal transition in hypopharyngeal carcinoma via the Notch1 signaling pathway. Exp Cell Res 2020; 386(2): 111746.[http://dx.doi.org/10.1016/j.yexcr.2019.111746] [PMID: 31778670]

[58] Khowal S, Wajid S. Role of Smoking-Mediated molecular events in the genesis of oral cancers. Toxicol Mech Methods 2019; 29(9): 665-85.[http://dx.doi.org/10.1080/15376516.2019.1646372] [PMID: 31345084]

[59] Guha N, Warnakulasuriya S, Vlaanderen J, Straif K. Betel quid chewing and the risk of oral and oropharyngeal cancers: a meta-analysis with implications for cancer control. Int J Cancer 2014; 135(6): 1433-43.[http://dx.doi.org/10.1002/ijc.28643] [PMID: 24302487]

[60] Boffetta P, Hayes RB, Sartori S, *et al.* Mouthwash use and cancer of the head and neck: a pooled analysis from the International Head and Neck Cancer Epidemiology Consortium. Eur J Cancer Prev 2016; 25(4): 344-8.[http://dx.doi.org/10.1097/CEJ.0000000000000179] [PMID: 26275006]

[61] Chattopadhyay I, Verma M, Panda M. Role of oral microbiome signatures in diagnosis and prognosis of oral cancer. Technol Cancer Res Treat 2019; 18: 1533033819867354.[http://dx.doi.org/10.1177/1533033819867354] [PMID: 31370775]

[62] Lafuente Ibáñez de Mendoza I, Maritxalar Mendia X, García de la Fuente AM, Quindós Andrés G, Aguirre Urizar JM. Role of Porphyromonas gingivalis in oral squamous cell carcinoma development: A systematic review. J Periodontal Res 2020; 55(1): 13-22.[http://dx.doi.org/10.1111/jre.12691] [PMID: 31529626]

[63] Singhvi HR, Malik A, Chaturvedi P. The role of chronic mucosal trauma in oral cancer: A review of literature. Indian J Med Paediatr Oncol 2017; 38(1): 44-50.[http://dx.doi.org/10.4103/0971-5851.203510] [PMID: 28469336]

[64] Montero PH, Patel SG. Cancer of the oral cavity. Surg Oncol Clin N Am 2015; 24(3): 491-508.[http://dx.doi.org/10.1016/j.soc.2015.03.006] [PMID: 25979396]

[65] Li Y, St John MAR, Zhou X, *et al.* Salivary transcriptome diagnostics for oral cancer detection. Clin Cancer Res 2004; 10(24): 8442-50.[http://dx.doi.org/10.1158/1078-0432.CCR-04-1167] [PMID: 15623624]

[66] Aro K, Kaczor-Urbanowicz K, Carreras-Presas CM. Salivaomics in oral cancer. Curr Opin Otolaryngol Head Neck Surg 2019; 27(2): 91-7.[http://dx.doi.org/10.1097/MOO.0000000000000502] [PMID: 30507690]

[67] Yao CMKL, Chang EI, Lai SY. Contemporary approach to locally advanced oral cavity squamous cell carcinoma. Curr Oncol Rep 2019; 21(11): 99.[http://dx.doi.org/10.1007/s11912-019-0845-8] [PMID: 31701240]

[68] Chai AWY, Lim KP, Cheong SC. Translational genomics and recent advances in oral squamous cell carcinoma. Semin Cancer Biol 2020; 61: 71-83.[http://dx.doi.org/10.1016/j.semcancer.2019.09.011] [PMID: 31542510]

[69] O'Sullivan B, Huang SH, Su J, *et al.* Development and validation of a staging system for HPV-related oropharyngeal cancer by the International Collaboration on Oropharyngeal cancer Network for Staging (ICON-S): a multicentre cohort study. Lancet Oncol 2016; 17(4): 440-51.[http://dx.doi.org/10.1016/S1470-2045(15)00560-4] [PMID: 26936027]

[70] de Martel C, Plummer M, Vignat J, Franceschi S. Worldwide burden of cancer attributable to HPV by site, country and HPV type. Int J Cancer 2017; 141(4): 664-70.[http://dx.doi.org/10.1002/ijc.30716] [PMID: 28369882]

[71] Argirion I, Zarins KR, Defever K, *et al.* Temporal changes in head and neck cancer incidence in Thailand suggest changing oropharyngeal epidemiology in the region. J Glob Oncol 2019; 5: 1-11.[http://dx.doi.org/10.1200/JGO.18.00219] [PMID: 30860955]

[72] Gupta B, Johnson NW, Kumar N. Global epidemiology of head and neck cancers: A continuing challenge. Oncology 2016; 91(1): 13-23.[http://dx.doi.org/10.1159/000446117] [PMID: 27245686]

[73] Globocan WHO. 2019.https://gco.iarc.fr/today/data/factsheets/cancers/3-Oropharynx-fact-sheet.pdf

[74] van Monsjou HS, Balm AJM, van den Brekel MM, Wreesmann VB. Oropharyngeal squamous cell carcinoma: a unique disease on the rise? Oral Oncol 2010; 46(11): 780-

5.[http://dx.doi.org/10.1016/j.oraloncology.2010.08.011] [PMID: 20920878]

[75]   Shi W, Kato H, Perez-Ordonez B, *et al.* Comparative prognostic value of HPV16 E6 mRNA compared with in situ hybridization for human oropharyngeal squamous carcinoma. J Clin Oncol 2009; 27(36): 6213-21.[http://dx.doi.org/10.1200/JCO.2009.23.1670] [PMID: 19884544]

[76]   Ndiaye C, Mena M, Alemany L, *et al.* HPV DNA, E6/E7 mRNA, and p16INK4a detection in head and neck cancers: a systematic review and meta-analysis. Lancet Oncol 2014; 15(12): 1319-31.[http://dx.doi.org/10.1016/S1470-2045(14)70471-1] [PMID: 25439690]

[77]   Agalliu I, Gapstur S, Chen Z, Wang T, Anderson RL, Teras L. Associations of oral α-, β-, and γ-human papillomavirus types with risk of incident head and neck cancer. JAMA Oncol. 2016 1; 2(5): 599–606.

[78]   van Gysen K, Stevens M, Guo L, *et al.* Validation of the 8th edition UICC/AJCC TNM staging system for HPV associated oropharyngeal cancer patients managed with contemporary chemo-radiotherapy. BMC Cancer 2019; 19(1): 674.[http://dx.doi.org/10.1186/s12885-019-5894-8] [PMID: 31288767]

[79]   Weinberger PM, Yu Z, Haffty BG, *et al.* Molecular classification identifies a subset of human papillomavirus--associated oropharyngeal cancers with favorable prognosis. J Clin Oncol 2006; 24(5): 736-47.[http://dx.doi.org/10.1200/JCO.2004.00.3335] [PMID: 16401683]

[80]   Chera BS, Amdur RJ, Green R, *et al.* Phase II trial of de-intensified chemoradiotherapy for human papillomavirus–associated oropharyngeal squamous cell carcinoma. J Clin Oncol 2019; 37(29): 2661-9.[http://dx.doi.org/10.1200/JCO.19.01007] [PMID: 31411949]

[81]   Globocan WHO. 2019.Http://gco.iarc.fr/today/data/factsheets/cancers/2-Salivary-glands-fact-sheet.pdf

[82]   Panwar A, Kozel JA, Lydiatt WM. Cancers of major salivary glands. Surg Oncol Clin N Am 2015; 24(3): 615-33.[http://dx.doi.org/10.1016/j.soc.2015.03.011] [PMID: 25979403]

[83]   Lewis AG, Tong T, Maghami E. Diagnosis and management of malignant salivary gland tumors of the parotid gland. Otolaryngol Clin North Am 2016; 49(2): 343-80.[http://dx.doi.org/10.1016/j.otc.2015.11.001] [PMID: 27040585]

[84]   Seethala RR, Stenman G. Update from the 4th Edition of the World Health Organization Classification of Head and Neck Tumours: Tumors of the Salivary Gland. Head Neck Pathol 2017; 11(1): 55-67.[http://dx.doi.org/10.1007/s12105-017-0795-0] [PMID: 28247227]

[85]   Yan K, Yesensky J, Hasina R, Agrawal N. Genomics of mucoepidermoid and adenoid cystic carcinomas. Laryngoscope Investig Otolaryngol 2018; 3(1): 56-61.[http://dx.doi.org/10.1002/lio2.139] [PMID: 29492469]

[86]   Lombardi D, Accorona R, Lambert A, *et al.* Long-term outcomes and prognosis in submandibular gland malignant tumors: A multicenter study. Laryngoscope 2018; 128(12): 2745-50.[http://dx.doi.org/10.1002/lary.27236] [PMID: 29756241]

[87]   Pan SY, de Groh M, Morrison H. A case-control study of risk factors for salivary gland cancer in Canada. J Cancer Epidemiol 2017; 2017: 4909214.[http://dx.doi.org/10.1155/2017/4909214] [PMID: 28133481]

[88]   Turner JH, Reh DD. Incidence and survival in patients with sinonasal cancer: a historical analysis of population-based data. Head Neck 2012; 34(6): 877-85.[http://dx.doi.org/10.1002/hed.21830] [PMID: 22127982]

[89]   Llorente JL, López F, Suárez C, Hermsen MA. Sinonasal carcinoma: clinical, pathological, genetic and therapeutic advances. Nat Rev Clin Oncol 2014; 11(8): 460-72.[http://dx.doi.org/10.1038/nrclinonc.2014.97] [PMID: 24935016]

[90]   Benninger MS. The impact of cigarette smoking and environmental tobacco smoke on nasal and sinus disease: a review of the literature. Am J Rhinol 1999; 13(6): 435-8.[http://dx.doi.org/10.2500/105065899781329683] [PMID: 10631398]

[91]   Binazzi A, Ferrante P, Marinaccio A. Occupational exposure and sinonasal cancer : a systematic review and meta-analysis. BMC Cancer 2015; 13;15: 49.[http://dx.doi.org/10.1186/s12885-015-1042-2]

[92]   Staffolani S, Manzella N, Strafella E, *et al.* Wood dust exposure induces cell transformation through EGFR-mediated OGG1 inhibition. Mutagenesis 2015; 30(4): 487-97.[http://dx.doi.org/10.1093/mutage/gev007] [PMID: 25711499]

[93]   Kılıç S, Kılıç SS, Kim ES, *et al.* Significance of human papillomavirus positivity in sinonasal squamous cell carcinoma. Int Forum Allergy Rhinol 2017; 7(10): 980-9.[http://dx.doi.org/10.1002/alr.21996] [PMID: 28859244]

[94]   Byrd JK, Clair JMS, El-Sayed I. AHNS Series: Do you know your guidelines? Principles for treatment of cancer of the paranasal sinuses: A review of the National Comprehensive Cancer Network guidelines. Head Neck 2018; 40(9): 1889-96.[http://dx.doi.org/10.1002/hed.25143] [PMID: 29952099]

[95]   Lee AWM, Foo W, Mang O, *et al.* Changing epidemiology of nasopharyngeal carcinoma in Hong Kong over

a 20-year period (1980-99): an encouraging reduction in both incidence and mortality. Int J Cancer 2003; 103(5): 680-5.[http://dx.doi.org/10.1002/ijc.10894] [PMID: 12494479]

[96] Globocan WHO. 2019.http://gco.iarc.fr/today/data/factsheets/cancers/4-Nasopharynx-fact-sheet.pdf

[97] Chen YP, Chan ATC, Le QT, Blanchard P, Sun Y, Ma J. Nasopharyngeal carcinoma. Lancet 2019; 394(10192): 64-80.[http://dx.doi.org/10.1016/S0140-6736(19)30956-0] [PMID: 31178151]

[98] Lee HM, Okuda KS, González FE, Patel V. Current perspectives on nasopharyngeal carcinoma. Adv Exp Med Biol 2019; 1164: 11-34.[http://dx.doi.org/10.1007/978-3-030-22254-3_2] [PMID: 31576537]

[99] Yi M, Cai J, Li J, et al. Rediscovery of NF-κB signaling in nasopharyngeal carcinoma: How genetic defects of NF-κB pathway interplay with EBV in driving oncogenesis? J Cell Physiol 2018; 233(8): 5537-49.[http://dx.doi.org/10.1002/jcp.26410] [PMID: 29266238]

[100] Chan KCA, Woo JKS, King A, et al. Analysis of plasma Epstein–Barr virus DNA to screen for nasopharyngeal cancer. N Engl J Med 2017; 377(6): 513-22.[http://dx.doi.org/10.1056/NEJMoa1701717] [PMID: 28792880]

[101] Ning JP, Yu MC, Wang QS, Henderson BE. Consumption of salted fish and other risk factors for nasopharyngeal carcinoma (NPC) in Tianjin, a low-risk region for NPC in the People's Republic of China. J Natl Cancer Inst 1990; 82(4): 291-6.[http://dx.doi.org/10.1093/jnci/82.4.291] [PMID: 2299678]

[102] World Health Organization International Agency for Research on Cancer2009. https://monographs.iarc.fr/wp-content/uploads/2018/06/mono94.pdf

[103] Riley CA, Marino MJ, Hawkey N, Lawlor CM, McCoul ED. Sinonasal tract inflammation as a precursor to nasopharyngeal carcinoma: a systematic review and meta-analysis. Otolaryngol Head Neck Surg 2016; 154(5): 810-6.[http://dx.doi.org/10.1177/0194599816629436] [PMID: 26908557]

[104] Chua MLK, Wee JTS, Hui EP, Chan ATC. Nasopharyngeal carcinoma. Lancet 2016; 387(10022): 1012-24.[http://dx.doi.org/10.1016/S0140-6736(15)00055-0] [PMID: 26321262]

[105] Xu C, Zhang S, Li WF, et al. Selection and validation of induction chemotherapy beneficiaries among patients with T3N0, T3N1, T4N0 nasopharyngeal carcinoma using Epstein-Barr Virus DNA : A joint analysis of real-world and clinical trial data. Front Oncol 2019; 9: 1343.[http://dx.doi.org/10.3389/fonc.2019.01343] [PMID: 31850226]

[106] Zhang H, Zou X, Wu L, et al. Identification of a 7-microRNA signature in plasma as promising biomarker for nasopharyngeal carcinoma detection. Cancer Med 2020; 9(3): 1230-41.[http://dx.doi.org/10.1002/cam4.2676] [PMID: 31856390]

[107] Lam WKJ, Chan JYK. Recent advances in the management of nasopharyngeal carcinoma. F1000 Research 2018; 7(F1000 Faculty Rev): 1829.

[108] Raghupathy R, Hui EP, Chan ATC. Epstein-Barr virus as a paradigm in nasopharyngeal cancer: from lab to clinic. Am Soc Clin Oncol Educ Book 2014; 34: 149-53.[http://dx.doi.org/10.14694/EdBook_AM.2014.34.149] [PMID: 24857071]

[109] Pellegriti G, Frasca F, Regalbuto C, Squatrito S, Vigneri R. Worldwide increasing incidence of thyroid cancer: update on epidemiology and risk factors. J Cancer Epidemiol 2013; 2013: 965212.[http://dx.doi.org/10.1155/2013/965212] [PMID: 23737785]

[110] Sinnott B, Ron E, Schneider AB. Exposing the thyroid to radiation: a review of its current extent, risks, and implications. Endocr Rev 2010; 31(5): 756-73.[http://dx.doi.org/10.1210/er.2010-0003] [PMID: 20650861]

[111] Harikrishna A, Ishak A, Ellinides A, et al. The impact of obesity and insulin resistance on thyroid cancer: A systematic review. Maturitas 2019; 125(March): 45-9.[http://dx.doi.org/10.1016/j.maturitas.2019.03.022] [PMID: 31133216]

[112] Howlader N, Noone AM, Krapcho M. SEER Cancer Statistics Review, 1975-2016, National Cancer Institute. Bethesda, MD, https://seer.cancer.gov/csr/1975_2016/, based on November 2018 SEER data submission, posted to the SEER web site, April 2019. https://seer. cancer.gov/csr/1975_22019.

[113] Choi YS, Kwon HJ, Kim BK, et al. A Case of medullary thyroid carcinoma with de novo V804M RET germline mutation. J Korean Med Sci 2013; 28(1): 156-9.[http://dx.doi.org/10.3346/jkms.2013.28.1.156] [PMID: 23341727]

[114] Cabanillas ME, Mcfadden DG, Durante C. Thyroid cancer. Lancet 2016; 3; 388(10061): 2783-95.[http://dx.doi.org/10.1016/S0140-6736(16)30172-6]

[115] Cancer Genome Atlas Research NetworkIntegrated genomic characterization of papillary thyroid carcinoma. Cell 2014; 159(3): 676-90.[http://dx.doi.org/10.1016/j.cell.2014.09.050] [PMID: 25417114]

[116] Kelly LM, Barila G, Liu P, et al. Identification of the transforming STRN-ALK fusion as a potential therapeutic target in the aggressive forms of thyroid cancer. Proc Natl Acad Sci USA 2014; 111(11): 4233-

8.[http://dx.doi.org/10.1073/pnas.1321937111] [PMID: 24613930]

[117] Haugen BR, Alexander EK, Bible KC, *et al.* 2015 American Thyroid Association management guidelines for adult patients with thyroid nodules and differentiated thyroid cancer: The American Thyroid Association guidelines task force on thyroid nodules and differentiated thyroid cancer. Thyroid 2016; 26(1): 1-133.[http://dx.doi.org/10.1089/thy.2015.0020] [PMID: 26462967]

[118] Bartolazzi A, Orlandi F, Saggiorato E, *et al.* Italian Thyroid Cancer Study Group (ITCSG)Galectin-3-expression analysis in the surgical selection of follicular thyroid nodules with indeterminate fine-needle aspiration cytology: a prospective multicentre study. Lancet Oncol 2008; 9(6): 543-9.[http://dx.doi.org/10.1016/S1470-2045(08)70132-3] [PMID: 18495537]

[119] Trimboli P, Virili C, Romanelli F, Crescenzi A, Giovanella L. Galectin-3 performance in histologic and cytologic assessment of thyroid nodules : A systematic review and meta-analysis. Int J Mol Sci 2017; 18(8): 1756.[http://dx.doi.org/10.3390/ijms18081756] [PMID: 28800068]

[120] Naoum GE, Morkos M, Kim B, Arafat W. Novel targeted therapies and immunotherapy for advanced thyroid cancers. Mol Cancer 2018; 17(1): 51.[http://dx.doi.org/10.1186/s12943-018-0786-0] [PMID: 29455653]

[121] Greco FA, Hainsworth JD. Introduction: unknown primary cancer. Semin Oncol 2009; 36(1): 6-7.[http://dx.doi.org/10.1053/j.seminoncol.2008.10.007] [PMID: 19179184]

[122] Rusthoven KE, Koshy M, Paulino AC. The role of fluorodeoxyglucose positron emission tomography in cervical lymph node metastases from an unknown primary tumor. Cancer 2004; 101(11): 2641-9.[http://dx.doi.org/10.1002/cncr.20687] [PMID: 15517576]

[123] Cianchetti M, Mancuso AA, Amdur RJ, *et al.* Diagnostic evaluation of squamous cell carcinoma metastatic to cervical lymph nodes from an unknown head and neck primary site. Laryngoscope 2009; 119(12): 2348-54.[http://dx.doi.org/10.1002/lary.20638] [PMID: 19718744]

[124] McDowell LJ, Young RJ, Johnston ML, *et al.* p16-positive lymph node metastases from cutaneous head and neck squamous cell carcinoma: No association with high-risk human papillomavirus or prognosis and implications for the workup of the unknown primary. Cancer 2016; 122(8): 1201-8.[http://dx.doi.org/10.1002/cncr.29901] [PMID: 26881928]

[125] Keller LM, Galloway TJ, Holdbrook T, *et al.* p16 status, pathologic and clinical characteristics, biomolecular signature, and long-term outcomes in head and neck squamous cell carcinomas of unknown primary. Head Neck 2014; 36(12): 1677-84.[http://dx.doi.org/10.1002/hed.23514] [PMID: 24115269]

[126] Mourad WF, Hu KS, Shasha D, *et al.* Initial experience with oropharynx-targeted radiation therapy for metastatic squamous cell carcinoma of unknown primary of the head and neck. Anticancer Res 2014; 34(1): 243-8.[PMID: 24403470]

[127] Sher DJ, Balboni TA, Haddad RI, *et al.* Efficacy and toxicity of chemoradiotherapy using intensity-modulated radiotherapy for unknown primary of head and neck. Int J Radiat Oncol Biol Phys 2011; 80(5): 1405-11.[http://dx.doi.org/10.1016/j.ijrobp.2010.04.029] [PMID: 21177045]

[128] Swerdlow SH, Campo E, Pileri SA, *et al.* The 2016 revision of the World Health Organization classification of lymphoid neoplasms. Blood 2016; 127(20): 2375-90.[http://dx.doi.org/10.1182/blood-2016-01-643569] [PMID: 26980727]

[129] Storck K, Brandstetter M, Keller U, Knopf A. Clinical presentation and characteristics of lymphoma in the head and neck region. Head Face Med 2019; 3;15(1): 1.[http://dx.doi.org/10.1055/s-0039-1686081]

[130] Weber AL, Rahemtullah A, Ferry JA. Hodgkin and non-Hodgkin lymphoma of the head and neck: clinical, pathologic, and imaging evaluation. Neuroimaging Clin N Am 2003; 13(3): 371-92.[http://dx.doi.org/10.1016/S1052-5149(03)00039-X] [PMID: 14631680]

[131] Hanna E, Wanamaker J, Adelstein D, Tubbs R, Lavertu P. Extranodal lymphomas of the head and neck. A 20-year experience. Arch Otolaryngol Head Neck Surg 1997; 123(12): 1318-23.[http://dx.doi.org/10.1001/archotol.1997.01900120068011] [PMID: 9413361]

[132] Shankland KR, Armitage JO, Hancock BW. Non-Hodgkin lymphoma. Lancet 2012; 380(9844): 848-57.[http://dx.doi.org/10.1016/S0140-6736(12)60605-9] [PMID: 22835603]

[133] Chihara D, Nastoupil LJ, Williams JN, Lee P, Koff JL, Flowers CR. New insights into the epidemiology of non-Hodgkin lymphoma and implications for therapy. Expert Rev Anticancer Ther 2015; 15(5): 531-44.[http://dx.doi.org/10.1586/14737140.2015.1023712] [PMID: 25864967]

[134] Morton LM, Sampson JN, Cerhan JR, *et al.* Rationale and Design of the International Lymphoma Epidemiology Consortium (InterLymph) Non-Hodgkin Lymphoma Subtypes Project. J Natl Cancer Inst Monogr 2014; 2014(48): 1-14.[http://dx.doi.org/10.1093/jncimonographs/lgu005] [PMID: 25174022]

[135] Cerhan JR, Kricker A, Paltiel O, *et al.* Medical history, lifestyle, family history, and occupational risk factors for diffuse large B-cell lymphoma: the InterLymph Non-Hodgkin Lymphoma Subtypes Project. J Natl

Cancer Inst Monogr 2014; 2014(48): 15-25.[http://dx.doi.org/10.1093/jncimonographs/lgu010] [PMID: 25174023]

[136] Slap GB, Connor JL, Wigton RS, Schwartz JS. Validation of a model to identify young patients for lymph node biopsy. JAMA 1986; 255(20): 2768-73.[http://dx.doi.org/10.1001/jama.1986.03370200070030] [PMID: 3701990]

[137] Florentine BD, Staymates B, Rabadi M, Barstis J, Black A. Cancer Committee of the Henry Mayo Newhall Memorial HospitalThe reliability of fine-needle aspiration biopsy as the initial diagnostic procedure for palpable masses: a 4-year experience of 730 patients from a community hospital-based outpatient aspiration biopsy clinic. Cancer 2006; 107(2): 406-16.[http://dx.doi.org/10.1002/cncr.21976] [PMID: 16773630]

[138] Hehn ST, Grogan TM, Miller TP. Utility of fine-needle aspiration as a diagnostic technique in lymphoma. J Clin Oncol 2004; 22(15): 3046-52.[http://dx.doi.org/10.1200/JCO.2004.02.104] [PMID: 15284254]

[139] Kwon M, Yim C, Baek HJ, et al. Ultrasonography-guided core needle biopsy of cervical lymph nodes for diagnosing head and neck lymphoma compared with open surgical biopsy: Exploration for factors that shape diagnostic yield. Am J Otolaryngol 2018; 39(6): 679-84.[http://dx.doi.org/10.1016/j.amjoto.2018.07.011] [PMID: 30055795]

[140] Pfreundschuh M, Trümper L, Österborg A, et al. MabThera International Trial GroupCHOP-like chemotherapy plus rituximab versus CHOP-like chemotherapy alone in young patients with good-prognosis diffuse large-B-cell lymphoma: a randomised controlled trial by the MabThera International Trial (MInT) Group. Lancet Oncol 2006; 7(5): 379-91.[http://dx.doi.org/10.1016/S1470-2045(06)70664-7] [PMID: 16648042]

[141] Torre LA, Bray F, Siegel RL, Ferlay J, Lortet-Tieulent J, Jemal A. Global cancer statistics, 2012. CA Cancer J Clin 2015; 65(2): 87-108.[http://dx.doi.org/10.3322/caac.21262] [PMID: 25651787]

[142] Hoeben A, Polak J, Van De Voorde L, Hoebers F, Grabsch HI, de Vos-Geelen J. Cervical esophageal cancer: a gap in cancer knowledge. Ann Oncol 2016; 27(9): 1664-74.[http://dx.doi.org/10.1093/annonc/mdw183] [PMID: 27117535]

[143] Newlands C, Currie R, Memon A, Whitaker S, Woolford T. Non-melanoma skin cancer: united kingdom national multidisciplinary guidelines. J Laryngol Otol 2016; 130(Suppl. S2): S125-32.

[144] Gandhi SA, Kampp J. Skin cancer epidemiology, detection, and management. Med Clin North Am 2015; 99(6): 1323-35.[http://dx.doi.org/10.1016/j.mcna.2015.06.002] [PMID: 26476255]

[145] Que SKT, Zwald F, Schmults C. Incidence, risk factors, diagnosis, and staging Cutaneous squamous cell carcinoma. J Am Acad Dermatol 2018; 78(2): 237-47.[http://dx.doi.org/10.1016/j.jaad.2017.08.059] [PMID: 29332704]

[146] Capalbo C, Belardinilli F, Filetti M, et al. Effective treatment of a platinum-resistant cutaneous squamous cell carcinoma case by EGFR pathway inhibition. Mol Clin Oncol 2018; 9(1): 30-4.[http://dx.doi.org/10.3892/mco.2018.1634] [PMID: 29977536]

[147] McGranahan N, Furness AJS, Rosenthal R, et al. Clonal neoantigens elicit T cell immunoreactivity and sensitivity to immune checkpoint blockade. Science 2016; 351(6280): 1463-9.[http://dx.doi.org/10.1126/science.aaf1490] [PMID: 26940869]

[148] Ouaz K, Robier A, Lescanne E, Bobillier C, Morinière S, Bakhos D. Cancer of the external auditory canal. Eur Ann Otorhinolaryngol Head Neck Dis 2013; 130(4): 175-82.[http://dx.doi.org/10.1016/j.anorl.2012.08.003] [PMID: 23845289]

[149] Bacciu A, Clemente IA, Piccirillo E, Ferrari S, Sanna M. Guidelines for treating temporal bone carcinoma based on long-term outcomes. Otol Neurotol 2013; 34(5): 898-907.[http://dx.doi.org/10.1097/MAO.0b013e318281e0a9] [PMID: 23507994]

[150] Leong SC, Youssef A, Lesser TH. Squamous cell carcinoma of the temporal bone: outcomes of radical surgery and postoperative radiotherapy. Laryngoscope 2013; 123(10): 2442-8.[http://dx.doi.org/10.1002/lary.24063] [PMID: 23553471]

[151] Lin CJ, Grandis JR, Carey TE, et al. Head and neck squamous cell carcinoma cell lines: established models and rationale for selection. Head Neck 2007; 29(2): 163-88.[http://dx.doi.org/10.1002/hed.20478] [PMID: 17312569]

[152] Curry JM, Sprandio J, Cognetti D, et al. Tumor microenvironment in head and neck squamous cell carcinoma. Semin Oncol 2014; 41(2): 217-34.[http://dx.doi.org/10.1053/j.seminoncol.2014.03.003] [PMID: 24787294]

[153] Plzák J, Bouček J, Bandúrová V, et al. The head and neck squamous cell carcinoma microenvironment as a potential target for cancer therapy. Cancers (Basel) 2019; 11(4): 440.[http://dx.doi.org/10.3390/cancers11040440] [PMID: 30925774]

[154] Bredell MG, Ernst J, El-Kochairi I, Dahlem Y, Ikenberg K, Schumann DM. Current relevance of hypoxia in head and neck cancer. Oncotarget 2016; 7(31): 50781-804.[http://dx.doi.org/10.18632/oncotarget.9549] [PMID: 27434126]

[155] Ries M, Loiola R, Shah UN, Gentleman SM, Solito E, Sastre M. The anti-inflammatory Annexin A1 induces the clearance and degradation of the amyloid-β peptide. J Neuroinflammation 2016; 13(1): 234.[http://dx.doi.org/10.1186/s12974-016-0692-6] [PMID: 27590054]

[156] Senchenkova EY, Ansari J, Becker F, et al. Novel role for the AnxA1-Fpr2/ALX signaling axis as a key regulator of platelet function to promote resolution of inflammation. Circulation 2019; 140(4): 319-35.[http://dx.doi.org/10.1161/CIRCULATIONAHA.118.039345] [PMID: 31154815]

[157] Chrysovergis A, S Papanikolaou V, Tsiambas E, et al. Caspase complex in laryngeal squamous cell carcinoma. J BUON 2019; 24(1): 1-4.[PMID: 30941944]

[158] Byzia E, Soloch N, Bodnar M, et al. Recurrent transcriptional loss of the PCDH17 tumor suppressor in laryngeal squamous cell carcinoma is partially mediated by aberrant promoter DNA methylation. Mol Carcinog 2018; 57(7): 878-85.[http://dx.doi.org/10.1002/mc.22808] [PMID: 29566279]

[159] Gastardelo TS, Cunha BR, Raposo LS, et al. Inflammation and cancer: role of annexin A1 and FPR2/ALX in proliferation and metastasis in human laryngeal squamous cell carcinoma. PLoS One 2014; 9(12): e111317.[http://dx.doi.org/10.1371/journal.pone.0111317] [PMID: 25490767]

[160] Peri S, Izumchenko E, Schubert AD, Slifker MJ, Ruth K, Serebriiskii IG. NSD1- A nd NSD2-damaging mutations define a subset of laryngeal tumors with favorable prognosis. Nat Commun 2017; 8(1): 1-9.[http://dx.doi.org/10.1038/s41467-017-01877-7] [PMID: 28232747]

[161] Xu E, Liang X, Ji Z, Zhao S, Li L, Lang J. Blocking long noncoding RNA MALAT1 restrained the development of laryngeal and hypopharyngeal carcinoma. Eur Arch Otorhinolaryngol 2020; 277(2): 611-21.[http://dx.doi.org/10.1007/s00405-019-05732-x] [PMID: 31792655]

[162] Dalianis T. Human papillomavirus and oropharyngeal cancer, the epidemics, and significance of additional clinical biomarkers for prediction of response to therapy (Review). Int J Oncol 2014; 44(6): 1799-805.[http://dx.doi.org/10.3892/ijo.2014.2355] [PMID: 24676623]

[163] Dogan S, Xu B, Middha S, et al. Identification of prognostic molecular biomarkers in 157 HPV-positive and HPV-negative squamous cell carcinomas of the oropharynx. Int J Cancer 2019; 145(11): 3152-62.[http://dx.doi.org/10.1002/ijc.32412] [PMID: 31093971]

[164] Nikiforov YE, Ohori NP, Hodak SP, et al. Impact of mutational testing on the diagnosis and management of patients with cytologically indeterminate thyroid nodules: a prospective analysis of 1056 FNA samples. J Clin Endocrinol Metab 2011; 96(11): 3390-7.[http://dx.doi.org/10.1210/jc.2011-1469] [PMID: 21880806]

[165] Alexander EK, Kennedy GC, Baloch ZW, et al. Preoperative diagnosis of benign thyroid nodules with indeterminate cytology. N Engl J Med 2012; 367(8): 705-15.[http://dx.doi.org/10.1056/NEJMoa1203208] [PMID: 22731672]

[166] Angell TE, Wirth LJ, Cabanillas ME, et al. Analytical and clinical validation of expressed variants and fusions from the whole transcriptome of thyroid FNA Samples. Front Endocrinol (Lausanne) 2019; 10: 612.[http://dx.doi.org/10.3389/fendo.2019.00612] [PMID: 31572297]

[167] Ryder M, Gild M, Hohl TM, et al. Genetic and pharmacological targeting of CSF-1/CSF-1R inhibits tumor-associated macrophages and impairs BRAF-induced thyroid cancer progression. PLoS One 2013; 8(1): e54302.[http://dx.doi.org/10.1371/journal.pone.0054302] [PMID: 23372702]

[168] French JD, Kotnis GR, Said S, et al. Programmed death-1+ T cells and regulatory T cells are enriched in tumor-involved lymph nodes and associated with aggressive features in papillary thyroid cancer. J Clin Endocrinol Metab 2012; 97(6): E934-43.[http://dx.doi.org/10.1210/jc.2011-3428] [PMID: 22466343]

[169] Buchbinder EI, Desai A. CTLA-4 and PD-1 pathways similarities, differences, and implications of their inhibition. Am J Clin Oncol 2016; 39(1): 98-106.[http://dx.doi.org/10.1097/COC.0000000000000239] [PMID: 26558876]

[170] Mehnert JM, Varga A, Brose MS, et al. Safety and antitumor activity of the anti-PD-1 antibody pembrolizumab in patients with advanced, PD-L1-positive papillary or follicular thyroid cancer. BMC Cancer 2019; 19(1): 196.[http://dx.doi.org/10.1186/s12885-019-5380-3] [PMID: 30832606]

[171] Alizadeh AA, Eisen MB, Davis RE, et al. Distinct types of diffuse large B-cell lymphoma identified by gene expression profiling. Nature 2000; 403(6769): 503-11.[http://dx.doi.org/10.1038/35000501] [PMID: 10676951]

[172] Rosenwald A, Wright G, Chan WC, et al. Lymphoma/leukemia molecular profiling projectThe use of molecular profiling to predict survival after chemotherapy for diffuse large-B-cell lymphoma. N Engl J Med 2002; 346(25): 1937-47.[http://dx.doi.org/10.1056/NEJMoa012914] [PMID: 12075054]

[173] Davis RE, Brown KD, Siebenlist U, Staudt LM. Constitutive nuclear factor kappaB activity is required for survival of activated B cell-like diffuse large B cell lymphoma cells. J Exp Med 2001; 194(12): 1861-74.[http://dx.doi.org/10.1084/jem.194.12.1861] [PMID: 11748286]

Histological Classification of Head and Neck Tumors

Sharifah Emilia Tuan Sharif[1], Anani Aila Mat Zin[1], [*]

[1] Department of Pathology, School of Medical Science, Universiti Sains Malaysia, Health Campus 16150, Kubang Kerian, Kelantan, Malaysia

Abstract

Head and neck constituency tumor display many types of cell depending on the lineages, which can develop in a variety of tumor types. Nodaway, all these types and variants of tumor have been recognized based on histomorphological features and their molecular behavior. The most updated and receptive classification is provided by the World Health Organization (WHO) and the American Joint Committee on Cancer (AJCC). In the chapter, the discussion will include the common neoplasm, which can occur in oropharynx, nasopharynx, sinonasal region, salivary gland, thyroid gland and other adjacent structures. A brief overview, clinical presentation, histomorphology, genetic profile and outcome/prognosis will be highlighted.

Keywords: Genetic profiling, Head and neck tumor, Miscellaneous tumor, Molecular, Morphology, Predictive factor, Prognostic, Salivary gland tumor, Tumor with and without squamous differentiation, WHO and AJCC classification.

---

[*] **Corresponding author Anani Aila Mat Zin:** Department of Pathology, School of Medical Science, Universiti Sains Malaysia, Health Campus 16150, Kubang Kerian, Kelantan, Malaysia; Tel: +60199624272; E-mail: ailakb@usm.my

INTRODUCTION

The head and neck areas have numerous specialized tissues giving rise to many types of malignancies. There are a few types and subtypes of lesions that will be described according to their histomorphology and molecular profiles, especially salivary gland, sinonasal tract, and oropharynx. Nasopharyngeal carcinoma had undergone a few classification changes. But, the most accepted classifications are from the World Health Organization (WHO). The same goes for the former in which the evolved classifications had been recognized by the WHO and American Joint Committee on Cancer (AJCC).

In this chapter, we focus on the most recent developments in the head and neck cancer classification. We will discuss the clinical features, pathological features, ancillary studies, prognostic and therapeutic considerations for each entity. These

cancers are further categorized by their histomorphological differentiation and the location of the head or neck in which they arise. These categories are described below, including the miscellaneous one.

HISTOPATHOLOGICAL CLASSIFICATION OF TUMOUR

Here, we discussed the histopathological classification based on histological features or differentiation (Fig. 1).

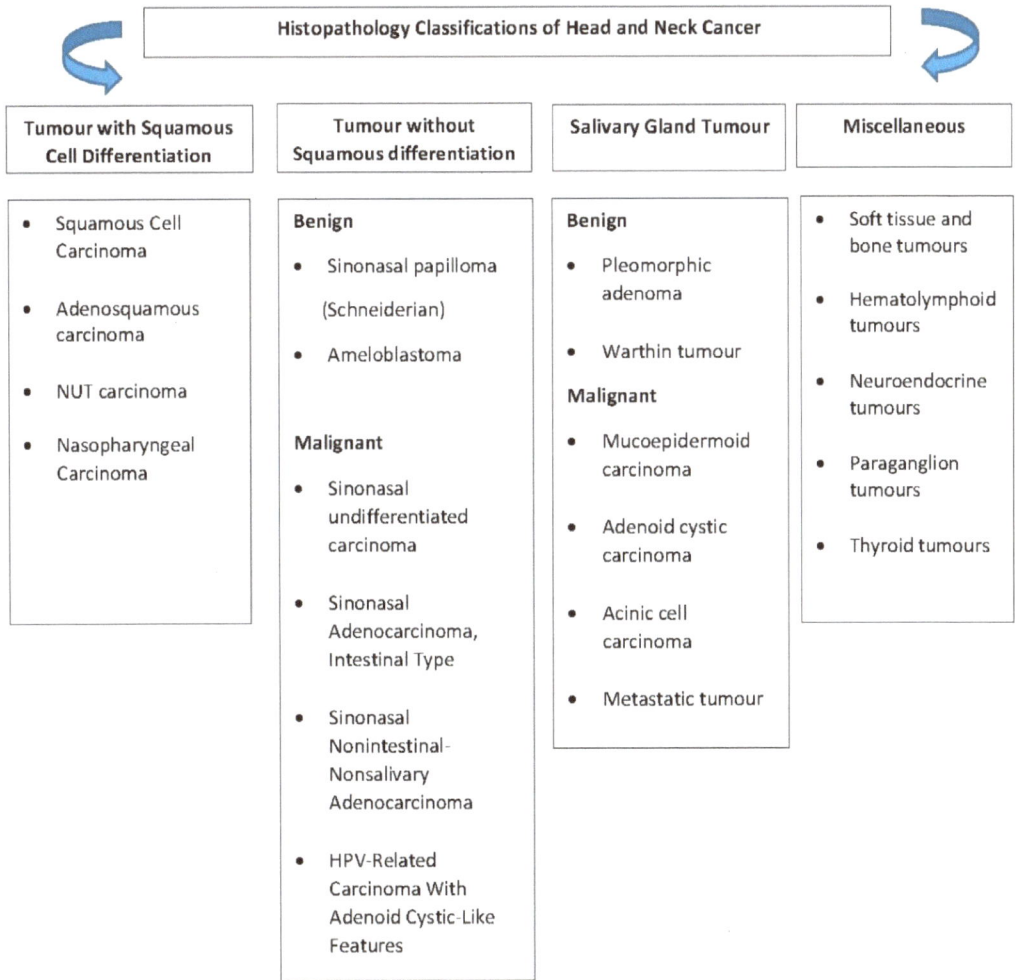

Histopathology Classifications of Head and Neck Cancer

Tumour with Squamous Cell Differentiation	Tumour without Squamous differentiation	Salivary Gland Tumour	Miscellaneous
• Squamous Cell Carcinoma • Adenosquamous carcinoma • NUT carcinoma • Nasopharyngeal Carcinoma	**Benign** • Sinonasal papilloma (Schneiderian) • Ameloblastoma **Malignant** • Sinonasal undifferentiated carcinoma • Sinonasal Adenocarcinoma, Intestinal Type • Sinonasal Nonintestinal-Nonsalivary Adenocarcinoma • HPV-Related Carcinoma With Adenoid Cystic-Like Features	**Benign** • Pleomorphic adenoma • Warthin tumour **Malignant** • Mucoepidermoid carcinoma • Adenoid cystic carcinoma • Acinic cell carcinoma • Metastatic tumour	• Soft tissue and bone tumours • Hematolymphoid tumours • Neuroendocrine tumours • Paraganglion tumours • Thyroid tumours

Fig. (1))
Classification of head and neck tumor.

1. Epithelial tumor with squamous differentiation.
2. Epithelial tumor without squamous differentiation.
3. Salivary gland tumors.
4. Miscellaneous – neuroendocrine carcinoma, hematolymphoid tumor, soft tissue and bone tumor, paraganglion tumors, thyroid neoplasm, *etc.*

EPITHELIAL TUMOUR WITH SQUAMOUS DIFFERENTIATION

Head and neck squamous cell carcinoma (HNSCC) and its variants are the most common types, usually developed in males of older age group. It develops from the lining of mucosa of the upper aerodigestive tract and is classified by its location; oral cavity/tongue, oropharynx, nasal cavity, and paranasal sinuses, nasopharynx, larynx or hypopharynx. Nasopharyngeal carcinoma (NPC) and other rarer tumor, such as NUT carcinoma, will also be discussed under this histopathological type.

Grossly, the tumor exhibits infiltrative exophytic or endophytic growth pattern with tan to white cut surface. The tumor can show variable degrees of ulceration, necrosis, and hemorrhage [1]. There are a few variants of HNSCC that depend on microscopic features and their associated etiologies will be discussed.

Keratinising Squamous Cell Carcinoma (KSCC)

It is the most common variant of HNSCC, which is most often described in head and neck malignancy.

Clinical Features

The presenting features vary depending on their location. Usually, they presented with non-specific symptoms, which include nasal obstruction and discharge, epistaxis, facial pain, a nasal mass, ulcer, or even eye-related symptoms [2].

Morphology

It is characterized by malignant squamous epithelial cell proliferation with evidence of keratinization and invasive growth pattern. Keratin pearl formation is common. Invasion into the stromal tissue is often accompanied by a desmoplastic changes, accompanied by chronic inflammatory cells (Fig. 2). In general, it is graded into well-, moderately-, and poorly differentiated. Well-differentiated SCC exhibits mild nuclear atypia with keratin pearls, whereas poorly differentiated SCC display highly pleomorphic and hyperchromatic cells, with numerous typical and atypical mitoses, minimal keratinization, and sometimes necrosis. In this case, the presence of intercellular bridges is an important diagnostic clue for squamous differentiation or origin. Most SCCs are moderately-differentiated, which exhibit features in between well-differentiated and poorly differentiated carcinoma. HNSCCs express most epithelial markers such as cytokeratin. However, in well-differentiated SCC, diagnosis can be made by H&E without additional stains. In poorly differentiated tumors, immunohistochemistry may play a role. HNSCCs are immunopositive for pan cytokeratin. CK5/CK6, p63 and p40 are excellent markers for squamous differentiation [3, 4].

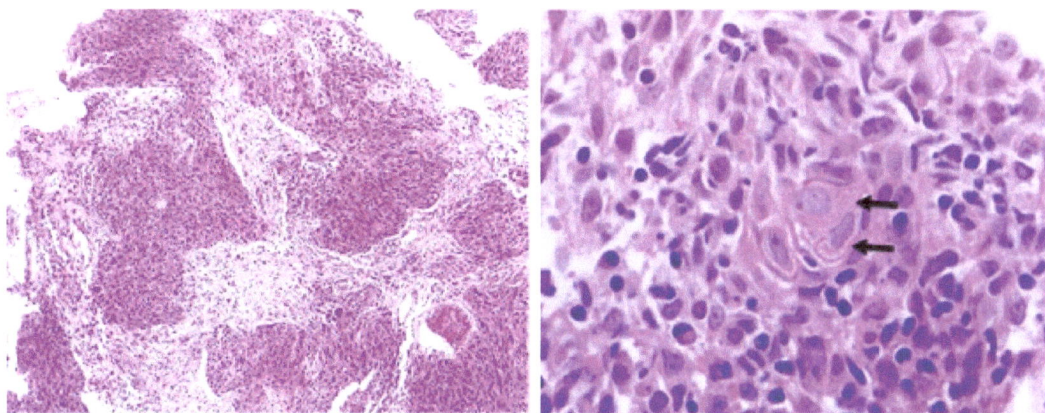

Fig. (2))

Keratinizing squamous cell carcinoma (KSCC). **Left (H&E 100X)**: Infiltrating tumours are seen arranged in large irregular sheets surrounded by desmoplastic stroma. **Right (H&E 400X)**: The intercellular bridges (arrow) is present.

Non-keratinizing Squamous Cell Carcinoma (NKSCC)

SCC exhibited a distinctive ribbon-like growth pattern with minimal maturation. It accounts for about 10 to 27% of sinonasal SCC; the maxillary sinus and nasal cavity are the most frequently involved. NKSCC in nasopharynx will be discussed separately. The risk factors are similar to KSCC or conventional SCC. However, about 30 to 50% of cases are reported to be associated with transcriptionally active high-risk HPV [1, 2].

Clinical Features

Patients' presentation, as described in KSCC is similar and non- specific.

Morphology

The tumor is variably exophytic or endophytic growth and friable with necrosis and haemorrhage. Microscopically, it shows submucosal tumor arranged in solid nests or anastomosing ribbons with pushing border, with minimal or no definite features of desmoplasia; thus, stromal invasion is difficult to confirm especially, in small biopsy sample. Papillary features can be seen and resembled urothelial carcinoma-like features. The cells usually show minimal or no keratinisation (Fig. 3). This tumor is INI1 or SMARCB1 positive tumor but negative for Neuroendocrine markers, S-100 and NUT1, and could differentiate with other differentials, including sinonasal undifferentiated carcinoma, neuroendocrine carcinoma, SMARCB-1 deficient carcinoma and NUT carcinoma (if there is an abrupt keratinization).

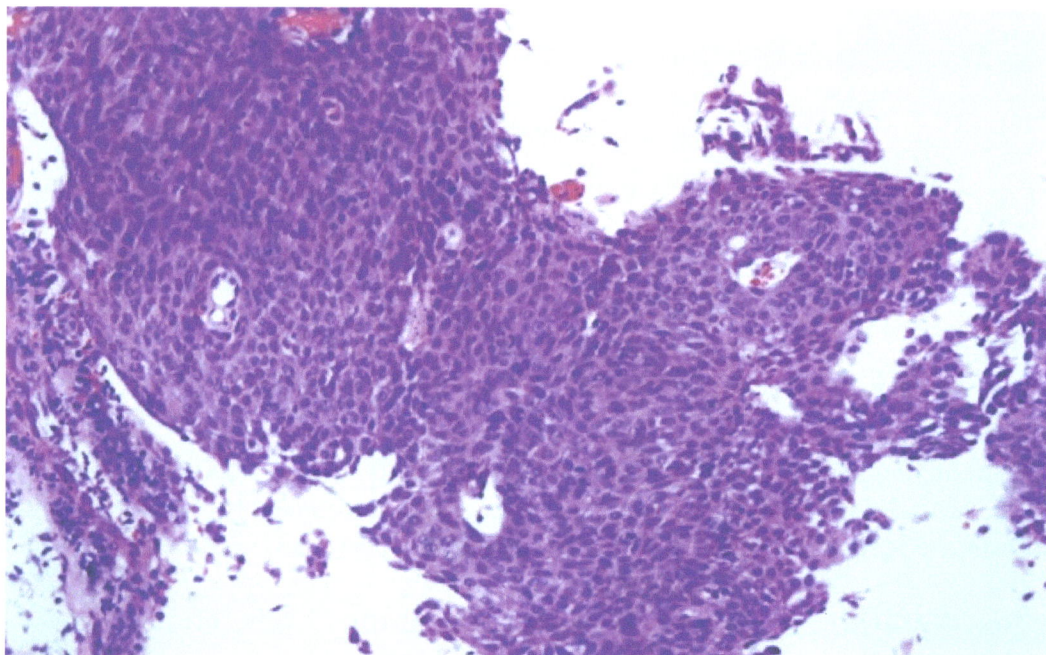

Fig. **(3))**
Sheets of malignant squamous epithelial cells with no evidence of keratinization (H&E x200).

Prognosis and Predictive Factors

The prognosis is better with the presence of HPV.They also shared similar distinctive mutational profiles of HPV-positive or negative tumors as in other parts of head and neck like an oropharynx [2, 5, 6].

Squamous Cell Carcinoma – HPV Positive

This type of carcinoma is also known as Oropharyngeal Squamous Cell Carcinoma (OPSCC). It is a distinct clinical entity, associated with high-risk HPV (OPSCC-HPV). Its high incidence of HPV-associated oropharyngeal carcinoma (more than 90% associated with HPV 16) has been firmly validated [7, 8]. The anatomical site of oropharynx, which is composed of lymphoid based mucosa is a target for viral-associated carcinoma. The incidence has increased for the past three decades and typically affect male, high socioeconomic status and associated with oral sex as a risk factor. The base of the tongue and palatine tonsils are the most frequent location for OPSCC-HPV [7].

Clinical Features

Typically, the patients came in at the advanced stage with cervical lymph nodes metastasis. The primary tumor is usually small and could be missed. This is the tumor that should be considered in a case of cervical lymph node metastasis of undetermined primary if the morphology correlates and HPV testing is positive.

Morphology

It shows features of non-keratinizing SCC; however, evidence of surface epithelium dysplasia is rarely identified. The tumor cells exhibit a high nuclear: cytoplasmic ratio, often resembled basaloid cells, grow in solid nests or lobules below the crypt epithelium, high mitosis/and apoptosis with necrosis. Evidence of keratinization is absent or inconspicuous. The tumor nests are embedded in the background of lymphoid stroma or penetrate it, renders more challenges in the histopathological diagnosis. There are morphological variants or spectrum of OPSCC-HPV, which include papillary, adenosquamous, lymphoepithelioma-like, sarcomatoid, and small cell features. The role of immunohistochemistry is important in this type of tumor to confirm the presence of HPV (p16) and to rule out the differentials, especially when it shows the morphologic variants mentioned above. HPV detection by molecular assays (*in situ* hybridization or/and PCR based assays) are used for confirmation. However, diffuse p16 immunoreactivity is sufficient as a reliable surrogate marker to confirm the presence of HPV in an appropriate morphology arising in the oropharynx. Molecular studies show HPV oncoproteins E6 and E7 inactivate p53 and RB by targeting them for protein degradation. Somatic mutations in *TFAF3* (immune regulator) and oncogenic *PIK3CA* mutation and gene amplification are unique and more common in this carcinoma, respectively.

Prognosis and Predictive Factor

OPSCC-HPV has a favorable prognosis and significantly better survival outcomes and lower risk of recurrence than HPV negative cancer. However, cigarette smoking could interfere with the prognosis and lead to unfavorable outcomes [7, 9].

Squamous Cell Carcinoma – HPV Negative

HPV-negative OPSCC is an OPSCC that lacks association with high-risk HPV, usually occuring in the older age group. The common site for this tumor is soft palatine. It shows similar morphological features of conventional SCC as described above. The immunohistochemistry for p16 is negative.

Molecular/genetic profile: Mutation of *TP53* is common. The differences between the HPV-positive OPSCC and HPV-negative OPSCC are summarized in Table 1.

Table 1 HPV-positive OPSCC and HPV-negative OPSCC (El-Naggar AK, Chan JKC, Grandis JR, Takata T, Slootweg PJ. WHO Classification of Head and Neck Tumors 4th edition. Lyon: International Agency for research on cancer 2017).

Characteristics	HPV-Positive OPSCC	HPV-Negative OPSCC
Age	50 to 56 years old	60 to 70 years old
Risk factors	Sexual behavior	Smoking and alcohol
Common sites	Base of tongue and palatine tonsils	Soft palatine
Clinical features	Advanced stage with lymph node metastasis	Neck mass, sore throat or dysphagia
Postulated origin	Reticulated epithelium of invaginated crypts	Surface epithelium
Morphology	Non-keratinizing SCC	Conventional SCC /KSCC
Dysplasia	Rare	Often present
Grading	Not applicable	As conventional SCC/KSCC
p16 immunohistochemistry	Positive	Negative
Overall Survival rate (3 years)	82%	57%
Prognosis	Favorable	Less favorable

Verrucous Carcinoma

Verrucous carcinoma (VC) is a non-metastasizing, slow-growing but locally invasive variant of well-differentiated SCC. The most common site of VC in the head and neck is the oral cavity followed by the larynx. The etiopathogenesis of VC of the head and neck has not been fully understood. It was generally believed that conventional SCC and VC share similar etiological factors [10], however, certain studies found results [11].

Morphology

Microscopically, it is composed of the thickened, club-shaped, projections, and invaginations of well-differentiated squamous epithelium with marked surface keratinization (church-spire keratosis). It lacks cytologic atypia and mitosis, which is usually confined to the basal cells layers, renders a potential pitfall in the diagnosis and could be misdiagnosed as a benign lesion. It usually invades into the stroma with a very well-defined pushing border, usually associated with the inflammatory response. The diagnosis should be made based on clinicopathological correlation to rule other possible differential diagnoses such as verrucous hyperplasia. The sufficient size of the sample is crucial for its orientation before rendering a definitive diagnosis. The role of molecular studies on VC is limited and mostly unknown.

Prognosis and Predictive Factor

The prognosis of VC is excellent, especially when it presents at an early stage. However, it is locally invasive and can lead to extensive destruction if left untreated. Hybrid VC (invasive SCC and VC) has the potential to metastasize and should be managed as conventional SCC [10].

Basaloid Squamous Cell Carcinoma

Basaloid squamous cell carcinoma (BSCC) is a rare and aggressive variant of cancer with distinct pathologic characteristics that mainly arises in the upper aerodigestive tract. Epiglottis, larynx, and hypopharynx (piriform sinus) and base of the tongue are among the common sites of involvement [12, 13]. and usually linked with tobacco use and alcohol consumption. *Human Papilloma Virus (HPV)* is usually absent in these anatomical sites [10].

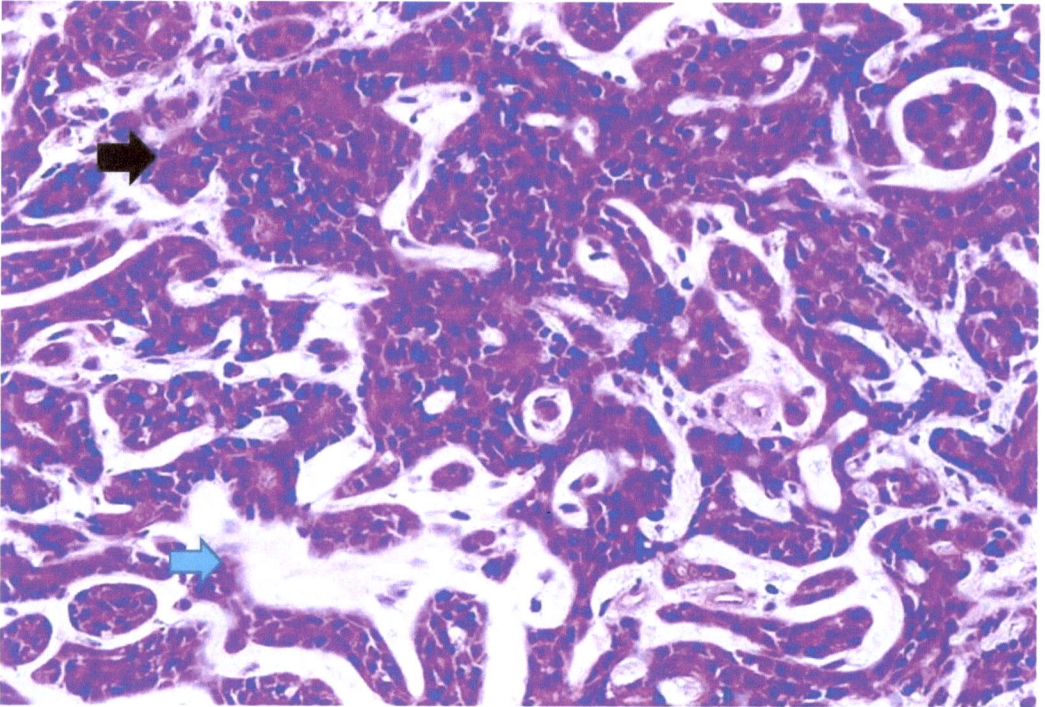

Fig. (4))

Basaloid squamous cell carcinoma exhibiting small crowded cells (black arrow) with hyperchromatic nuclei, minimal cytoplasm within the hyalinised stroma (blue arrow) (H&E x200).

Morphology

It consists of basaloid and conventional squamous components. They are arranged in nests or cords of small crowded cells with minimal cytoplasm, hyperchromatic nuclei. Comedo-necrosis, prominent stromal hyalinization and peripheral palisading, small cystic spaces and mitotic activity are the common findings (Fig. 4). The differential diagnosis includes neuroendocrine carcinoma, adenoid cystic carcinoma, and adenosquamous carcinoma. Immunohistochemistry is strongly positive for p63 and p40 (diffuse pattern) and negative for neuroendocrine markers (synaptophysin and chromogranin). Adenoid cystic carcinoma shows a lack of squamous differentiation (partial p63 positivity). HPV-related oropharyngeal basaloid SCC are morphologically similar with laryngeal and hypopharyngeal BSCC [10].

Prognosis and Predictive Factor

Most of the investigators found that BSCC in laryngeal/hypopharyngeal sites are more aggressive and commonly presented at the advanced stage with lymph nodes metastasis (50-70%) and a higher risk of distant metastasis [4, 13]. It has a poorer prognosis than conventional SCC [7].

Papillary Squamous Cell Carcinoma

It is an another distinct variant of SCC that usually presents as a soft, friable, polypoid, exophytic to papillary tumor, and ranges from 0.2 to 4.0 cm [14]. It usually arises from a thin stalk, however, the broad-based lesions have also been described. On top of tobacco and alcohol consumption, recent evidence found that PSCC is also associated with HPV, especially in the oropharynx and sinonasal tract [14, 15].

Morphology

It is characterized by a papillary growth pattern, with thin fibrovascular cores covered by epithelial cells or immature basaloid cells with high grade dysplasia and minimal or no maturation. The assessment of stalk invasion or involvement will be difficult especially in superficial biopsies.

Prognosis and Predictive Factor

It has a better prognosis and is usually presented at an early stage. It also has a low metastatic potential. However, HPV-negative tumor has a poorer prognosis than HPV-positive oropharynx PSCC [15].

Spindle Cell Squamous Cell Carcinoma

Spindle cell squamous cell carcinoma (SCSCC) is a rare variant of SCC, accounting for less than 1% of all laryngeal malignancies. It affects elderly patients with male predominant. The most frequent site is the larynx, especially glottis. It is usually linked with tobacco and alcohol consumption. Radiation-induced SCSCC has also been described as an etiological agent. HPV is invariably negative in SCSCC of larynx and hypopharynx. The patient presented with airway obstruction due to polypoid mass protruding into the airway, often with surface ulceration [16].

Morphology

Microscopically, the tumor is composed of predominantly pleomorphic and hyperchromatic spindle-shaped cells, arranged in a haphazard pattern, which resembled sarcoma. However, it derived from squamous epithelial cells and exhibited the epithelial-mesenchymal transition. The remnant of dysplastic squamous epithelium usually is seen. Heterologous mesenchymal differentiation such as malignant bone, cartilage, or skeletal muscle is reported in 7 to 15% of cases [16]. The role of immunohistochemistry is important in this case to differentiate SCSCC with the true sarcoma, which is even rarer. The former is positive for epithelial markers *i.e.*, pan-cytokeratin, EMA, p63, and p40. Molecular studies or genetic profile is similar to poorly differentiated SCC [17].

Prognosis and Predictive Factors

Even though the tumor is pleomorphic and appears sarcomatoid, the patient usually presented at an early stage and stage-to-stage prognosis is comparable with the conventional SCC. Since the tumor is usually exophytic and polypoid, it is resectable and has the best prognosis [16].

Adenosquamous Carcinoma (ASC)

It is a malignant tumor arising from the surface epithelium exhibiting both squamous and glandular differentiation. It is a rare tumor, usually in old age (6th to 7th decade of life), with male predisposition. It is associated with alcohol and heavy smoking but ASC from larynx and hypopharynx are not related to HPV infection. The common sites involved include larynx and a few cases reported from hypopharynx [18].

Clinical Features

Patients presented with hoarseness of voice, sore throat, dysphagia, hemoptysis, or neck mass [19].

Morphology

The mass usually exophytic polypoid mass with mucosal ulceration similar to SCC. Microscopically, it shows biphasic morphology, with both squamous and glandular differentiation. Both components are distinct and located in proximity is an important diagnostic clue.

Metastatic ASC may exhibit only one component. The tumor is p63 positive in squamous component and Carcinoembryonic antigen (CEA), CK7, and low molecular weight CK positive in the glandular component. The cells are CK20 negative.

Prognosis and Predictive Factors

It is more aggressive than conventional SCC, prone to recurrence and dissemination. Lymph node metastasis is as high as 75% and about 25% develop distant metastasis, mostly to the lung [19].

NUT Carcinoma

It is a poorly differentiated carcinoma (often with evidence of squamous differentiation), defined by the presence of nuclear protein in testis (NUT) gene (*NUTM1)* rearrangement. The tumors are generally midline. It was also called as NUT midline carcinoma or t(5; 19) carcinoma. It is a rare tumor in the aerodigestive tract in which the actual incidence is unknown [20]. About 65% of cases were noted in the nasal cavity and paranasal sinuses but rare cases were reported in oropharynx, orbital, nasopharynx, larynx, epiglottis, and salivary glands [21]. There is no association with virus-induced carcinogenesis such as HPV or EBV and environmental factors like smoking, *etc.*

Clinical Features

Non-specific symptoms like nasal obstruction, pain, nasal discharge, epistaxis, or eye-related symptoms like proptosis caused by a rapidly growing mass.

Morphology

It shows features of undifferentiated carcinoma or poorly differentiated squamous cell carcinoma. The hallmark features are the presence of moderate-sized monomorphic cells with vesicular nuclei having pale to clear glycogenated cytoplasm and an abrupt island of keratinization embedded within the sea of poorly differentiated cells. Mitoses are brisk and necrosis is common. However, the diagnosis will only be confirmed by the demonstration of NUT rearrangement. An equivocal diagnosis could be made by the presence of diffuse (more than 50%) nuclear staining with NUT monoclonal antibody immunohistochemistry [1, 22]. **Genetic profile** is defined by the rearrangement of nuclear protein in testis, *NUTM1.* In most cases (70%) NUTM1 on chromosome 15q14 fused with *BRD4,* 6% fused with *BRD3* or *WHSC1L1 (NSD3)* creating chimeric genes that encode NUT fusion proteins [1, 21, 23]. **Prognosis** is poor with a median survival of 9.8 months (3 to 11 months) [23].

Nasopharyngeal Carcinoma

The "nasopharyngeal carcinoma", is defined as malignant tumor arising from the nasopharynx that shows evidence of squamous differentiation by ultrastructure or light microscopy. It is sub-divided to 1) non-keratinizing [further sub-categorized as undifferentiated or differentiated], 2) keratinizing types, and 3) basaloid SCC. This classification system is published in the latest WHO classification (4th edition, 2017) (Table 2); and retained similar classification as published in the 3rd edition (2005).

Table 2 Histopathological Classification of NPC (*Chan J.K.C., Slootweg P.J. Petersson B.F, Bell D, El-Mofty S.K, Gillison M. Nasopharyngeal carcinoma. In: Adel K.El-Naggar, John K.C. Chan, Jennifer R. Grandis, Takashi Takata, Pieter J.Slootweg. Editors WHO Classification of Head and Neck Tumors. 4th edition. Lyon: International Agency for research on cancer, 2017*).

Characteristics	Non-keratinizing Squamous Cell Carcinoma (NK-NPC)	Keratinizing Squamous Cell Carcinoma (K-NPC)	Basaloid Squamous Cell Carcinoma
Epidemiology	It is rare among Caucasians, however, it has a distinctive ethnic and geographic distribution to Southern China and Asia and [24].		
Etiology/risk factors	• High association with Epstein Barr Virus (EBV) infection [25].	• Smoking and alcohol play a major role. • Usually not associated with Epstein Barr Virus (EBV).	• High-incidence ethnic group – may associated with EBV positive.
Morphology	Two histological variants 1) Differentiated. 2) Undifferentiated. However, there is no clinical or prognostic significance [24]. **Undifferentiated Variant**: The tumor cells are arranged in syncytial sheets with indistinct cell border, composed of large, round to oval vesicular nuclei, large central nucleoli and scanty eosinophilic to amphophilic cytoplasm. (Fig. 5).	Similar features with other HNSCC. It shows obvious squamous differentiation with evidence of keratinization *i.e.* keratin pearls, individual keratinization and intercellular bridges. The stroma often shows marked	It is similar with other BSCC in other head and neck region.

		desmoplastic reaction.	
Morphology	**Differentiated Variant:** It shows stratification or pavement arrangement, resembling transitional cell carcinoma of bladder. The tumor cells are smaller with fairly well-defined cell border. Vague intercellular bridges and occasional keratinized cells can be observed. The nuclei is conspicuous. The lymphoplasma cells is variable in both variants and lack of desmoplastic reaction.		
Prognosis	-	Locally aggressive tumor, with less tendency for lymph node or distant metastasis [24, 26]. Poorer respond to radiotherapy, worse prognosis as compared to non-keratinizing subtype.	It has better prognosis than basaloid neoplasm at other area of head and neck [24, 27].

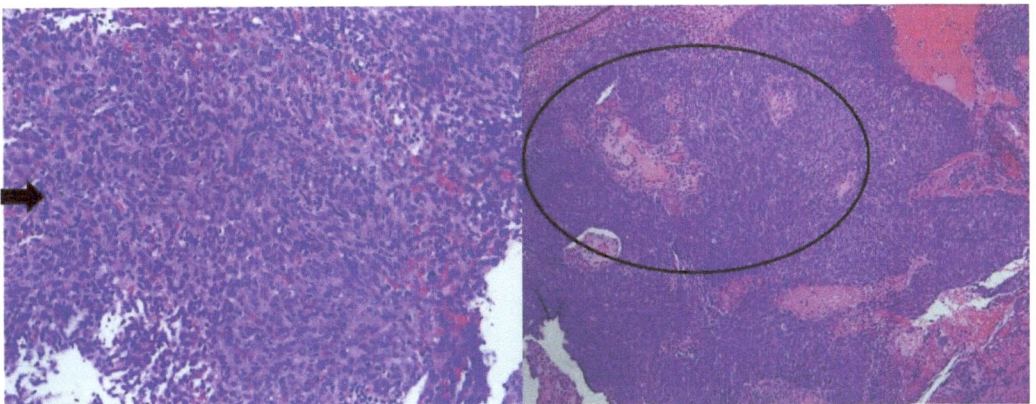

Fig. **(5))**
Non-keratinizing Nasopharyngeal carcinoma (undifferentiated variant). The cells are large, round to oval vesicular nuclei, large central nucleoli and scanty eosinophilic to amphophilic cytoplasm **(black arrow)**, arranged in syncytial sheets **(in circle)** (H&Ex200).

EPITHELIAL TUMOUR WITHOUT SQUAMOUS DIFFERENTIATION

Sinonasal Papilloma (Schneiderian)

Sinonasal papilloma is a benign epithelial tumor which arising from the oral mucosa tract lining cells. The incidence of occurrence is about 5% of total head and neck neoplasm. It also can affect in all age groups.

Precursor/Risk Factors

One of the risk factors for inverted papilloma is history of exposure to organic solvents [28]. No definite proof of HPV and P16 association have been identify in the lesions [29]. An exophytic papilloma increase evidence etiology related to HPV [30]. No evidence of HPV association seen in oncocytic type papilloma [31].

Morphology

It is divided into three type growth pattern as endophytic, exophytic and mixed (oncocytic) [31]. Endophytic type arises from lateral nasal cavity and sinuses with thickened squamous epithelial. Meanwhile, the exophytic type usually growth at nasal septum. Oncocytic type shows mixed exophytic and/or endophytic growth which occur at lateral nasal cavity and sinuses.

Histologically, the inverted type exhibits endophytic growth of markedly thickened squamous epithelial proliferation growing downward admixed mucocytes and mucous cysts (Figs. 6 and 7).

The exophytic type also shows similar histomorphology features as endophytic type.Thirdly, oncocytic type displays proliferation of columnar epithelial cells with abundant granular eosinophilic cytoplasm. The tumor also composed of goblet and mucous cells. However, the malignant transformation is rarely observed.

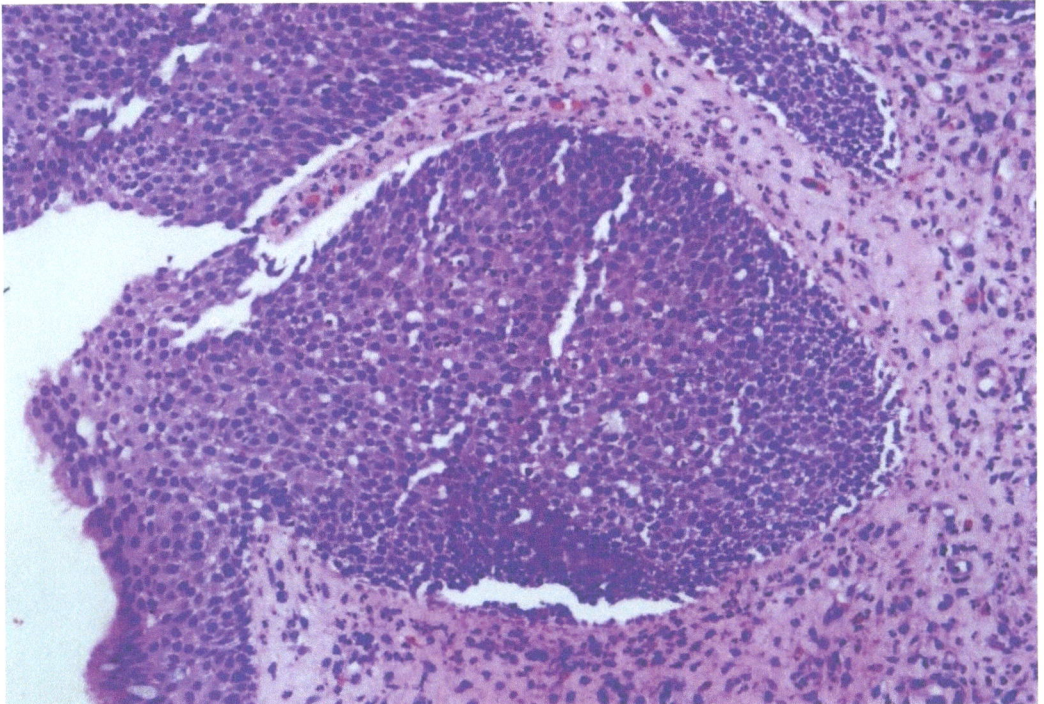

Fig.   **(6))**
Inverted type exhibits endophytic growth with marked thickened squamous epithelium admixed with mucocytes and mucous cysts.

Molecular/Genetic Profile

Inverted papilloma have high EGFR gene prevalence [32].

Prognosis and Predictive Factors

The outcome is influence by the tumor type and the evidence of tumor cells infiltration. Prognosis depends on the histological type, the degree of invasion and the extent of tumor. The treatment of choices will be a complete or wide surgical removal to avoid recurrence.

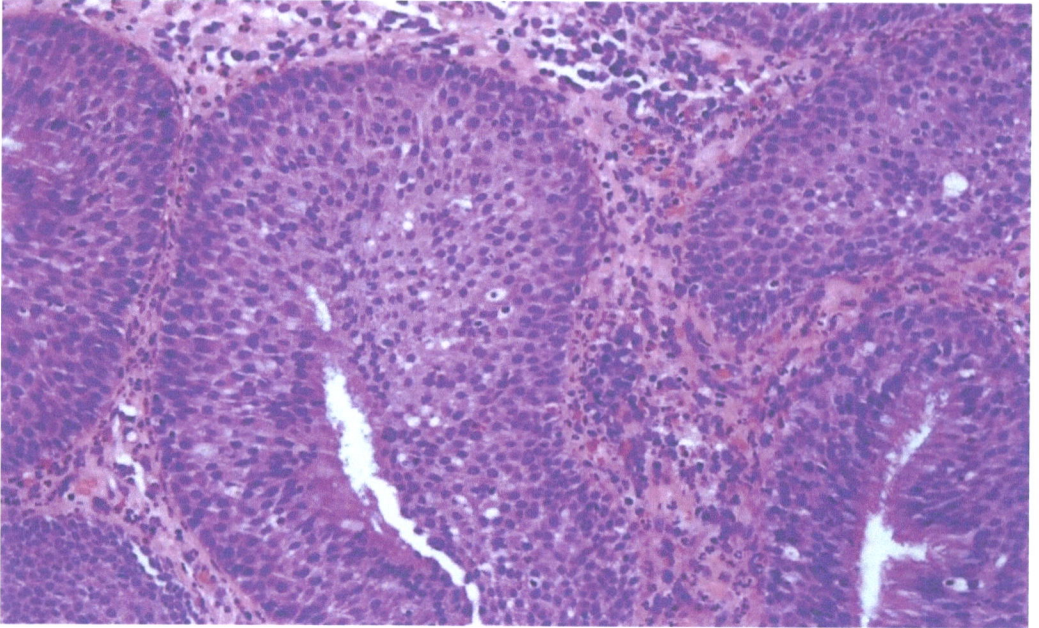

Fig.   **(7))**
Inverted type exhibits endophytic growth with downward epithelial proliferation pattern.

Ameloblastoma

It is a locally aggressive benign epithelial odontogenic neoplasm arising from sinonasal cavity or maxillary sinus, with potential extension into adjacent areas.

Clinical Features

It is present as late presentation in elderly which predominantly in male > female (4:1). The symptoms are nonspecific, including unilateral enlarging mass, sinusitis, nasal obstruction, and epistaxis. It can be associated with an impacted tooth.

Morphology

Polypoidal and solid to cystic mass is the commonest presentation. Unicystic ameloblastoma presents as a single cystic lesion with thickening that can fill the entire lumen.

There are many histologic types; however plexiform, ameloblastic, and acanthomatous are most common in sinonasal tract. The tumor cells can be spindle shaped, basaloid, granular, or show squamous (acanthomatous) differentiation.

Basal cells are arranged in anastomosing strands (plexiform pattern) with reverse polarity of basal columnar cells (a.k.a. Vickers-Gorlin change) with subnuclear vacuolization. Loosely arranged stellate reticulum, which can become cystic can be seen centrally. But pleomorphism and mitoses are rare.

Molecular/Genetic Profile

BRAF V600E has been the most common mutation [33].

Prognosis/Predictive Factors

A complete surgical excision with adequate margin is recommend with long term close follow- up. BRAF-targeted treatment is an option along with surgery in a few aggressive tumor cases [33, 34].

Sinonasal Undifferentiated Carcinoma

It is extremely rare which affect all age range. This tumor is very malignant whereby the pathogenesis is still unknown.

Precursor/Risk Factor

The etiologic agents are not known. But the Human Papilloma Virus (HPV) was found in some of the cases evidence by P16 staining and molecular testing.

Morphology

The tumor is very aggressive with multifocal site involvement. The symptoms last in a short duration. The exophytic mass usually large with more than 4cm and having ill- defined margins [35]. Histologically, the tumor is hypercellular composed of pleomorphic poorly differentiated cells. The pattern of proliferation includes nest, solid, trabecular and sheet (Fig. 8). The tumor cells may having lymph-vascular invasion and neurotropism with increase mitotic figures with extensive area of tumor necrosis with no squamous or glandular differentiation. The tumor are positive for cytokeratin but variable staining for synaptophysin, chromogranin and p63.

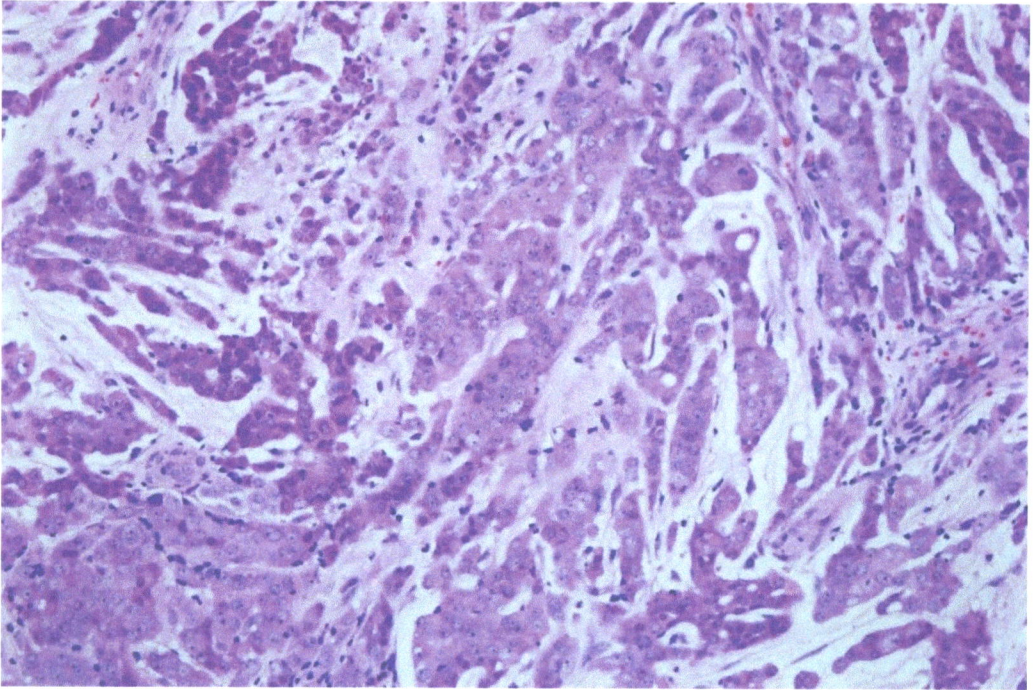

Fig.   (8))
Hypercellular proliferation of high-grade undifferentiated malignant cells with varied growth, including trabecular, sheet-like and cord pattern.

Molecular/Genetic Profile

CD117 is strongly expressed but no gene have been amplified [36]. However, SOX2 gene is amplified in one third of tumors [37].

Prognosis/Predictive Factors

The prognosis is very poor. Chemotherapy is a mode of treatment with good response rate [38]. Patient survival is significantly better with primary surgery resection [39].

Sinonasal Adenocarcinoma, Intestinal Type

Malignant sinonasal tract tumor arising from glandular epithelial that mimic intestinal type adenocarcinoma.

Precursor/Risk Factors

The incidences is increase in shoe and furniture workers. But, may occur sporadically.

Morphology

It arise in sinonasal tract, ethmoid sinus, nasal cavity (inferior and middle turbinates), and maxillary sinus. Most sporadic cases occur in maxillary antrum.

Histologically, they are divided by tumor growth pattern. The colonic type (40%) composed of tubular and glandular pattern, papillae is rarely seen (Fig. 9). The papillary type (18%) exhibits papillary pattern with few tubular glands and while the solid type (20%) characterized by solid and trabecular growth with isolated tubule formation. Uncommon, mucinous type shows nest of cells, single glands, signet ring cells, or well-formed glands filled by mucus and extracellular mucin pools. Immunohistochemically, CK20 (almost 86% of cases) and CDX-2 positivity.

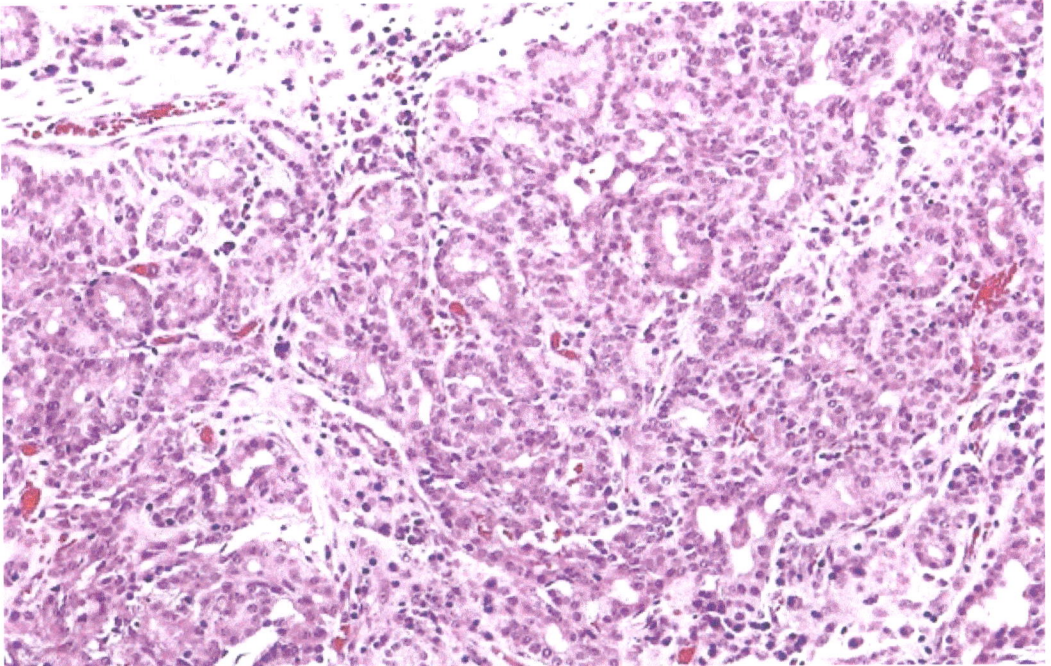

Fig. (9))
The colonic type exhibits tubular and glandular growth pattern.

Molecular/Genetic Profile

KRAS mutations occur in 10-40% of cases [40]. The tumor have no microsatellites instability and mismatch repair protein [41]. Aberrant p53 expression in more than half of all cases [42].

Prognosis/Predictive Factors

All ITACs are highly fatal. Surgical removal adjuncts with radiotherapy is the treatment. The 5-year cumulative survival rate is ~ 40%, with most deaths occurring within 3 years. However, there is no prognostically difference between occupational exposed and sporadic ITACs.

SALIVARY GLAND TUMOUR

Salivary gland neoplasm comprises about 5% of head and neck tumor whereby the mass swelling is the commonest presentation [43]. Histologically, the lesion shows variable histomorphological growth and cells pattern. Some of them may have overlapping feature which can present in both benign and malignant condition [44].

Microscopic Anatomy of Salivary Glands

The salivary gland has a basic secretory unit called acini which composed of secretory cells surrounded by a duct. The secretory unit consists of acinus cells, myoepithelial cells, intercalated duct, striated duct and excretory duct [45].

Neoplasm of Salivary Glands

Neoplastic lesion can be subdivided as benign and malignant based on its cell origin either epithelial or non-epithelial. Majority of tumor are occur in parotid gland follow by minor type salivary gland and submandibular gland [45].

Benign and Malignant Epithelial Neoplasm

The World Health Organization (WHO) in 2005 classified benign tumors into 13 subtypes and malignant tumors into 24 subtypes in Table **3** [46]. The tumors are heterogenous composed of epithelial and myoepithelial components. Parotid gland also is the commonest metastatic site for head and neck tumor especially squamous cell carcinoma type.

Table 3 World Health Organization classification of epithelial salivary glands neoplasms (Barnes L. Pathology and genetics of head and neck tumors. International Agency for research on cancer 2005; In press).

Benign Epithelial Neoplasms	Malignant Epithelial Neoplasms
Pleomorphic	Mucoepidermoid carcinoma

adenoma Warthin tumor Myoepithelioma Basal cell adenoma Oncocytoma Canalicular adenoma	Adenoid cystic carcinoma Acinic cell carcinoma Polymorphous low-grade adenocarcinoma Epithelial-emyoepithelial carcinoma Clear cell carcinoma not otherwise specified
Sebaceous adenoma Lymphadenoma Sebaceous Non sebaceous Ductal papilloma Inverted papilloma Intra-ductal papilloma Sialoadenoma papilliferum Cystadenoma	Basal cell adenocarcinoma Sebaceous carcinoma Sebaceous lymphadenocarcinoma Cystadenocarcinoma Low-grade cribriform cystadenocarcinoma Mucinous adenocarcinoma Oncocytic carcinoma Salivary duct carcinoma Adenocarcinoma, not otherwise specified Myoepithelial carcinoma Carcinoma ex-pleomorphic adenoma Carcinosarcoma Metastasizing pleomorphic adenoma Metastatic Squamous cell carcinoma Small cell carcinoma Large cell carcinoma Lymphoepithelial carcinoma Sialoblastoma

Pleomorphic Adenoma

The commonest salivary gland tumor is found in parotid gland. It is present as a painless growing mass.

Precursor/Risk Factors

The origin of the neoplasm is unknown with uncertain histogenesis. However, history of radiation exposure is a risk.

Morphology

Pleomorphic adenoma is a well circumscribed mass which rarely exceed 6 cm in widest diameter. The lesion is encapsulated, rounded and having pushing growth pattern into adjacent gland tissue. On sectioning, they exhibits grey white surface with chondromyxoid area.

The epithelial components composed of ductal or myoepithelial cells arranged in acini, tubules or sheets pattern. These components are intermingled with mesenchymal components such as myxoid and chondroid or bony island (Fig. 10). In some area, there is sheet of myoepithelial cells with foci of mature squamous epithelium. However, no features of malignancy seen such as dysplasia or increased mitotic figures seen.

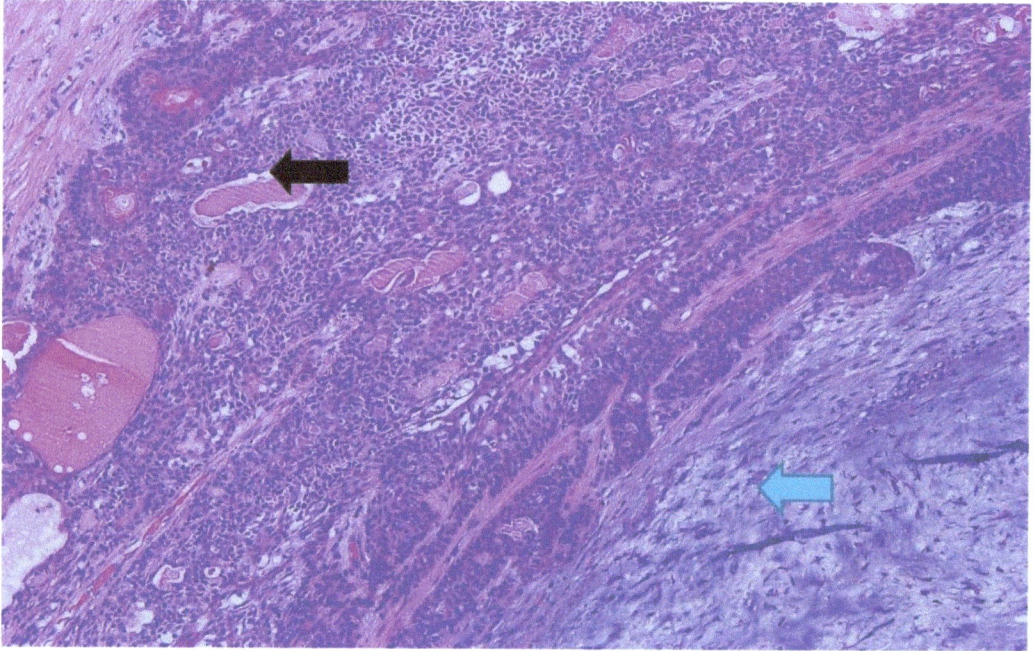

Fig. **(10))**
A pleomorphic adenoma composed of epithelial elements resembling ductal cells or myoepithelial cells **(black arrow)** are disposed in duct formations, acini, irregular tubules, strands, or sheets of cells and the mesenchymal elements are typically dispersed within a loose myxoid tissue containing islands of chondroid **(blue arrow)**.

Molecular/Genetic Profile

About 70% of Pas show translocations and rearrangements result in gene fusions involving PLAG1 and HMGA2 [47, 48]. These two genes fusion are only encounter in PA and carcinoma ex PA and may be used as biomarkers to distinguish PA from its mimickers [49].

Prognosis/Predictive Factors

Therefore, no significant differences of tumor prognosis influence by dominant component. The recurrence rate and malignant behavior are low in PAs [50].

Warthin Tumor (Papillary Cystadenoma Lymphomatosum)

Warthin tumor is the second common benign tumor also synonym as adenolymphoma. About 10 percent are bilateral and present as solid cystic mass uniquely in parotid gland. Ten percent are bilateral and there is an association with smoking [51].

It commonly arises in parotid gland and affect predominantly in older man. About 10 percent, they are bilateral and multifocal.

Precursor/Risk Factors

The histogenesis of these tumors is unclear. Some suggest these tumors arise from the aberrant lymphoid tissue in the parotid gland. Smokers have a higher risk getting the tumor.

Morphology

The tumors are encapsulated, round to oval mass, arising in superficial parotid gland. They are easily palpable with average size from 2 to 5 cm in diameter. On sectioning, tumor shows a pale gray surface with cystic or cleft-like spaces filled with mucin or serous fluid.

Microscopically, these cystic are lined by a double layer of neoplastic epithelial cells resting on a dense lymphoid stroma having prominent germinal centers. The spaces are frequently narrowed by polypoid projections of the lymphoepithelial elements. The epithelial lining cells is palisade of columnar cells having an abundant, granular, eosinophilic cytoplasm, conveying an oncocytic appearance. Foci of squamous metaplasia are noted.

Prognosis/Predictive Factors

Complete surgical removal with adequate margin is the treatment [52]. The recurrence rates is low and rarely transform to malignancy.

Mucoepidermoid Carcinoma

The most common malignant neoplasm in salivary glands. About 50 percent, the tumor occur in the major glands, mostly in the parotid gland. These tumor are composed of mixtures of squamous cells, mucus-secreting cells, and intermediate cells (Fig. 11).

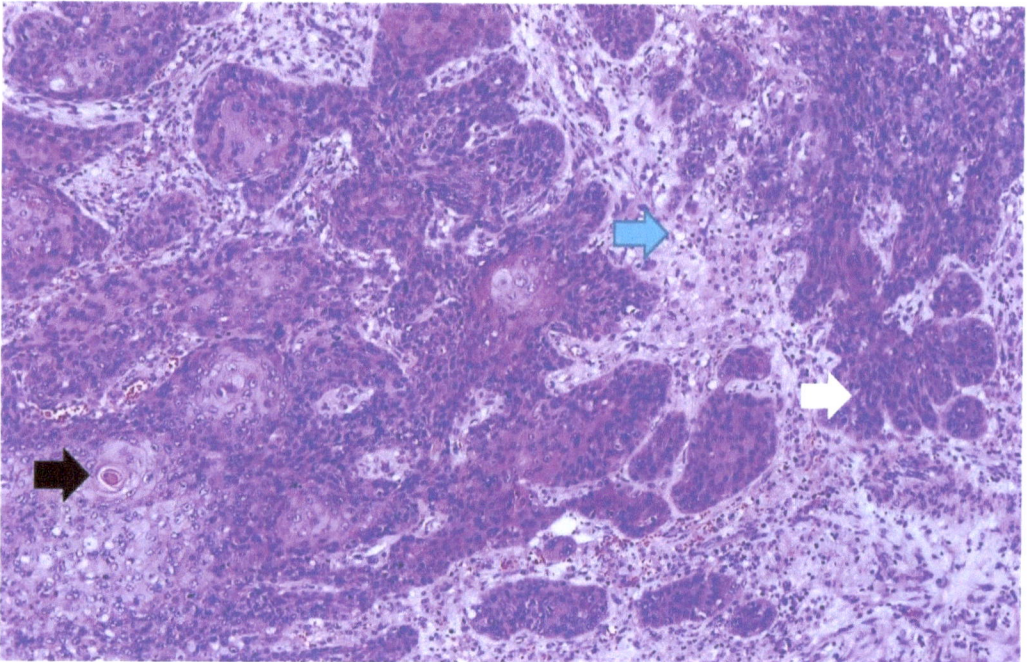

Fig. (11))

These neoplasms are composed of variable mixtures of squamous cells **(black arrow)**, mucus-secreting cells **(blue arrow)**, and intermediate cells (white arrow).

Morphology

The tumor can be large up to 8 cm in diameter. They are circumscribed, but have lack well-defined capsules and are often having infiltrative at some area. On sectioning, the tumor shows pale and gray-white with small foci of mucin-containing cysts. Mucoepidermoid carcinoma are subdivided as low, intermediate, or high grade. The histology shows squamous, mucous, or intermediate cells in cords, sheets, or cystic archictures.

Molecular/Genetic Profile

Many of MEC are having t (11; 19)(q21;p31) translocation and CRTC1-MAML2 gene fusion [53]. Tumor associated with these gene fusion tends to be low-intermediate grade. However, clinical implication of this fusion is unknown.

Prognosis and Predictive Factors

The prognosis of these tumor depending on their grade. The majority of tumors are low or intermediate grade, are treated surgically and have a good prognosis.

Low-grade tumors may invade locally but rarely metastasize .The 5-year survival rate is high, more than 90%. In contrast, intermediate-high grade tumors are invasive and difficult to excise and so recur in about 25% to 30% of cases and, in 30% of cases, disseminate to distant sites. The 5-year survival rate of these tumors is only 50% and increased metastatic potential.

Adenoid Cystic Carcinoma

The tumor is relatively uncommon tumor of malignant salivary gland tumors. However, it arise quite frequent in minor salivary gland. The tumors have a predilection for perineural spread and may associated with nerve palsy.

Morphology

Grossly, it is present as a firm, grey-white, non-capsulated mass. But, hemorrhage and necrosis are rare.

Histology, it exhibits tubular and cribriform pattern with variable solid components. The cribriform pattern characterized by nests of tumor cells by sharply punched-out spaces filled with basophilic matrix (Figs. 12 and 13). The tubular pattern is composed of bilayered tubules with true lumina. The solid growth pattern is sheets of tumor cells without lumen formation.

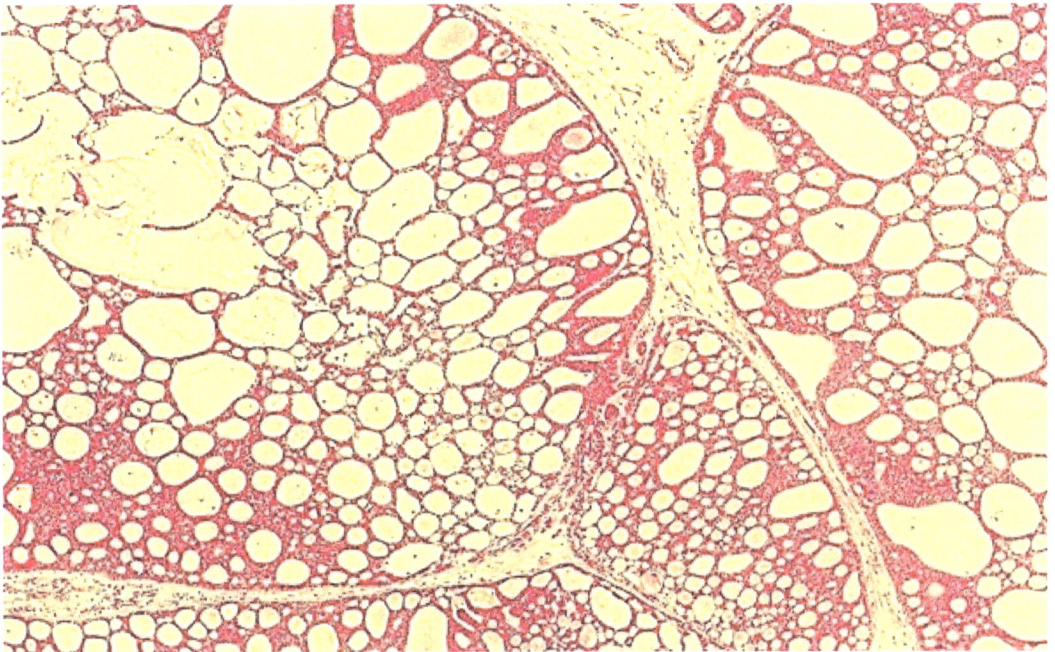

Fig. (12))
A tubular and cribriform structures with variable solid components.

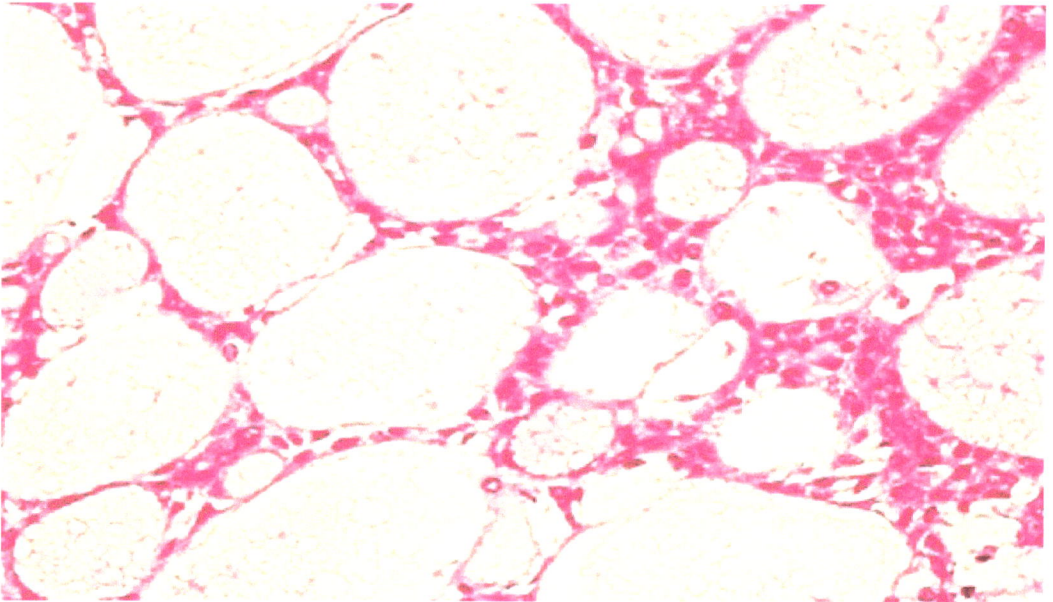

Fig. (13))

The cribriform pattern characterized by nests of tumor cells by sharply punched-out spaces filled with basophilic matrix.

Genetic and Prognosis

More than 80 percent the tumor having MYB or mYBL1 oncogenes fusion. Whereby losses of 1p and 6q are associated with poor prognosis. Overall, the survival rate is 50-70% and the local recurrence rate is high [54].

Acinic Cell Carcinoma

The tumor commonly arise in the parotid gland presented with slow-growing mass. Tender, bilateral glands involvement and facial nerve palsy are the signs. They tend to metastasize to the adjacent cervical lymph nodes.

Morphology

Majority the tumors are fairly circumscribed with solitary nodules of varying size. The tumor is composed of cells resembling the normal serous acinar cells of salivary glands (Fig. 14). The acinar cells are large and polygonal with basophilic granular cytoplasm and eccentric round nuclei (Fig. 15). The granular cytoplasm is positive for periodic acid-Schiff (PAS) stain while acinar cells positive for DOG1 and SOX10 stains.

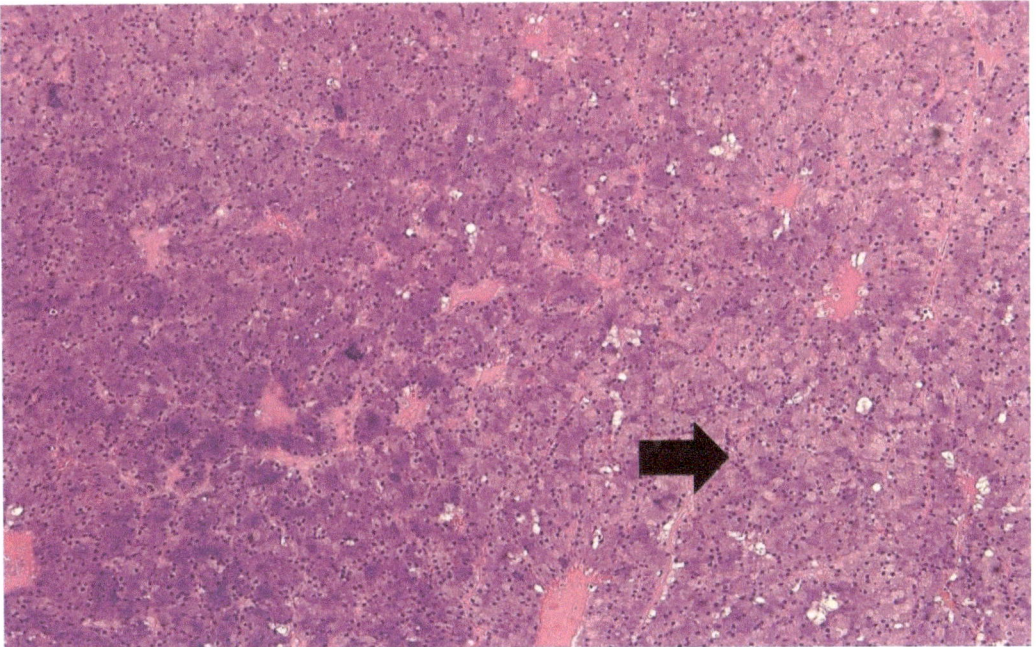

Fig. (14))
The acinic cell tumor is composed of cells resembling the normal serous acinar cells (black arrow) of salivary glands.

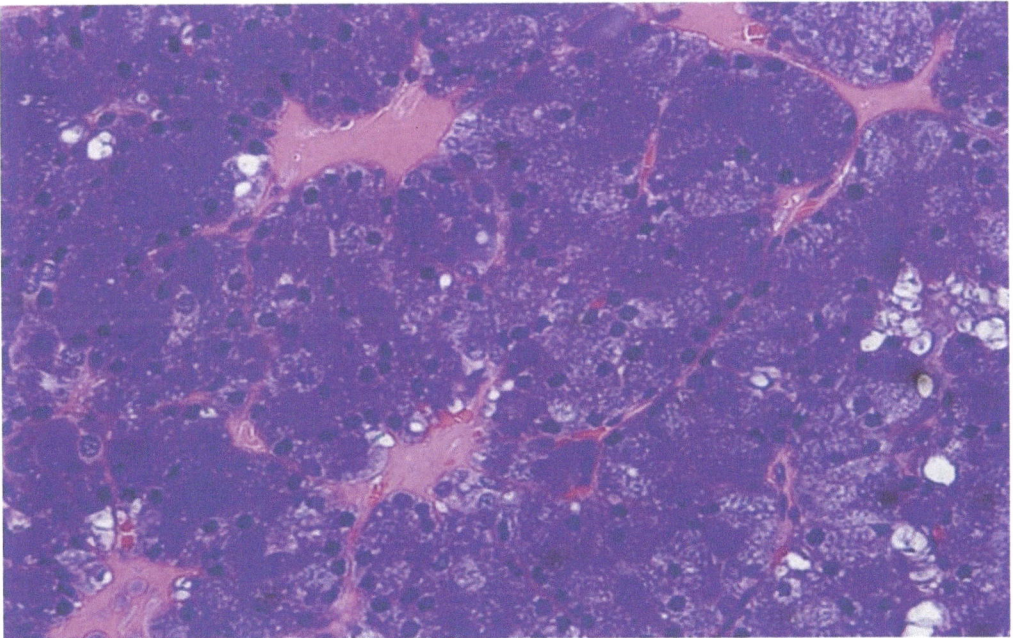

Fig. (15))
The acinar cells are large and polygonal with basophilic granular cytoplasm and eccentric round nuclei.

Prognosis and Predictive Factors

The survival rate is 20% with a recurrence rate is high [55, 56] Poor outcome risks include larger tumor size, involvement of deep loop of parotid gland and incomplete surgical margin.

MISCELLANEOUS TUMOR

Soft Tissue Tumors and Bone Tumors

Benign and malignant primary bone and soft tissue lesions of the head and neck are rare. It remains as diagnostic challenges to pathologist due to its rarity especially with the complex anatomy of the head and neck. Most of these tumors resembled their counterparts arising elsewhere in the body. There are, however, several entities that are largely restricted to the head and neck, which deserve special attention and worth to be highlighted.

Soft Tissue Tumors

Biphenotypic Sinonasal Sarcoma

It is also known as low-grade sinonasal sarcoma with neural and myogenic features which has a distinct histological, IHC, and molecular features (PAX3-MAML3] gene fusion). The tumor has a predilection to females with the mean age is 52 years (24-85 years). It is a slowly growing but locally invasive tumor. Multiple sites in the sinonasal tracts are common. The superior aspect of the nasal cavity and ethmoid sinus are usually involved which may extend to the orbit and cribriform plate.

Morphology: It is a poorly circumscribed tumor composed of spindle cells arranged in a herringbone-fascicular pattern. The cells exhibit ovoid and elongated nuclei with minimal atypia. Rare mitosis is encountered. Proliferation of the overlying epithelium has been reported in majority of cases. Immunohistochemically shows diffuse positivity for S-100, co-expression with SMA and/or related muscle markers, a minority of cases showing focal immunoreactivity for desmin, EMA and keratin.

**Genetic and Prognosis**: It is characterized by a chromosomal translocation t (2; 4)(q35; q31.1) which resulted in PAX3-MAML3 gene fusion (most commonly) [1]. Local recurrence is high (almost 50%) within 9 years follow-up after initial treatment. However, neither metastasis nor death has been reported [57, 58].

Nasopharyngeal Angiofibroma

Nasopharyngeal angiofibroma is a rare, benign neoplasm, accounts less than 0.5% of all head and neck tumors. It is a locally aggressive tumor, which occur almost exclusively in males during adolescence [24, 59]. There is evidence of hormonal dependency in which the tumor cells frequently expressed androgen receptor. The female patient, if involved, androgen insensitivity syndrome should be excluded [24]. Despite its name, most tumors arise from the posterolateral wall of the nasal cavity in the area of the sphenopalatine foramen. Tumors may extend into the paranasal sinuses, soft tissues, and cranial cavity [57].

Clinical Features: Patients usually presented with nasal obstruction, epistaxis, mass, or discharge. The radiological findings of anterior bowing of the posterior wall of the maxillary antrum (Holman-Miller sign) are characteristic and angiography which identifies feeding vessels (usually maxillary artery) is diagnostic and warrant embolization pre-surgical procedure and diagnostic biopsy may not be necessary due to its risk of life-threatening hemorrhage.

Morphology: Microscopically, it has two components which are vascular and stromal tissue. The vessels are thin to thick-walled lined by endothelial cells. The stroma consists of bipolar to stellate shape fibroblastic cells, arranged around these vessels. The background is collagenous, edematous, and paucicellular with scattered mast cells. The endothelium is highlighted by CD31 and CD34 immunohistochemistry. The stromal cells show nuclear expression of androgen receptor and Beta-catenin.

Genetic Profile: It is characterized by chromosomal gains [24]. Loss of Y chromosome with a gain of the X chromosome is frequently found. Somatic mutation in exon 3 of the beta-catenin gene is demonstrated in about 75% of cases. It has been reported to be associated with familial adenomatous polyposis [24, 60].

Prognosis: It depends on the size and extend of tumor and completeness of surgery, and about 5 to 25% case had recurred. The sarcomatous transformation has been reported in association with radiotherapy. Spontaneous regression after puberty can rarely occur [24, 57].

Spindle Cell/Pleomorphic Lipoma

It typically occurs in the neck and trunk of the elderly, predominantly males. It is characterized by an admixture of mature adipocytes and spindled cells. The presence of multinucleated floret cells is seen in pleomorphic lipoma which represents the morphological continuum. The median age is 55 years.

Clinical Features: Patients are usually presented as a long-standing subcutaneous mass in the posterior neck, back, and shoulder. Other less common sites include face, forehead, scalp, buccal-perioral area, and upper arm. The tumor is firmer (depends on the spindle cell component) than the usual lipoma.

Morphology: The tumor often has a firmer texture than the ordinary lipoma. Microscopically it is composed of an admixture of two components (mature adipocytes) and spindle cell components (Fig. **16**). One of the components could be the predominant component. The spindle cells are mostly blended, with rare mitosis. Characteristic thick ropy collagen is common (Fig. **17**). Scattered mast cells are seen in the background. The spindle cell components are strongly positive for CD34 immunohistochemistry and negative for S-100 protein. These two IHC are helpful markers, especially in spindle cell dominated variant. Genetically, it has unbalanced karyotypes, mostly hypodiploid with multiple partial losses. It is a benign lesion with local excision is usually adequate [57, 61].

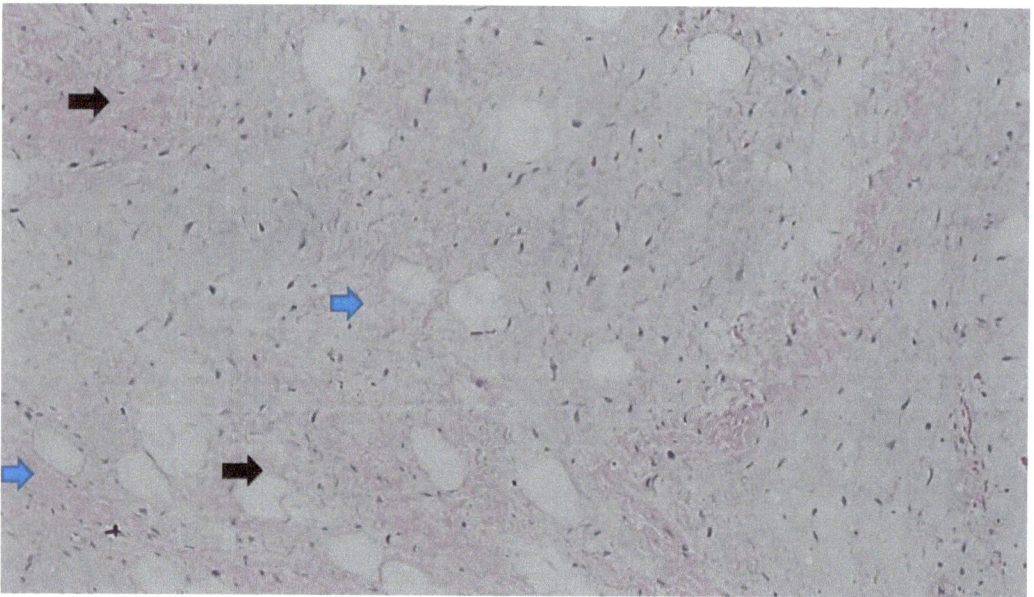

Fig.   **(16))**
Spindle cell lipoma characterized by admixture of adipocytes **(blue arrow)** and spindle cells **(black arrow)** (H&EX100).

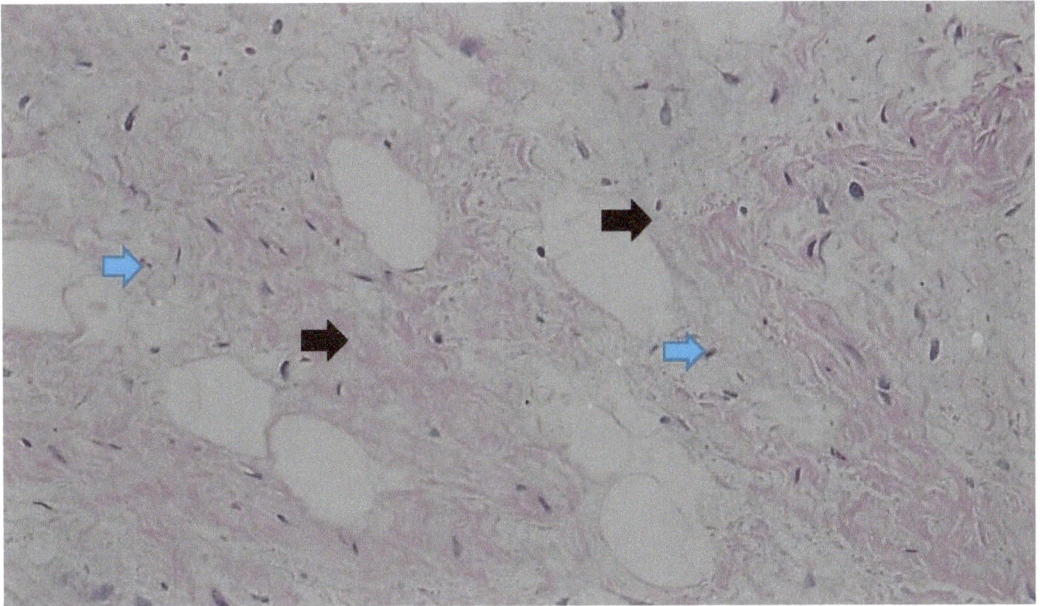

Fig. (17))
Characteristic ropey collagen **(blue arrow)** and mast cells **(black arrow)** in the background.

Bone Tumors

Osteosarcoma

Osteosarcoma (OS) is a malignant tumor of the bone, commonly be found in children and adolescents. It usually arises from the metaphysis of the long bones (femur, tibia, humerus), followed by jaw bone (6% of cases) which develops 10 to 20 years later than the former [62]. The mandible and maxilla are the most frequently affected head and neck sites for osteosarcoma, followed by the paranasal sinuses and skull [57].

Clinical Features: The symptoms are usually non-specific which include pain, swelling, or even loosening of teeth.

Morphology: Microscopically the tumor cells are spindled to round pleomorphic with highly atypical nuclei. The degree of vascularization varies from scant to abundant. These tumor cells produce neoplastic osteoid (a precursor of bone) which is present within a sarcomatous stroma (Fig. 18). Conventional OS is mostly high- grade tumor, periosteal OS is of intermediate-grade and low-grade central and parosteal OS are low-grade subtypes. Maxillofacial OS predominantly of low-grade central subtype. Among the conventional OS, Chondroblastic OS is relatively more common in the jawbones and may mimic chondrosarcoma. Genetic susceptibility shows increased risk to develop OS in a few rare tumor syndromes include Li-Fraumeni Syndrome, retinoblastoma, Werner syndrome, and Rothmund-Thomson syndrome.

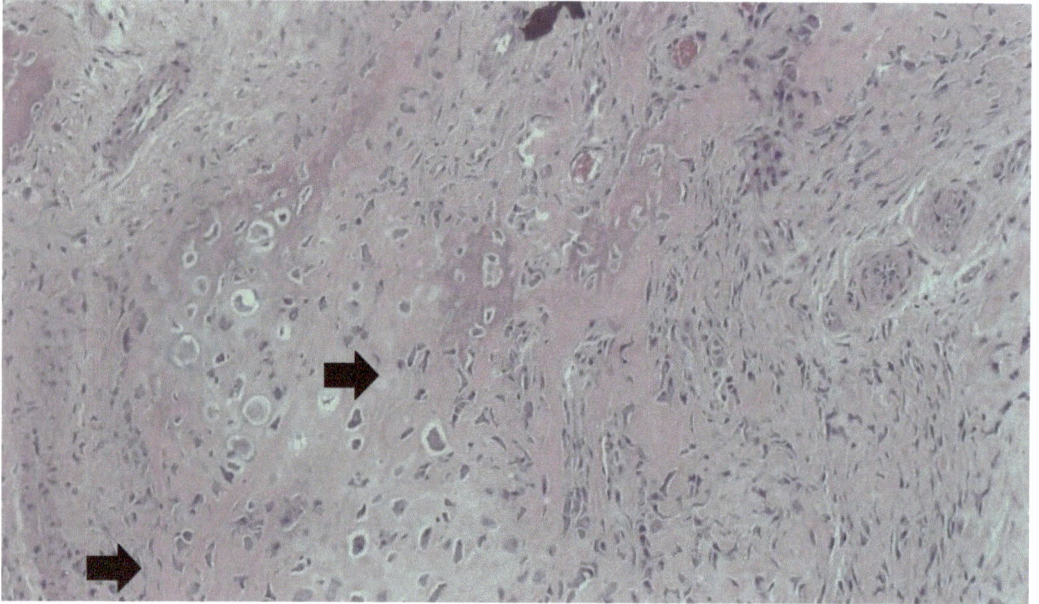

Fig.   **(18))**
Pleomorphic tumor cells produce malignant osteoid **(arrow)** in osteosarcoma.

Prognosis and Predictive Factors: OS of the jaw has a more favorable outcome. It metastasizes less frequently and later in the disease course (6 to 21% of cases). The clear resected margin is the most important prognostic factor with a good 10-years survival rate (>80%) [63]. Low-grade OS is usually cured by complete resection with a clear margin. However, extragnathic OS of the skull and facial bones behave more aggressively as in other conventional OS at the periphery and generally treated by surgery and chemotherapy [62, 64].

Chondrosarcoma

Chondrosarcoma is a malignant bone tumor that produces a cartilaginous matrix. It accounts for 20% of primary malignant bone tumors and about 5-10% are located in the head and neck. The most common location is larynx, followed by the maxilla, mandible, and base of the skull. Chondrosarcomas are the most common type of laryngeal sarcoma and the second most common type of sarcoma arising from the bone in the head and neck. It occurs at any age but has a slight predilection to middle-aged men [65]. Calcification is common and may be helpful in making a diagnosis using radiographs.

**Clinical Features**: As other head and neck tumors, the symptoms are non-specific and it depends on the site of origin.

**Morphology**: Grossly it often exhibits lobular architecture with glistening bluish-grey cut surface. The microscopic diagnostic clue is the entrapment of pre-existing trabecular bone and/or cortical permeation by the neoplastic cartilages with osteodestructive growth pattern. A thorough search on osteoid deposits is required to exclude chondroblastic osteosarcoma. Chondrosarcoma is graded based on cellularity, nuclear pleomorphism, and mitosis into 3 grades, which are well-differentiated (grade I), moderately differentiated (grade II), and poorly differentiated (grade III) lesions.

Genetic Profile

About 49 to 61% of cases exhibit _IDH1/IDH2_ mutations. Prognosis depends on the histologic grade and complete resection with clear surgical margins [65].

Mesenchymal Chondrosarcoma is a biphasic malignant tumor composed of small round cells (Fig. 19) and islands of differentiated hyaline cartilage commonly encountered in the younger age group (second to fourth decades of life). The craniofacial bones especially jaws are the most commonly affected.

Genetic Profile

Typically show HEY1-NCOA2 fusions but _IDH1/IDH2_ mutations are absent._**Prognosis**_: Overall is favorable, however, late metastasis can occur after years or decades [65, 66].

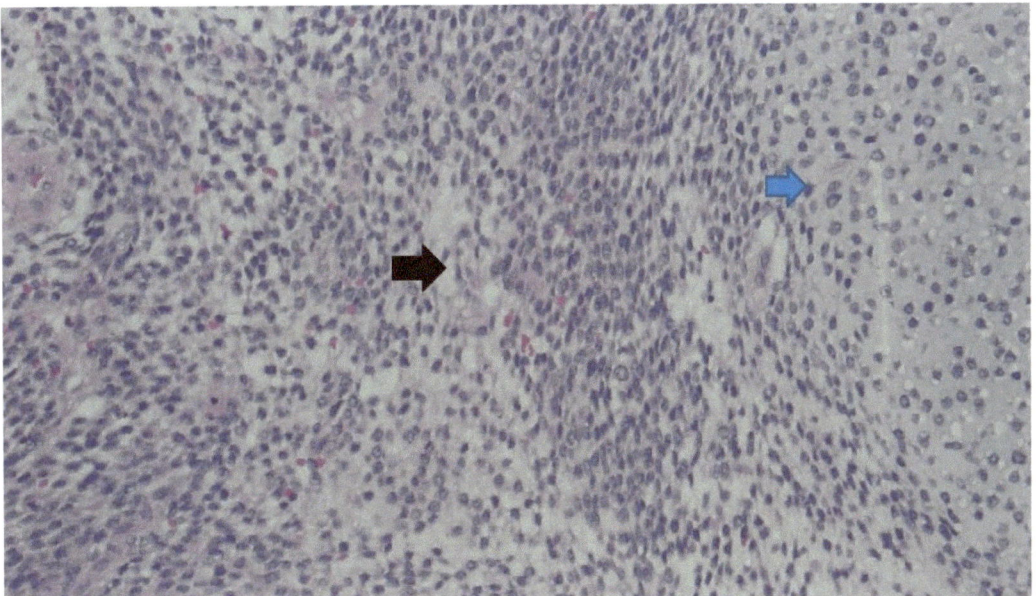

Fig.   **(19))**
Mesenchymal Chondrosarcoma; a biphasic tumor with small round mesenchymal cells **(black arrow)** admixed with island of hyaline cartilage **(blue arrow)**.

Chordoma

It is a malignant tumor with notochord differentiation. It is a rare tumor with about 32-42% arising from cranium especially the base of the skull. In affects any age, with male predominance. The most common location is clivus, which may extend into the nasopharynx and nasal cavity. The patient presented with CNS symptoms including headache, cranial nerve palsy depends on the structure involved.

Morphology:

It is a destructive bone lesion, consists of cords and lobules of physaliphorous cells in the myxoid stroma with intersecting fibrous septae (Fig. **20**). The cells are large, having abundant vacuolated (bubbly) cytoplasm, uniform nuclei with variable pleomorphism. It typically expressed Cytokeratin, EMA, S-100, and brachyury immunohistochemistry.

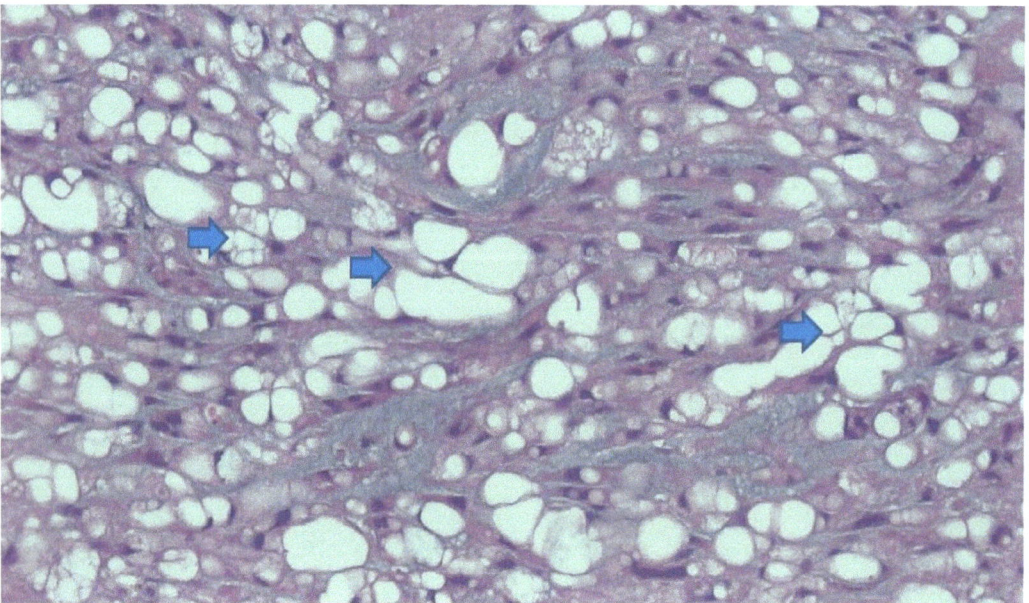

Fig.   **(20))**
Chordoma with characteristic large physalipharous cells **(arrow)** with abundant vacuolated cytoplasm (H&E x200).

Prognosis:

It depends on the surgical resection margins, which rarely could be cleared in the cranial sites. The survival rate for 3, 5 and 10 years are about 80.9%, 73.5% and 58.7%, respectively [67, 68].

Hematolymphoid Tumours

Lymphoma constitutes about 3 to 5% of total head and neck malignancies, and account for 2.5% of total lymphoma affecting the lymphatic tissue of human [69, 70]. It is the 3rd most common malignancy after SCC and adenocarcinoma [71]. The common location and its tumor are summarized in Table 4.

Table 4 **Head and neck hematolymphoid tumors and sites of common involvement (Alfouzan AF. Head and Neck cancer pathology: Old world *vs.* new world disease. Nigeria Journal of Clinical Practice, 2019).**

Head and Neck	Most Common Hematolymphoid Tumor
Nasal cavity, paranasal sinuses and skull base, Nasopharynx	• Extranodal NK/T-Cell Lymphoma
	• Extraosseous plasmacytoma
	• Diffuse Large B-Cell Lymphoma
	-
Larynx and trachea	-
• MALT Lymphoma	-
Oral cavity and mobile tongue	• Extramedullary Myeloid sarcoma
	• CD30-positive T-Cell lymphoproliferative disorder
	• Plasmablastic Lymphoma
	• Langerhans Cell Histiocytosis
Oropharynx	• Hodgkin Lymphoma
	• Burkitt Lymphoma
	• Follicular Lymphoma
	• Mantle Cell Lymphoma
	• T-Lymphoblastic leukaemia/ lymphoma
	• Follicular dendritic cell sarcoma
Salivary gland tumors	• MALT lymphoma
Odontogenic and maxillofacial bone	• Solitary plasmacytoma

Oral and perioral areas, especially in Waldeyer's ring (ring of lymphoid tissue arising in palatine tonsils, nasopharynx, oropharyngeal wall, and base of the tongue), are among the common sites of involvement, in which it originates from B and T lymphocytes and Natural Killer (NK) cells at variable stage of maturation [69].

It can be classified as Hodgkin Lymphoma [HL] and Non-Hodgkin Lymphoma (NHL) as proposed by WHO, however, about 75% of cases are NHL [72]. Lymphoma usually affects immunocompromised patients and viral infection, which includes EBV or HIV plays a role in carcinogenesis. Cervical lymphadenopathy is the most common presenting features. It could also be presented as a mass in the oral cavity or mucosa. We only discussed in detail of 2 types of lymphoma, due to its aggressiveness but early diagnosis is important for a better prognosis Extranodal NK/T cell lymphoma, nasal type (ENKTL) and CD30-positive T-cell lymphoproliferative disorder because it is could be missed or masked by a non-neoplastic inflammatory condition in this area.

Extranodal NK/T Cell Lymphoma, Nasal Type (ENKTL)

Extranodal NK/T cell lymphoma, nasal type (ENKTL) is an aggressive extranodal non-Hodgkin lymphoma, with cytotoxic phenotype and associated with EBV. It is common in East Asia and Latin America but with increasing incidence in the United States [73]. It was also known as lethal midline granuloma or angiocentric lymphoma. The actual etiology is unknown. However, EBV infection plays a role in carcinogenesis. Environmental factors like pesticide exposure, living near incinerators might be the risk factors.

Clinical Features: Patients may have nasal septum or palate perforation due to the tumor infiltrations, it may spread into the nearby structures like orbital or skin. The paranasal sinuses tumor presented with features of chronic sinusitis with 10-20% of cases with lymph nodes metastasis [74].

Morphology: It infiltrates the nasal tissue in a diffuse pattern, frequently with angiocentric and angioinvasive pattern with extensive coagulative necrosis and apoptosis. The atypical lymphoid cells are small to large size, having an irregularly folded nuclei, granular chromatin and conspicuous nucleoli with abundant pale or clear cytoplasm. Perivascular and intravascular destructive infiltrates with fibrinoid changes of blood vessels even without invasion are common. Sometimes prominent inflammatory infiltrate may mimic an inflammatory process. IHC: The tumor cells express CD3, cytotoxic markers. CD56 is more frequently expressed in tumors with NK-cell origin. ENKTL is positive for EBER (EBV-encoded small RNA) by *in-situ* hybridisation. Cases with similar phenotype but negative for EBV are considered as peripheral T-Cell Lymphoma, NOS [74, 75].

Genetic Profile: Strong EBV association and ethnic predisposition suggest a genetic defect in the host immune to the viral infection. It also shows a complex genetic alteration with numerous chromosomal gains and losses [74]. The most commonly deleted chromosomal region is at 6q21-23 that contains many tumor suppressor genes. It has a distinctive genetic signature shared by NK-cell and

T-cell origin. Recurrent mutations of tumor suppressor genes which including *TP53* are frequent.

Prognosis and Predictive Factors: EBV itself downregulates the host microRNA profiles and promotes cell proliferation which predicts poor prognosis. The amount of EBV DNA in plasma is a substitute biomarker with diagnostic and prognostic significance. With the current regime, durable remission is achievable in about 70-80% and 50% of stage I / II cases and stage III/IV cases, respectively [74‑76].

CD30-positive T-Cell Lymphoproliferative Disorder

It is a neoplastic proliferation of large, CD30-positive T cells, arising in the oral cavity or occasionally in other mucosal sites of the head and neck region. It is important to differentiate this lesion with its mimickers which are the reactive inflammatory conditions in the oral cavity or secondary involvement by systemic anaplastic large cell lymphoma. It is a male predominance, which commonly affects adults in the 6th decade of life.

Clinical Features: It is usually presented with ulcerative mass lesions. This lesion may have spontaneous regression.

Morphology: It shows a morphological spectrum of the primary cutaneous lesion. They are large atypical lymphoid cells, exhibiting the hallmark cells of anaplastic large cell lymphoma, arranged in diffuse or sheet-like pattern (Fig. 21). The background may have mixed inflammatory cells rich in eosinophils or neutrophils. This is the common pitfall where it should demonstrate strong and uniform CD30 positive large cells to differentiate it with reactive inflammatory lesions. CD4 is more frequently expressed than CD8 T-cell marker, as well as cytotoxic markers. EMA may be positive but EBV, ALK, and CD56 are negative.

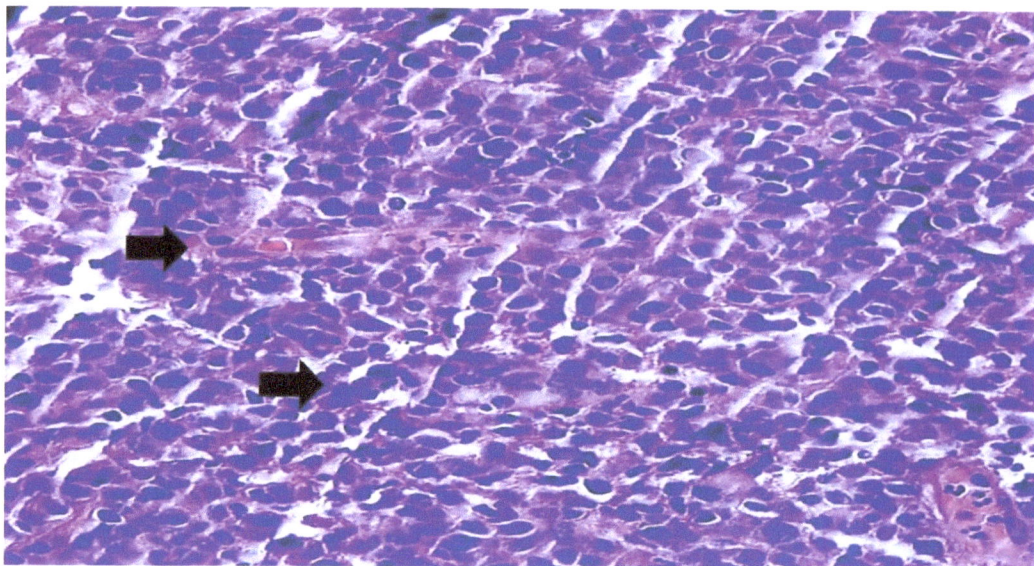

Fig. **(21))**

Atypical large neoplastic lymphoid cells **(black arrow)** infiltration in diffuse pattern.

__Genetic Profile__: Clonal gene rearrangement has been detected in most of the cases.

__Prognosis__: is good in which most cases show complete resolution with local therapy with or without chemotherapy. Spontaneous regression is occasionally encountered [74, 77].

Neuroendocrine Carcinoma

It is a carcinoma with evidence of neuroendocrine differentiation. It is commonly described in subglottic larynx (>90%) with low-grade disease and sinonasal (the most common involved location included ethmoid sinuses followed by a nasal cavity, maxillary and sphenoid sinuses) with mostly high grade [78].

Laryngeal Neuroendocrine Carcinomas

The commonest is moderately differentiated neuroendocrine carcinoma followed by poorly differentiated neuroendocrine carcinoma (SmCC and LCNEC). It is common in the middle-aged, male patients. It is associated with heavy tobacco used. An association with HPV has been identified in poorly differentiated tumor [79].

Clinical Features: Patients may be presented with hoarseness or dysphagia or airway obstruction, and rarely with paraneoplastic syndrome.

Morphology: A well-differentiated tumor shows a typical organoid pattern of well-differentiated tumor, grow in nests, cords or trabeculae pattern, composed of cells with round to oval-shaped with moderate to ample cytoplasm, with minimal atypia. Mitosis is rare (< 2 per 10 high power fields) and necrosis is absent. The moderately differentiated tumor has more nuclear atypia, mitosis (2 to 10/10 high power fields), and necrosis. The typical evenly distributed salt and pepper chromatin pattern of the nuclear are seen. Rosettes are commonly be found. Immunohistochemistry shows neuroendocrine differentiation highlighted by at least 1 neuroendocrine marker as mentioned above. Prognosis seems to be good with 5-year SR is about 80%. About 30% reported cases with recurrence and metastasis [78, 79]

Sinonasal Neuroendocrine Carcinomas

It accounts for about 3% of sinonasal tumors, commonly involved middle-aged to older men. Rarely associated with active high-risk HPV infection and previous radiation.

Clinical Features: Patients presented with non-specific symptoms like sinusitis, nasal obstruction or discharge, or even with metastatic symptoms (lungs, liver, and bone).

Morphology: It is a highly infiltrative poorly differentiated carcinoma with 2 types; small cell neuroendocrine carcinoma (SmCC) and Large Cell Neuroendocrine carcinoma (LCNEC). The cells are small monomorphic (SmCC) to large pleomorphic cells (LCNEC) exhibit prominent nucleoli. Typical salt and pepper chromatin pattern may be seen. Frequent perineural and lymphovascular invasion, mitosis >10 mitosis /10 high power fields) and necrosis are the features of the poorly differentiated tumor. They are strongly positive for neuroendocrine markers (at least 1 marker), Synaptophysin, Chromogranin, NSE, or CD56.

Prognosis: An overall 5-year survival rate is about 50-65% with better prognosis in sphenoid tumor (~80%) when managed with surgery and chemoradiotherapy especially for LCNEC. 770, 1428, 2462. About 70% of laryngeal high-grade NEC presented with advanced stage, with regional and distant metastasis, with very low 5 years SR of 5 to 20% [78, 80].

Paraganglion Tumours

Paraganglioma is one of the tumors with the highest degree of heritability, up to 40% of the cases are associated with germline mutation with known gene susceptibility [81]. Those patients with paraganglioma are advised to have clinical genetic testing, even though it appears like a sporadic tumor clinically. There are 4 types of paranglion tumors in head and neck, namely Carotid, Laryngeal, Middle ear (previously known as jugulotympanic), and Vagal paraganglioma. The latest 4th edition WHO Classifications also replaced the term "malignant paraganglioma" to paraganglioma with metastasis or metastasizing paraganglioma (Table 5).

Table 5 **Major mutated genes involved in hereditary head and neck paraganglioma (HNPGL).**

Gene	Syndrome	Chromosome	Inheritance	Risk of Metastasis	PCC	Thoraco-Abdominal PGL	Other Syndromic Lesions
SDHD	PGL1/CSS	11q23	AD-PT	4%	14-53%	12-39%	RCC, GIST, PA
SDHAF2	PGL2/CSS	11q12.2	AD-PT	Low	-	-	-
SDHC	PGL3/CSS	1q23.3	AD	3%	<3%	Very rare	RCC, GIST
SDHB	PGL4/CSS	1p36.3	AD	23%	<18-28%	52-84%	RCC, GIST, PA
SDHA	PGL5/CSS	5p15.33	AD	Low	Rare	+	RCC, GIST, PA
VHL	VHL	3p25-26	AD	4%	10-34%	Rare	RCC, HB
RET	MEN2	10q11.2	AD	<5%	50%	Rare	MTC, HPT, GNM
NF1	NF1	17q11.2	AD	1-5%	1-5%	Rare	NF,PNST, SOM, Lisch nodules, GIST
TMEM127	Non-syndromic	2q11.2	AD	+	+	+	-

Dominant; AD-PT Autosomal Dominant with paternal transmission, CSS Carney-

Stratakis Syndrome (Paraganglioma PGL and Gastrointestinal Stromal Tumor AD Autosomal GIST), GNM Ganglioneuromatosis, HPT Hyperparathyroidism, MEN2 Multiple Endocrine Neoplasm Type 2, MTC Medullary Thyroid Carcinoma, NF neurofibroma, PA Pituitary Adenoma, PCC Pheochromocytoma, PGL 1-5 paraganglioma syndrome types 1-5, PNST Peripheral nerve sheath tumour, RCC Renal cell carcinoma, SOM Duodenal somatostatinoma, VHL Von Hippel-Lindau disease [82].

Thyroid Neoplasm

It can be divided as benign (follicular adenoma) and malignant such papillary, follicular, anaplastic and medullary carcinoma.

Follicular Adenoma

Clinical Feature: A benign, encapsulated neoplasm of thyroid follicular epithelial cells. Account about 3-5% of adults. Most presented in 5th-6th decades which female to male ratio (4-5:1). The lesion is painless, slow-growing thyroid nodule/mass mobile, discrete, smooth nodules that move with thyroid.

Etiology/Pathogenesis: A well-known causes are iodine deficiency and environmental exposure such radiation (γ radiation specifically).

Other uncommon causes are include Cowden disease; is a multiple hamartoma syndrome with germline mutations of PTEN tumor suppressor gene (located on 10q23), resulting in loss of PTEN function and Carney complex; an autosomal dominant disease caused by germline mutations in PRKAR1A gene [83].

Morphology: A solitary, well delineated from adjacent parenchyma with encapsulated tumor surrounded by variable thick fibrous connective tissue capsule. The presence of smooth muscle-walled vessels in fibrosis help to confirm the capsule. The tumor architecture and cytologic appearance distinct from surrounding parenchyma cells which exhibit cuboidal to polygonal cells with dark round nuclei of follicular cells. Variable architecture can be presence such as solid (embryonal), trabecular, microfollicular (fetal), normofollicular, macrofollicular, insular, and papillary patterns.

Molecular/Genetic Profile: RAS mutations (specifically NRAS); BRAF; RET/PTCH1 and NCOA4; PAX8/PPARG have been detected [84].

Treatment/Prognosis: Surgical approaches whereby lobectomy treatment of choice with excellent long-term outcome.

Malignant Thyroid Neoplasm

Malignant thyroid carcinoma according to its clinical, risk factors, morphology, molecular profile and prognosis is explained in Table 6.

Table 6 Malignant thyroid carcinoma according to its clinical, risk factors, morphology, molecular profile and prognosis.

Criteria	Papillary Carcinoma	Follicular Carcinoma	Anaplastic Carcinoma	Medullary Carcinoma
Clinical features	•Malignant epithelial tumor showing the evidence of follicular cell differentiation and can be characterized by the distinctive nuclear features •Accounts for vast majority which is 85% of all malignant thyroid neoplasms • The female to male ratio is about 4:1.	• Accounts for approximately 10% of primary thyroid malignancies which is 0.8/100,000 persons per year • 5th and 6th decades with female to male (2-2.5:1) • Shows asymptomatic, solitary, slowly enlarging, painless and palpable thyroid mass.	• Malignant thyroid neoplasm is highly aggressive that composed of undifferentiated cells • Elderly, majority > 65 years at diagnosis • Rapidly expanding the neck mass with long history of the thyroid disease.	• Malignant C-cell-derived tumor with RET gene germline mutations • Sporadic which is 5th to 6th decades; the familial: 3rd decade • Serum calcitonin and CEA levels are elevated • Cervical lymph node metastases shows 50% • The sporadic tumors are solitary and unilateral • Familial tumors are bilateral and multifocal.
Etiology/risk factor	• Ionizing radiation exposure	Pre-existing malignant or benign thyroid disease in	• Pre-existing malignant or benign	• MEN2A and 2B known as the

	• Pre-existing benign thyroid disease; Solitary nodule that associated with 28x increased risk • Hereditary which is 5-10x increased risk in 1st-degree relatives of patients with the papillary carcinoma • Familial adenomatous polyposis (FAP): APC germline mutations	nearly all cases	thyroid disease in nearly all cases	strong inherited association • C-cell hyperplasia is the precursor of medullary carcinoma
Morphology	•Discrete, ill-defined mass with an irregular or infiltrative border • The gritty or the dystrophic calcification is common Histology .	• Thicker and have more irregular capsule than adenoma • Parenchyma, capsule and tumor zone should be submitted Histology • Either vascular or capsular invasion is enough for the diagnosis [86, 87].	• Fleshy to firm mass that typically complete replacing the thyroid Parenchyma and the mean size is 6 cm Histology • Extrathyroidal extension and lymph-vascular invasion shows a significant necrosis and	• Usually well-defined but poorly formed a capsule that consist with infiltration • It's involve the middle to upper, lateral portion of lobes .

				haemorrhage.
Morphology	• Multiple patterns shows such as solid, papillary, micro- or macrofollicular and trabecular. • Intratumor and sclerotic fibrosis • Consist of Psammoma bodies • Nuclear features are include an overlapping, crowding with high nuclear to cytoplasmic ratio, nuclear chromatin clearing, nuclear grooves and have intranuclear cytoplasmic inclusions • Many variants that are most common which are the follicular and oncocytic macrofollicular, IHC	• Microfollicles, trabecular, solid, cystic, insular • Nuclei are small in size and round with regular smooth contours • Variants consist of widely invasive, oncocytic, clear cell IHC •Positive:Thyroglobulin, TTF-1, CK7 Thicker and have more irregular capsule than adenoma • Parenchyma, capsule and tumor zone should be submitted to Histology • Either vascular or capsular invasion is enough for the diagnosis [86, 87] • Microfollicles, trabecular, solid, cystic, insular • Nuclei are small in size and round with regular smooth contours • Variants consist of widely invasive, oncocytic, clear cell IHC •Positive:Thyroglobulin, TTF-1, CK7.	• Variety of patterns that consist of Sheet-like, angiomatoid, storiform and fascicular • Poorly differentiated cells which are the polygonal, pleomorphic, giant, squamoid, epithelioid and spindle • Marked pleomorphism which increased the mitotic figures that include an atypical forms and pyknotic cells IHC • Cytokeratins and pax-8 which is a nuclear staining were up to 80% of cases • The TTF-1 and Thyroglobulin are usually lost.	• Firm and rubbery cut surface which is rarely soft consistency • The gritty is due to finely granular calcifications Histology • Necrosis or haemorrhage are usually absent • There are many patterns which consist of Organoid, insular and solid sheets that are separated by hyalinised fibrovascular stroma • Amyloid stromal accumulation is consist of 70% to 80% of cases. • Round or oval, spindled to plasmacytoid cells • Stippled, fine and uniform nuclear chromatin

			IHC • Positive: keratin, Calcitonin, chromogranin, synaptophysin, CEA-P,TTF-1.
• The HBME-1, galectin-3 and MSG1 (CITED-1) are more sensitive and specific [85].			
Molecular/Genetic profile	• BRAF gene mutations are known as the most common genetic alterations in the TPC.	• Gene rearrangements of PPARG and RAS gene in a 50% of FC.	• RAS family, BRAF mutations, ALK fusions alteration are typically occur [88].	• Increase in function that activating germline mutation of RET gene which is usually point mutation that involving 10q11.2.
Prognosis/Predictive factor	• Surgery is a choice of treatment despite an extent of surgery which are the lobectomy, subtotal thyroidectomy, or total thyroidectomy that remains controversial • Radiation • Great long-term clinical outcome consist of over 98% 20-year survival with less	• Surgery whether the lobectomy or thyroidectomy with radioablative iodine • 20-year survival are 97% minimally invasive and 50% widely invasive • Excellent long-term prognosis • Adverse prognostic factors • Age over 45 years old • Extrathyroidal extension (ETE) • Tumour size over 4 cm • Distant metastasis showing up.	• This local disease shows rapidly progressive • There's a lot of patients that diagnosed have a lymph node disease -Require many type of treatment • Overall prognosis:-statistically, 95% are dying from the disease and the median survival is 3 months.	• 5-years and 10-years survival rates are 65-90% and 45-85%, respectively depending on the disease stage [88].

	0.2% mortality.			

CONCLUSION

Head and neck tumor diagnosis is always a challenge due to its limited biopsy sample and non-specific clinical presentation. However, the histomorphology of a particular tumor is similar regardless of the location in the head and neck. This chapter covers the pathology of head and neck cancer based on their differentiation. The advancement in the ancillary test, such as the immunohistochemistry and molecular pathology, and updated classifications, and the discoveries that have emerged in disease pathogenesis and an understanding of the etiological factors of these cancers are discussed.

CONSENT FOR PUBLICATION

Not applicable.

CONFLICT OF INTEREST

The authors confirm that the content of this chapter has no conflict of interest.

ACKNOWLEDGEMENTS

Declared none.

REFERENCES

[1]   Slootweg PJ, Chan JKC, Stelow EB. Tumours of the nasal cavity, paranasal sinuses and skull base. WHO Classification of Head and Neck Tumours (4th edn.) 4th edn.201714-61.

[2]   Llorente JL, López F, Suárez C, Hermsen MA. Sinonasal carcinoma: clinical, pathological, genetic and therapeutic advances. Nat Rev Clin Oncol 2014; 11(8): 460-72.[http://dx.doi.org/10.1038/nrclinonc.2014.97] [PMID: 24935016]

[3]   Dabbs D. Diagnostic Immunohistochemistry 2006.

[4]   Rousseau A, Badoual C. Head and Neck: Squamous cell carcinoma: an overview. Paris: Atlas of Genetics and Cytogenetics in Oncology and Haematology 2011. Available from: http://atlasgeneticsoncology.org/Tumors/HeadNeckSCCID5078.html

[5]   López F, Llorente JL, García-Inclán C, *et al.* Genomic profiling of sinonasal squamous cell carcinoma. Head Neck 2011; 33(2): 145-53.[http://dx.doi.org/10.1002/hed.21417] [PMID: 20848437]

[6]   Chung CH, Guthrie VB, Masica DL, *et al.* Genomic alterations in head and neck squamous cell carcinoma determined by cancer gene-targeted sequencing. Ann Oncol 2015; 26(6): 1216-

23.[http://dx.doi.org/10.1093/annonc/mdv109] [PMID: 25712460]

[7] Adel K, El Naggar, John KC, Grandis JR, Takata T, Slootweg PJ. WHO Classification of Head and Neck Tumours (4th edition.), 4th edition.2017.

[8] Gillison ML, D'Souza G, Westra W, *et al.* Distinct risk factor profiles for human papillomavirus type 16-positive and human papillomavirus type 16-negative head and neck cancers. J Natl Cancer Inst 2008; 100(6): 407-20.[http://dx.doi.org/10.1093/jnci/djn025] [PMID: 18334711]

[9] Bishop JA, Lewis JS, Jr, Rocco JW, Faquin WC. HPV-related squamous cell carcinoma of the head and neck: An update on testing in routine pathology practice. Semin Diagn Pathol 2015; 32(5): 344-51.[http://dx.doi.org/10.1053/j.semdp.2015.02.013] [PMID: 25724476]

[10] Zidar N, Cardesa A, Gillison M, Helliwell T, Hile J, Nadal A. Verrucous squamous cell carcinoma. Tumours of the hypopharynx, larynx, trachea and parapharangeal space. In: El-Naggar AK, Chan JKC, Grandis JR, Takata T, Slootweg PJ, eds. WHO Classification of Head and Neck Tumours (4th.) El-Naggar AK, Chan JKC, Grandis JR, Takata T, Slootweg PJ. 4th.201781-104.

[11] Odar K, Kocjan BJ, Hošnjak L, Gale N, Poljak M, Zidar N. Verrucous carcinoma of the head and neck - not a human papillomavirus-related tumour? J Cell Mol Med 2014; 18(4): 635-45.[http://dx.doi.org/10.1111/jcmm.12211] [PMID: 24350715]

[12] Banks ER, Frierson HF, Jr, Mills SE, George E, Zarbo RJ, Swanson PE. Basaloid squamous cell carcinoma of the head and neck. A clinicopathologic and immunohistochemical study of 40 cases. Am J Surg Pathol 1992; 16(10): 939-46.[http://dx.doi.org/10.1097/00000478-199210000-00003] [PMID: 1384369]

[13] Ereño C, Gaafar A, Garmendia M, Etxezarraga C, Bilbao FJ, López JI. Basaloid squamous cell carcinoma of the head and neck: a clinicopathological and follow-up study of 40 cases and review of the literature. Head Neck Pathol 2008; 2(2): 83-91.[http://dx.doi.org/10.1007/s12105-008-0045-6] [PMID: 20614328]

[14] Suarez PA, Adler-Storthz K, Luna MA, El-Naggar AK, Abdul-Karim FW, Batsakis JG. Papillary squamous cell carcinomas of the upper aerodigestive tract: a clinicopathologic and molecular study. Head Neck 2000; 22(4): 360-8.[http://dx.doi.org/10.1002/1097-0347(200007)22:4<360::AID-HED8>3.0.CO;2-W] [PMID: 108620 19]

[15] Mehrad M, Carpenter DH, Chernock RD, *et al.* Papillary squamous cell carcinoma of the head and neck: clinicopathologic and molecular features with special reference to human papillomavirus. Am J Surg Pathol 2013; 37(9): 1349-56.[http://dx.doi.org/10.1097/PAS.0b013e318290427d] [PMID: 23797720]

[16] Thompson LD, Wieneke JA, Miettinen M, Heffner DK. Spindle cell (sarcomatoid) carcinomas of the larynx: a clinicopathologic study of 187 cases. Am J Surg Pathol 2002; 26(2): 153-70.[http://dx.doi.org/10.1097/00000478-200202000-00002] [PMID: 11812937]

[17] Choi HR, Roberts DB, Johnigan RH, *et al.* Molecular and clinicopathologic comparisons of head and neck squamous carcinoma variants: common and distinctive features of biological significance. Am J Surg Pathol 2004; 28(10): 1299-310.[http://dx.doi.org/10.1097/01.pas.0000138003.46650.dc] [PMID: 15371945]

[18] Masand RP, El-Mofty SK, Ma XJ, Luo Y, Flanagan JJ, Lewis JS, Jr. Adenosquamous carcinoma of the head and neck: relationship to human papillomavirus and review of the literature. Head Neck Pathol 2011; 5(2): 108-16.[http://dx.doi.org/10.1007/s12105-011-0245-3] [PMID: 21305368]

[19] Keelawat S, Liu CZ, Roehm PC, Barnes L. Adenosquamous carcinoma of the upper aerodigestive tract: a clinicopathologic study of 12 cases and review of the literature. Am J Otolaryngol 2002; 23(3): 160-8.[http://dx.doi.org/10.1053/ajot.2002.123462] [PMID: 12019485]

[20] Solomon LW, Magliocca KR, Cohen C, Müller S. Retrospective analysis of nuclear protein in testis (NUT) midline carcinoma in the upper aerodigestive tract and mediastinum. Oral Surg Oral Med Oral Pathol Oral Radiol 2015; 119(2): 213-20.[http://dx.doi.org/10.1016/j.oooo.2014.09.031] [PMID: 25434692]

[21] Bauer DE, Mitchell CM, Strait KM, *et al.* Clinicopathologic features and long-term outcomes of NUT midline carcinoma. Clin Cancer Res 2012; 18(20): 5773-9.[http://dx.doi.org/10.1158/1078-0432.CCR-12-1153] [PMID: 22896655]

[22] Haack H, Johnson LA, Fry CJ, *et al.* Diagnosis of NUT midline carcinoma using a NUT-specific monoclonal antibody. Am J Surg Pathol 2009; 33(7): 984-91.[http://dx.doi.org/10.1097/PAS.0b013e318198d666] [PMID: 19363441]

[23] Hellquist H, French CA, Bishop JA, *et al.* NUT midline carcinoma of the larynx: an international series and review of the literature. Histopathology 2017; 70(6): 861-8.[http://dx.doi.org/10.1111/his.13143] [PMID: 27926786]

[24] Chan JKC, Slootweg PJ, Petersson BF, Bell D, El-Mofty SK, Gillison M. Nasopharyngeal carcinoma. In: El-Naggar AK, Chan JKC, Grandis JR, Takata T, Slootweg PJ, eds. WHO Classification of Head and Neck

Tumours (4th.) El-Naggar AK, Chan JKC, Grandis JR, Takata T, Slootweg PJ. 4th.201765-76.

[25] Adham M, Kurniawan AN, Muhtadi AI, *et al.* Nasopharyngeal carcinoma in Indonesia: epidemiology, incidence, signs, and symptoms at presentation. Chin J Cancer 2012; 31(4): 185-96.[http://dx.doi.org/10.5732/cjc.011.10328] [PMID: 22313595]

[26] Reddy SP, Raslan WF, Gooneratne S, Kathuria S, Marks JE. Prognostic significance of keratinization in nasopharyngeal carcinoma. Am J Otolaryngol 1995; 16(2): 103-8.[http://dx.doi.org/10.1016/0196-0709(95)90040-3] [PMID: 7540805]

[27] Wan SK, Chan JK, Lau WH, Yip TT. Basaloid-squamous carcinoma of the nasopharynx. An Epstein-Barr virus-associated neoplasm compared with morphologically identical tumors occurring in other sites. Cancer 1995; 76(10): 1689-93.[http://dx.doi.org/10.1002/1097-0142(19951115)76:10<1689::AID-CNCR2820761003>3.0.CO;2-9] [PMID: 8625035]

[28] d'Errico A, Pasian S, Baratti A, *et al.* A case-control study on occupational risk factors for sino-nasal cancer. Occup Environ Med 2009; 66(7): 448-55.[http://dx.doi.org/10.1136/oem.2008.041277] [PMID: 19153109]

[29] Cheung FM, Lau TW, Cheung LK, Li AS, Chow SK, Lo AW. Schneiderian papillomas and carcinomas: a retrospective study with special reference to p53 and p16 tumor suppressor gene expression and association with HPV. Ear Nose Throat J 2010; 89(10): E5-E12.[http://dx.doi.org/10.1177/014556131008901002] [PMID: 20981655]

[30] Syrjänen K, Syrjänen S. Detection of human papillomavirus in sinonasal papillomas: systematic review and meta-analysis. Laryngoscope 2013; 123(1): 181-92.[http://dx.doi.org/10.1002/lary.23688] [PMID: 23161522]

[31] Gaffey MJ, Frierson HF, Weiss LM, Barber CM, Baber GB, Stoler MH. Human papillomavirus and Epstein-Barr virus in sinonasal Schneiderian papillomas. An *in situ* hybridization and polymerase chain reaction study. Am J Clin Pathol 1996; 106(4): 475-82.[http://dx.doi.org/10.1093/ajcp/106.4.475] [PMID: 8853035]

[32] Boukheris H, Curtis RE, Land CE, Dores GM. Incidence of carcinoma of the major salivary glands according to the WHO classification, 1992 to 2006: a population-based study in the United States. Cancer Epidemiol Biomarkers Prev 2009; 18(11): 2899-906.[http://dx.doi.org/10.1158/1055-9965.EPI-09-0638] [PMID: 19861510]

[33] Brown NA, Rolland D, McHugh JB. Activating FGFR2-RAS-BRAF mutatons in ameloblastoma. Clin Cancer Res 2014; (20)517-26.

[34] Sweeney RT, McClary AC, Myers BR, *et al.* Identification of recurrent SMO and BRAF mutations in ameloblastomas. Nat Genet 2014; 46(7): 722-5.[http://dx.doi.org/10.1038/ng.2986] [PMID: 24859340]

[35] Philips CD, Futterer SF, Lipper MH, Levine PA. Sinonsal undifferentiated carcinoma: CT and MR imaging of an uncommon neoplasm of the nasal cavity. Radiology 1997; (202)477-80.[http://dx.doi.org/10.1148/radiology.202.2.9015077]

[36] Chernock RD, Perry A, Pfeifer JD, Holden JA, Lewis JS, Jr. Receptor tyrosine kinases in sinonasal undifferentiated carcinomas--evaluation for EGFR, c-KIT, and HER2/neu expression. Head Neck 2009; 31(7): 919-27.[http://dx.doi.org/10.1002/hed.21061] [PMID: 19283847]

[37] Rodic N, Maleki Z. Cytomorphologic findings of Schneiderian papilloma: a case report. Diagn Cytopathol 2012; 40(12): 1100-3.[http://dx.doi.org/10.1002/dc.21711] [PMID: 21548118]

[38] Bossi P, Saba NF, Vermorken JB, *et al.* The role of systemic therapy in the management of sinonasal cancer: A critical review. Cancer Treat Rev 2015; 41(10): 836-43.[http://dx.doi.org/10.1016/j.ctrv.2015.07.004] [PMID: 26255226]

[39] Reiersen DA, Pahilan ME, Devaiah AK. Meta-analysis of treatment outcomes for sinonasal undifferentiated carcinoma. Otolarngol Head Neck Surg 2012; (147)7-14.[http://dx.doi.org/10.1177/0194599812440932]

[40] Franchi A, Innocenti DR, Palomba A, *et al.* Low prevalence of K-RAS, EGF-R and BRAF mutations in sinonasal adenocarcinomas. Implications for anti-EGFR treatments. Pathol Oncol Res 2014; 20(3): 571-9.[http://dx.doi.org/10.1007/s12253-013-9730-1] [PMID: 24338245]

[41] Martínez JG, Pérez-Escuredo J, López F, *et al.* Microsatellite instability analysis of sinonasal carcinomas. Otolaryngol Head Neck Surg 2009; 140(1): 55-60.[http://dx.doi.org/10.1016/j.otohns.2008.10.038] [PMID: 19130962]

[42] Franchi A, Palomba A, Fondi C, *et al.* Immunohistochemical investigation of tumorigenic pathways in sinonasal intestinal-type adenocarcinoma. A tissue microarray analysis of 62 cases. Histopathology 2011; 59(1): 98-105.[http://dx.doi.org/10.1111/j.1365-2559.2011.03887.x] [PMID: 21668475]

[43] Ameli F, Baharoom A, Md Isa N, Noor Akmal S. Diagnostic challenges in fine needle aspiration cytology of salivary gland lesions. Malays J Pathol 2015; 37(1): 11-8.[PMID: 25890608]

[44] Zerpa Zerpa V, Cuesta Gonzáles MT, Agostini Porras G, Marcano Acuña M, Estellés Ferriol E, Dalmau

Galofre J. [Diagnostic accuracy of fine needle aspiration cytology in parotid tumours]. Acta Otorrinolaringol Esp 2014; 65(3): 157-61.[http://dx.doi.org/10.1016/j.otorri.2013.12.002] [PMID: 24598025]

[45] Spiro RH. Salivary neoplasms: overview of a 35-year experience with 2,807 patients. Head Neck Surg 1986; 8(3): 177-84.[http://dx.doi.org/10.1002/hed.2890080309] [PMID: 3744850]

[46] Barnes L, Eveson JW, Reichart P, Sidransky D. Pathology and genetics of head and neck tumours. World Health Organization Classification of Tumours 2005.

[47] Geurts JM, Schoenmakers EF, Röijer E, Aström AK, Stenman G, van de Ven WJM. Identification of NFIB as recurrent translocation partner gene of HMGIC in pleomorphic adenomas. Oncogene 1998; 16(7): 865-72.[http://dx.doi.org/10.1038/sj.onc.1201609] [PMID: 9484777]

[48] Geurts JM, Schoenmakers EF, Röijer E, Stenman G, Van de Ven WJ, van de Ven WJM. Expression of reciprocal hybrid transcripts of HMGIC and FHIT in a pleomorphic adenoma of the parotid gland. Cancer Res 1997; 57(1): 13-7.[PMID: 8988031]

[49] Katabi N, Ghossein R, Ho A, et al. Consistent PLAG1 and HMGA2 abnormalities distinguish carcinoma ex-pleomorphic adenoma from its de novo counterparts. Hum Pathol 2015; 46(1): 26-33.[http://dx.doi.org/10.1016/j.humpath.2014.08.017] [PMID: 25439740]

[50] Gnepp DR. Malignant mixed tumors of the salivary glands: a review. Pathol Annu 1993; 28(Pt 1): 279-328.[PMID: 8380049]

[51] Teymoortash A, Werner JA, Moll R. Is Warthin's tumour of the parotid gland a lymph node disease? Histopathol 2011; (59)143-5.[http://dx.doi.org/10.1111/j.1365-2559.2011.03891.x]

[52] Espinoza S, Felter A, Malinvaud D, et al. Warthin's tumor of parotid gland: Surgery or follow-up? Diagnostic value of a decisional algorithm with functional MRI. Diagn Interv Imaging 2016; 97(1): 37-43.[http://dx.doi.org/10.1016/j.diii.2014.11.024] [PMID: 25543869]

[53] Jee KJ, Persson M, Heikinheimo K, et al. Genomic profiles and CRTC1-MAML2 fusion distinguish different subtypes of mucoepidermoid carcinoma. Mod Pathol 2013; 26(2): 213-22.[http://dx.doi.org/10.1038/modpathol.2012.154] [PMID: 23018873]

[54] Coca-Pelaz A, Rodrigo JP, Bradley PJ, et al. Adenoid cystic carcinoma of the head and neck--An update. Oral Oncol 2015; 51(7): 652-61.[http://dx.doi.org/10.1016/j.oraloncology.2015.04.005] [PMID: 25943783]

[55] Patel NR, Sanghvi S, Khan MN, Husain Q, Baredes S, Eloy JA. Demographic trends and disease-specific survival in salivary acinic cell carcinoma: an analysis of 1129 cases. Laryngoscope 2014; 124(1): 172-8.[http://dx.doi.org/10.1002/lary.24231] [PMID: 23754708]

[56] Ellis GL, Corio RL. Acinic cell adenocarcinoma. A clinicopathologic analysis of 294 cases. Cancer 1983; 52(3): 542-9.[http://dx.doi.org/10.1002/1097-0142(19830801)52:3<542::AID-CNCR2820520326>3.0.CO;2-A] [PMID: 6861091]

[57] Dickson BC. Advances in head and neck pathology. An update on mesenchymal tumors of the head and neck. Diagn Histopathol 2014; 20(8): 308-15.[http://dx.doi.org/10.1016/j.mpdhp.2014.06.005]

[58] Lewis JT, Oliveira AM, Nascimento AG, et al. Low-grade sinonasal sarcoma with neural and myogenic features: a clinicopathologic analysis of 28 cases. Am J Surg Pathol 2012; 36(4): 517-25.[http://dx.doi.org/10.1097/PAS.0b013e3182426886] [PMID: 22301502]

[59] Boghani Z, Husain Q, Kanumuri VV, et al. Juvenile nasopharyngeal angiofibroma: a systematic review and comparison of endoscopic, endoscopic-assisted, and open resection in 1047 cases. Laryngoscope 2013; 123(4): 859-69.[http://dx.doi.org/10.1002/lary.23843] [PMID: 23483486]

[60] Ferouz AS, Mohr RM, Paul P. Juvenile nasopharyngeal angiofibroma and familial adenomatous polyposis: an association? Otolaryngol Head Neck Surg 1995; 113(4): 435-9.[http://dx.doi.org/10.1016/S0194-5998(95)70081-1] [PMID: 7567017]

[61] Miettinen MM, Mandhl N. Spindle cell/Pleomorphic lipoma. In: Fletcher CDM, Bridge AB, Hogendoorn PCW, Mertens F, eds. WHO classification of Soft Tissue and Bone Tumours (4th.) Fletcher CDM, Bridge AB, Hogendoorn PCW, Mertens F. 4th.201329-30.

[62] Baumhoer D, Lopes M, Raubenheimer E. Osteosarcoma. In: El-Naggar AK, Chan JKC, Grandis JR, Takata T, Slootweg PJ, Eds. WHO Classification of Head and Neck Tumours 4th Lyon: International Agency for research on cancer 2017. pp. 244-46.

[63] Guadagnolo BA, Zagars GK, Raymond AK, Benjamin RS, Sturgis EM. Osteosarcoma of the jaw/craniofacial region: outcomes after multimodality treatment. Cancer 2009; 115(14): 3262-70.[http://dx.doi.org/10.1002/cncr.24297] [PMID: 19382187]

[64] Jasnau S, Meyer U, Potratz J, et al. Craniofacial osteosarcoma Experience of the cooperative German-Austrian-Swiss osteosarcoma study group. Oral Oncol 2008; 44(3): 286-

94.[http://dx.doi.org/10.1016/j.oraloncology.2007.03.001] [PMID: 17467326]

[65]   Baumhoer D, Casirajhi O, Hunt JL. Malignant maxillofacial bone and cartilage tumours. In: El-Naggar AK, Chan JKC, Grandis JR, Takata T, Slootweg PJ, eds. WHO Classification of Head and Neck Tumours (4th.) El-Naggar AK, Chan JKC, Grandis JR, Takata T, Slootweg PJ. 4th.2017243-44.

[66]   Vencio EF, Reeve CM, Unni KK, Nascimento AG. Mesenchymal chondrosarcoma of the jaw bones: clinicopathologic study of 19 cases. Cancer 1998; 82(12): 2350-5.[http://dx.doi.org/10.1002/(SICI)1097-0142(19980615)82:12<2350::AID-CNCR8>3.0.CO;2-W] [PMID: 9635527]

[67]   Baumhoer D, Bullediek J, Nicolai P. Notochordal tumours. In: El-Naggar AK, Chan JKC, Grandis JR, Takata T, Slootweg PJ, eds. WHO Classification of Head and Neck Tumours (4th.) El-Naggar AK, Chan JKC, Grandis JR, Takata T, Slootweg PJ. 4th.201776.

[68]   Flanagan AM, Yamaguchi T. Chordoma In: Fletcher CDM, Bridge AB, Hogendoorn PCW, Mertens F, eds. WHO classification of Soft Tissue and Bone Tumours (4th.) Fletcher CDM, Bridge AB, Hogendoorn PCW, Mertens F. 4th.2013328-29.

[69]   Alfouzan AF. Head and Neck cancer pathology: Old world *vs* new world disease. Nig J Clin Pract 2019; (22): 1-8.

[70]   Essadi I, Ismaili N, Tazi E. Primary lymphoma of the head and neck: two case reports and review of the literature. Cases J 2008; 30; 1(1): 426.[http://dx.doi.org/10.1186/1757-1626-1-426]

[71]   Cooper JS, Porter K, Mallin K, *et al.* National Cancer Database report on cancer of the head and neck: 10-year update. Head Neck 2009; 31(6): 748-58.[http://dx.doi.org/10.1002/hed.21022] [PMID: 19189340]

[72]   Ambinder AJ, Shenoy PJ, Nastoupil LJ, Flowers CR. Using primary site as a predictor of survival in mantle cell lymphoma. Cancer 2013; 119(8): 1570-7.[http://dx.doi.org/10.1002/cncr.27898] [PMID: 23341329]

[73]   Haverkos BM, Pan Z, Gru AA, *et al.* Haverkos, Zenggang Pan, Alejandro A. Gru. Extranodal NK/T-cell lymphoma, nasal type [ENKTL-NT]: An update on epidemiology, clinical presentation, and natural history in North American and European cases. Curr Hematol Malig Rep 2016; 11(6): 514-27.[http://dx.doi.org/10.1007/s11899-016-0355-9] [PMID: 27778143]

[74]   Chuang SS, Ferry JA, El-Naggar AK, *et al.* Editors WHO Classification of Head and Neck Tumours 4th edition 201752-5.

[75]   Elaine S, Jaffe ES, Nicolae A, Pittaluga S. Peripheral T-cell and NK-cell lymphomas in the WHO classification: pearls and pitfalls. Mod Pathol 2013; 26(1): 71-87.[PMID: 22899286]

[76]   Komabayashi Y, Kishibe K, Nagato T, Ueda S, Takahara M, Harabuchi Y. Downregulation of miR-15a due to LMP1 promotes cell proliferation and predicts poor prognosis in nasal NK/T-cell lymphoma. Am J Hematol 2014; 89(1): 25-33.[http://dx.doi.org/10.1002/ajh.23570] [PMID: 23963825]

[77]   Wang W, Cai Y, Sheng W, Lu H, Li X. The spectrum of primary mucosal CD30-positive T-cell lymphoproliferative disorders of the head and neck. Oral Surg Oral Med Oral Pathol Oral Radiol 2014; 117(1): 96-104.[http://dx.doi.org/10.1016/j.oooo.2013.10.002] [PMID: 24332333]

[78]   Perez-Ordonez B, Bishop JA, Gnepp DR, Hunt JL, Thompson LDR. Neuroendocrine carcinoma. Editors WHO Classification of Head and Neck Tumours (4th edition.) 4th edition.201795-100.

[79]   van der Laan TP, Plaat BE, van der Laan BF, Halmos GB. Clinical recommendations on the treatment of neuroendocrine carcinoma of the larynx: A meta-analysis of 436 reported cases. Head Neck 2015; 37(5): 707-15.[http://dx.doi.org/10.1002/hed.23666] [PMID: 24596175]

[80]   Ferlito A, Rinaldo A. Small cell neuroendocrine carcinoma of the larynx: a preventable and frustrating disease with a highly aggressive lethal behavior. ORL J Otorhinolaryngol Relat Spec 2003; 65(3): 131-3.[http://dx.doi.org/10.1159/000072249] [PMID: 12925812]

[81]   Dahia PL. Pheochromocytoma and paraganglioma pathogenesis: learning from genetic heterogeneity. Nat Rev Cancer 2014; 14(2): 108-19.[http://dx.doi.org/10.1038/nrc3648] [PMID: 24442145]

[82]   Chan JKC, Kimura N, Capella C. Paraganglion tumours. In: El-Naggar AK, Chan JKC, Grandis JR, Takata T, Slootweg PJ, eds. WHO Classification of Head and Neck Tumours (4th.) El-Naggar AK, Chan JKC, Grandis JR, Takata T, Slootweg PJ. 4th.2017274-84.

[83]   Beaudenon-Huibregtse S, Alexander EK, Guttler RB, *et al.* Centralized molecular testing for oncogenic gene mutations complements the local cytopathologic diagnosis of thyroid nodules. Thyroid 2014; 24(10): 1479-87.[http://dx.doi.org/10.1089/thy.2013.0640] [PMID: 24811481]

[84]   Hunt JL. Molecular alterations in hereditary and sporadic thyroid and parathyroid diseases. Adv Anat Pathol

2009; 16(1): 23-32.[http://dx.doi.org/10.1097/PAP.0b013e3181915f7d] [PMID: 19098464]

[85] Fischer S, Asa SL. Application of immunohistochemistry to thyroid neoplasms. Arch Pathol Lab Med 2008; 132(3): 359-72.[PMID: 18318579]

[86] Serra S, Asa SL. Controversies in thyroid pathology: the diagnosis of follicular neoplasms. Endocr Pathol 2008; 19(3): 156-65.[http://dx.doi.org/10.1007/s12022-008-9031-5] [PMID: 18548351]

[87] Baloch ZW, LiVolsi VA. Our approach to follicular-patterned lesions of the thyroid. J Clin Pathol 2007; 60(3): 244-50.[http://dx.doi.org/10.1136/jcp.2006.038604] [PMID: 16798933]

[88] Ricardo VL, Robert YO, Gunter K, Juan R. WHO Classification of Tumours of Endocrine Organs (4th Edition.), 4th Edition.2017.

Inflammation, Risk Factors and Etiopathogenesis of Head and Neck Cancer

Norhafiza Mat Lazim*

Department of Otorhinolaryngology-Head and Neck Surgery, School of Medical Sciences, Universiti Sains Malaysia, Health Campus 16150, Kubang Kerian 16150, Kelantan, Malaysia

Abstract

Head and neck malignancy is a critical disease across the globe as its incidence is on the rise. This malignancy comprises the oral cavity, oropharynx, larynx, nasal cavity, paranasal sinus, nasopharynx, salivary glands, and thyroid malignancies. Multiple known risk factors have been strongly associated with the majority of these malignancies. Importantly, the majority of these known risk factors are intricately involved in the inflammation and its ecosystem. Of note, inflammation cascades and inflammatory markers play a dominant role in the pathogenesis of head and neck malignancy. Thus, it is crucial to understand the true process of each identified risk factor and its related inflammation process in the etiopathogenesis of head and neck malignancy. This can serve as an effective platform for the future development of potential agents for screening, prevention, and treatment of head and neck malignancy. This chapter will discuss the significant risk factors of head and neck malignancy and highlight the spectrum of inflammation process that governs the basis of carcinogenesis and its etiopathogenesis.

Keywords: Alcohol, Dietary factor, Epstein Barr virus (EBV), Head and neck malignancy, Human papilloma virus (HPV), Inflammatory markers, Nasopharyngeal carcinoma, Smoking.

* **Corresponding author Norhafiza Mat Lazim:** Department of Otorhinolaryngology-Head and Neck Surgery, School of Medical Sciences, Universiti Sains Malaysia, Health Campus 16150, Kubang Kerian 16150, Kelantan, Malaysia; Tel: +60199442664, +6097676418, Fax: +6097676424; E-mail: norhafiza@usm.my

INTRODUCTION

Head and neck malignancy is paramount as it involves a critical anatomic region that plays an important role in humans' basic functioning. Its incidence is on the rise with some geographical variations. It affects both the adult and pediatric patients population. In addition, there are some ethnic and racial differences among patients afflicted with this disease. However, the majority of head and neck malignancies share common etiopathogenesis and risk factors. For instance, the human papilloma virus (HPV) is closely related to oropharyngeal carcinoma,

tongue carcinoma, laryngeal carcinomas, and salivary glands carcinoma. Epstein Barr virus (EBV) is a significant risk factor for nasopharyngeal carcinoma, lymphoma and sinonasal carcinoma. The other risk factors include smoking tobacco products, drinking alcoholic beverages, dietary factors, factory and chemicals products, wood dust and other environmental carcinogens.

It is estimated that 75% of head and neck squamous cell carcinoma (HNSCC) in the US is due to cigarette smoking and alcohol consumption. This is also true for other parts of the world, where alcohol and cigarette smoking remain the dominant risk factors for human malignancy. This is attributed to many carcinogenic substances that are found in cigarettes and alcohol. The mucosal contact with this carcinogenic substance plays a critical role in the carcinogenesis of head and neck cancer. Laryngeal carcinoma is commonly associated with cigarette smoking, whereas oral cavity carcinoma is related to alcohol consumption. There are other factors include genetic alteration, individuals biometabolism and epigenetic changes that interact with the carcinogenic agents in promoting carcinogenesis and lead to HNSCC development and progression [1]. This can be true for other geographical locations also, such as the Indian subcontinent, where the majority of the population are heavy smokers and alcohol drinkers.

Dietary factors such as consumption of salty fish, smoked seafood and pickled vegetables are also significant risk factors for the development of head and neck malignancy especially nasopharyngeal carcinoma (NPC). NPC is prevalent at certain geographic locations like South China, South East Asia, Northern Africa, Artic and selected Mediterranean countries. These are attributed to different dietary and lifestyle habits. The risk factors can have synergistic effects where for instance, the dietary factor and familial inheritance can act in combination and increase the risk of the selected population to four times of having NPC instead of two-fold. At the other end of the spectrum, oral cavity carcinoma is associated with betel nut chewing and reversed smoking. Reversed smoking is commonly practiced in the Indian population and this has been linked to carcinoma of the hard palate. In this scenario, the carcinogens from the cigarette smoke have direct and close contact with the hard palate.

Other than the dietary factors, the oncogenic viruses such as EBV and HPV have emerged as crucial risk factors. It also dictates the treatment strategy and prognosis of selected HNSCC patients. Numerous research works have been performed on these two critical viruses and will continue in the future. This will enable better management and treatment outcomes of patients with HNSCC. NPC also is strongly associated with EBV where the virus serology has been utilized as a diagnostic tool at the majority of head and neck surgical oncology centers worldwide. The other immunomarkers of EBV are also under intense investigation by many scientists in order to come up with novel diagnostic and therapeutic targets.

Clinical presentation of head and neck malignancy varies, and it depends on the anatomical site and structures involvement, the tumor size, the specific pathology of the tumor as well as the patient's factors such as an immune response. Some of the significant symptoms include odynophagia, dysphagia, throat pain, trismus, airway obstruction, epistaxis, hearing impairment, facial nerve paralysis, hoarseness, and so forth. Oral cavity and oropharyngeal carcinoma tend to cause odynophagia and dysphagia, whereas laryngeal and hypopharyngeal carcinoma can lead to fatal airway obstruction. Epistaxis and trismus are significant features of sinonasal carcinoma and facial nerve paralysis can be due to parotid glands malignancy. All these symptoms and signs can give clues for nearby structure's involvement and can be used as part of the clinical staging for each type of HNSCC.

EPIDEMIOLOGY AND SURVIVAL RATES OF HEAD AND NECK MALIGNANCY

As aforementioned, certain head and neck malignancy types are prevalent at certain geographic locations. This is attributed to factors namely dietary consumption, lifestyle habits, environmental pollutants as well as genetic inheritance. In the last decades, we can observe an improve the overall survival rate of patients with HNSCC, and this differs for various subtypes of head and neck cancer. However, this is partly true only for certain geographic locations due to factors such as better facilities and expertise, and the availability of a strong rehabilitation team and support system at a specific center. Importantly, if we see statistics in the European country, 5-year survival rates for oral and pharyngeal cancers have also improved over the years [2]. These can be partly due to limited local logistic factors for instance the facility, instrumentation, expertise, funds, and so forth. The patient's compliance due to lack of awareness and education, a low socioeconomic background also contributes to the overall survival of HNSCC patients.

These can be partly due to limited local logistic factors, for instance, the facility, instrumentation, expertise, funds, and so forth. The patient's compliance due to lack of awareness and education, and the low socioeconomic background also contributes to the overall survival of HNSCC patients. In addition, HNSCC patients are known to have high rates of recurrent disease and distant metastasis. The incidence of second primary malignancy in the head and neck region is also a common phenomenon and is associated with poor prognosis and a high risk of early death [3, 4]. Thyroid malignancy has been strongly associated with secondary primary especially in those patients who had received radiation as treatment [5, 6]. Children with head and neck cancer also are at risk of developing second primary [7]. Generally, the recurrent cases are challenging to treat due to the fact that the patients already had chemoradiation, which causes significant tissue fibrosis and imposes significant sequelae if patients had to undergo salvage surgery. The dissection during surgery will be difficult due to fibrotic tissues, the distorted normal anatomy of neurovascular structures, as well as the risk of bleeding is also high.

HNSCC with second primary malignancy patients had poorer survival rates compared to those without secondary malignancy [2, 8]. The risk factors for the development of second primary malignancy include the older age group of patients, oropharyngeal carcinoma as primary, and alcohol drinker [9, 10]. These second primary cancers are observed to be highly prevalent in the Caucasian population in contrast to Asian, Blacks, or Hispanic ethnicity. Genetic aberration and familial inheritance may also play a critical role in the development of second primary malignancies.

Different kinds of literature quote different incidences of head and neck malignancy. Tsai *et al.* stated that globally, Taiwan is one of the countries with the highest incidences of HNSCC, especially in the East Asia region. Low prevalence areas of HNSCC can be observed in Latin America and European countries. HPV-related oropharyngeal carcinoma is on the rise in the developed countries and also in Taiwan [11, 12]. The study reported that the

HNSCC incidence is in reducing trends in most of the western countries but with an increased incidence of HPV positive tumors, especially in northern Europe and North America [12, 13]. Globally, the incidence of oropharyngeal squamous cell carcinomas (OPSCC) also is on the rise and is strongly associated with HPV as a risk factor [14, 15].

Aldalwg *et al.* documented that in 2008, a quarter of total cases of OPSCC were tested with positive HPV. Differences in geographical location, socioeconomic and culture contribute to the differences in the epidemiology of OPSCC [16]. The incidence of OPSCC has been reported to be low in countries like South America, Africa, and Asia in contrast to Australia, North America, and Europe, which have high reported cases. In America, the vaccination program against HPV is becoming critical as the incidence of HPV-positive oropharyngeal cancer is on the rise [17]. The HPV positive OPSCC is commonly seen in nonsmoker patients and a history of multiple sexual partners increases the risks [18]. The difference in the epidemiology of head and neck cancer partially imparts on the treatment and diagnostic facilities available at specific head and neck oncology centers. Some centers may excel in the management of oral cavity and oropharyngeal malignancy, whereas other institutions may develop an effective therapeutic approach for thyroid and salivary glands malignancies. The countries with a high prevalence of OPSCC have made great progress in the treatment protocol and treatment outcomes of these subsets of patients.

Recently, there has been a dramatic increase in the works of literatures focusing on HPV driven head and neck malignancies. The surge of research and clinical trials on HPV related malignancies has extra advantages and added up to the current scientific database. This is vital for the management and prevention of head and neck malignancies globally. Related techniques and procedures for the identification of HPV status also have evolved with the advancement in molecular analysis and genomic imprinting. Most of the literatures data documented that HPV positive OPSCC is highest in the region of Northern Europe and Northern America. The HPV also has been implicated in other head and neck tumor carcinogenesis such as the oral cavity cancer and laryngeal cancer, but with much less percentage.

The availability of recent procedures and test kit have made the diagnosis of OCSCC effective, with a subsequent increment of incidence of OSCC has been recorded, especially in a subset of patients with OPSCC. Importantly, both p16 and HPV E6 and E7 were detected positive for 80% of patients with positive HPV DNA [13].

RISK FACTORS OF HEAD AND NECK MALIGNANCY AND ROLES OF INFLAMMATION

The majority of risk factors involved in the development of head and neck malignancy are strongly associated with inflammation. The inflammation is the initial insults that induce significant mucosal changes with the presence of numerous substances and molecules which interact with each other in promoting carcinogenesis and subsequently lead to the malignant tumor formation. Heterogeneous patterns in incidence rates, trends, and etiologic factors for HNSCC can be observed across the geographic regions worldwide. The majority of head and neck malignancy is caused by tobacco and alcohol use and selected types are strongly associated with oncogenic viruses such as HPV and EBV infection, dietary habits, chemical carcinogens, and environmental pollutants such as wood dust and so forth. Most of these inciting agents cause remarkable pathologic changes that lead to the inflammation process and its cascade which subsequently progress to malignancy. Myriad significant humoral and molecular events take place in the tissues and epithelial which are confounded by multiple

processes of angiogenesis, vascularization, fibroblast formation, and granulation that ensure the vitality of cancerous cells.

Numerous aforementioned carcinogens, in addition to their tumorigenic properties, may also possess pro-invasive and pro-metastatic abilities. These essential properties of the cancerous cell are versatile and require complex interaction within the tumor microenvironment and its ecosystem. For instance, significant carcinogenic sources are strongly linked to the lifestyle habits and pollutants in the environment, such chemical carcinogens, wood dust exposure, alcohol consumption, and dietary habits, it is imperative to ensure the public know and aware of their harmful habit. The screening and health-oriented educational programs targeting community at risk are essential in order to reduce the risk and improve the detection rate of HNSCC. Importantly, some of these risk factors are preventable by applying a simple protective method. For example, an individual who worked at the wood factory is at risk of developing sinonasal malignancy. These can be easily lessened by educating these people to wear a protective mask and gloves.

It is prudent to investigate the true biology of human cancer by conducting research and so forth. Malignant cells possess multiple properties, some of which are not yet fully comprehended by scientists and researchers. Multiple processes and interactions exist in the cancer frameworks and its eco-system due to oncogenic stimuli that persist for years. To illustrate, considering the carcinomas, most of the oncogenic transformations begin with for instance the E-cadherin involvement. The E-cadherin downregulation, which binds the quiescent and well-differentiated epithelial cells, is the early process in carcinogenesis. Subsequently, the epithelial cells are converted to the mesenchymal cell known as epithelial-mesenchymal transition (EMT). Several recent studies stated that exposure to environmental carcinogens would accelerate the transition [19]. At the same time, others claimed that high dose exposure to carcinogenic stimuli would double up the carcinogenesis process and malignant transformation, such as in the case of smoking cigarettes.

Smoking as A Risk Factor for Head and Neck Malignancy

Smoking is a hazardous lifestyle habit, yet millions of populations acquire this fatal habit inclusive of that female population. Now with the changing pace in digital media and electronics, smoking also has become a serious trend and cultures that are practiced among teenagers and young school goers. The prevalence rate of cigarette smoking is comparatively higher in males than in females [13]. There is also a geographical difference in the incidence of smoking across the globe with higher trends are seen in southern Europe. There is probably not much data on the youngsters and students who smoke cigarettes, but the figures are alarming. This is particularly true in the region of South East Asia which includes Malaysia, Thailand, Philippines, Singapore, Indonesia, Vietnam, and so forth, where smoking is observed is heavily practiced in young students.

As we all aware, cigarette smoking is a well-known risk factor for cancer of the head and neck with a well-defined dose-response relationship for rates of use and duration of consumption of the cigarette. Indeed, the number of cigarettes and the duration of use are critical in determining the development of malignancy. In several epidemiological studies, the classification of degree cigarette smoking has been defined as the smoking of fewer than 10 cigarettes per day. However, for some, region this number can be considered as a heavy smoker. The higher number of cigarettes is linked to for example, to an increased risk of laryngeal cancers, compared with the other head and neck subsites. As stated by Berthiller *et al.* that the finding of laryngeal cancer and smoking association is critical where cigarette smoking is a significant risk factor for the carcinoma of the larynx than oral cavity carcinoma, especially among those who is non-alcohol drinkers [20]. The region of the study conducted plays a role in yielding the outcomes and findings of any given study. In India, the majority of middle age and elderly population practices reversed smoking, and this has been strongly related to oral cavity carcinoma particularly hard palate carcinoma (Fig. 1).

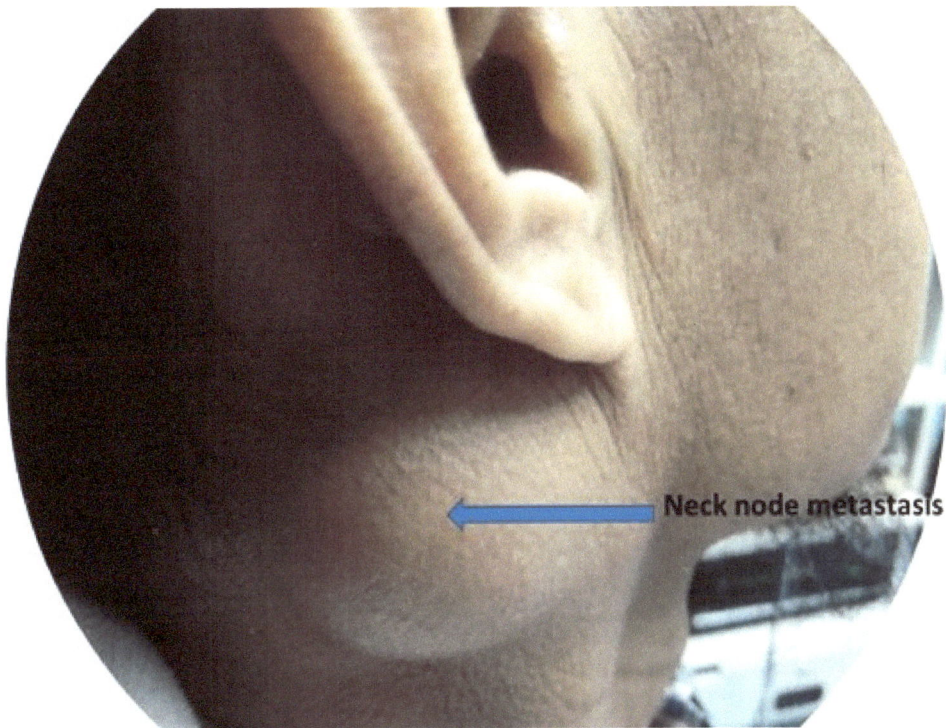

Fig. **(1))**

Right neck nodes metastases at level V from hard palate carcinoma.

Smoking is associated with carcinogenic particles, namely tobacco-specific nitrosamines (TSNA) and polycyclic aromatic hydrocarbons (PAH). These two components are recognized to play an important role in the development of HNSCC. Khariwala *et al.* recently reported that TSNA related DNA adduct is higher in the smoker patients with oral cavity carcinoma than those smokers without cancer [21]. This TSNA and PAH cause changes in the tissues with resultant secretions of multiple molecules such as peptides, chemokines, proteases, growth factors, and so forth. These components are part of the inflammation reactions to the carcinogenic stimuli that will persist and accumulate with time. Additionally, the study also documented that the tobacco- specific nitrosamines (TSNA) include the 4-(methylnitrosamino)-1-(3-pyridyl)-1-butanone (NNK) and *N*'-nitrosonornicotine (NNN) which can be easily detected in urinary excretes of a smoker. Khariwala *et al.* stated that the risks of developing esophageal and lung cancers are proportionately related to the level of urinary levels of NNN and NNK biomarkers, respectively. Their previous study also showed that the risk of HNSCC is highly associated with uptake of NNN [21]. This can be explained by the inflammatory substances that are produced in response to PAH and TSNA derived from the cigarettes. Several smokeless products are added to the tobacco in order to increase the nicotine absorption such as snuffs, betel quid, and areca nut [22]. All of these in long term promote the process of carcinogenesis, malignant mass formation and subsequently can also result in metastasis.

Alcohol and Its Roles in Head and Neck Malignancy

Alcohol consumption is another important factor that induces chronic inflammation. This is true, especially in chronic alcohol drinkers. The amount and duration of alcohol consumption determine the effects on carcinogenic events. Additionally, the individual body metabolism also plays a significant role. Patients who have a slow metabolism of ethanol may a dose-response relationship between alcohol and head and neck malignancy-risk that is different from that in individuals with normal ethanol metabolism. Alcohol cessation is known to reduce head and neck malignancy risk, although it is unclear whether this risk reduction depends on the previous level of alcohol intake before the. In the analysis by Huang *et al.* they found out that alcohol showed a positive dose-response relationship with head and neck malignancy risk, with the oropharyngeal and hypopharyngeal are at the highest risk. Importantly, alcohol intake has a significant impact on the prognosis of the larynx and pharyngeal cancer, especially if patients had radiation in contrast to patients who had surgery [23]. Liquor had a higher positive association with head and neck malignancy risk [24]. Alcohol dehydrogenase (ADH) is responsible for the production of acetaldehyde, the potent carcinogenic agent in ethanol. The metabolism of acetaldehyde to acetate which is non-toxic is *via* aldehyde dehydrogenase (ALDH) to non- toxic acetate.

Critically, the gene polymorphisms of ethanol metabolism influence the individual susceptibility to alcohol carcinogenic effects by regulating the speed of metabolism of the ethanol. This also depends on the interaction of inflammatory molecules. Reactive oxygen species are produced from the metabolism of alcohol. The reactive oxygen species enhance the stimulation of inflammatory markers like nuclear factor-κB (NF- κB). Additionally, the metabolism of alcohol also causes hypoxia, which is a strong inducer of the inflammatory response. All of these will eventually lead to a complex process that is linked to the progression of cancer. Patient with alcoholic liver disease has higher circulating inflammatory cytokines and it has been shown that inflammation related to alcohol can trigger pathways and markers that increase the risk of tumorigenesis [25].

It is well established that the frequency and the amount of alcohol and tobacco consumption are significant risk factors for head and neck malignancy. Over 80% of head and neck malignancy cases are due to overconsumption of cigarette smoke and alcohol. Only a small percentage of head and neck cancer cases are not directly linked to these social habits. The other contributing risk factors include the dietary, environmental pollutants, genetic, and the recent emergence of HPV [26].

Human Papilloma Virus (HPV) as a Risk Factor for Head and Neck Malignancy

Recent changes in the recent human cancer landscapes include the discovery of new oncogenic viruses that are highly potent. This includes HPV, EBV, and HTLV. There has been a surge in current literature on the association of HPV and head and neck malignancy. This is in relation to the oropharyngeal, oral cavity, and laryngeal carcinoma. The status of HPV positivity significantly affects the prognosis, treatment outcomes, and survival of selective head and neck malignancy patients. Generally, for instance, a positive HPV oropharyngeal cancer is a male and non-smoker and is associated with a better prognosis. Of note, how this virus causes human malignancy is paramount to be critically analyzed. Mesri *et al.* stated that the HPV alone would not be sufficient to cause carcinogenesis, without the interactions with other critical factors [27]. The HPV most likely represents one of the initial steps or the oncogenic hits required for the multiple complex processes for cancer formation.

For malignant transformation to take place, numerous other additional factors are required such as chemical carcinogens, immunosuppression and chronic inflammation [27]. Essentially, chronic inflammation is also a critical element in the virus infection and transformation to cancer formation. Other equally important factors are immunodeficient and genetic aberrations. It seems that these factors act in combination in a complex and delicate environment with multiple stimuli that promotes the carcinogenesis to take place and persists. Fig. (**2**) showed buccal carcinoma, which is highly associated with chronic inflammation.

HPV is a spherical DNA virus that has been known for years causing cervical cancer. To date, it has been consistently shown that this virus has a causal role in oropharyngeal cancer formation. The HPV-associated OPSCC is a unique tumor which has different epidemiology, clinical presentation, molecular features, and management protocol. The prognosis of this subset of patients is also different. The majority of patients are male, younger, and non-smokers. This group of patients has a better prognosis, even though most of them present with higher stage tumors [12]. This again highlights how chronic inflammation indeed induced tumorigenesis. Numerous other evidences that show the significant role of viruses in initiating inflammation and causing carcinogenesis.

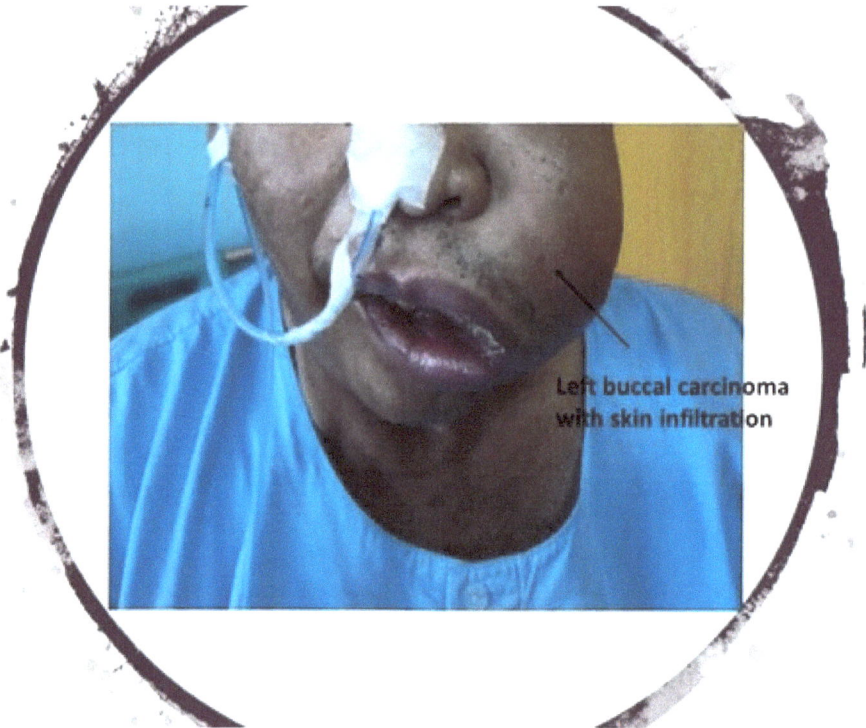

Fig. (2))
Aggressive Left Buccal Carcinoma.

Recent scientific data globally has implicated significant infections with HPV in the pathogenesis of head and neck malignancy. It has been reported that approximately 25% of all head and neck malignancy are positive for HPV-DNA, with 90–95% of those positive for HPV type 16. Cole *et al.,* have reported that HPV type 16 seropositivity is associated with an approximately four-fold increased risk of head and neck malignancy [28]. The detection of HPV varies considerably across head and neck malignancy sub-sites, where the HPV positive cases are much higher in the oropharynx and tonsil compared to the larynx and oral cavity [28]. Additionally, there were different reports of HPV positive HNSCC with different rates for oropharynx, oral cavity, and larynx subsites [29]. This heterogeneous prevalence rate is likely to be attributed to the difference in the environment and other lifestyle factors that are well-known risk factors for head and neck malignancy. With regard to HPV type distribution, HPV16 prevalence accounted for 82% of all HPV DNA positive cases and was higher for OPC (>90%) than for other cancer types. The reported cases of HPV positive OPSCC have increased in recent years and mostly occurred at the base of the tongue and tonsillar region. In the majority of cases, the HPV DNA belongs to HPV 16 subtypes, which again is predominantly associated with OPSCC than other head and neck subsites [13]. HPV positive cancer express mRNA E6/E7 transcripts and perturbations of the *Rb* tumor suppressor pathway as well as the tight coupling of viral transcription to HPV DNA integration point to the critical and fundamental roles for HPV in cellular transformation [30].

Even though, cervical cancer and oropharyngeal cancer share the same carcinogenic stimuli of the HPV, the oropharyngeal and oral cavity are exposed to many other insults like alcohol and tobacco as well as carcinogenic nitrosamine from the dietary habits that placed more complex process involved. The heterogeneity of the HPV positive OPSCC in its molecular characteristic, biology, and clinical presentations may attributed to the various expression of viral oncogene and the amount of viral load [31].

Detail study showed that there are different risk factors involved in the pathogenesis of HPV positive head and neck cancer than HPV negative head and neck cancer. It was revealed that patients with HPV positive cancer belong to:

1. Younger patients with higher education backgrounds
2. Patients with higher economic status
3. Patients who had more life-time sexual partner
4. Caucasians
5. Patient with no history of cigarette smoking and alcohol consumption.

In addition, it is observed that the incidence of HPV-positive cancer will dramatically increase in coming years as the lifestyles of younger generations are prone to be involved in sexual debut at an earlier age, having multiple sexual partners, and engaged in oral sex especially in the western countries [29]. The practice of oral sex increases the HPV infection in the head and neck subsites of the oral cavity and oropharyngeal region. A higher number of HPV infection has been reported in men in contrast to women, which may be partly attributed to the fact that men giving oral sex to HPV infected partners [32].

Critically, the HPV positive tumors have distinct morphology compares to the keratinizing squamous cell carcinoma and undifferentiated carcinoma. These subsets of patients have a better prognosis compared to HPV-negative cancers. As far as investigation is concerned, nowadays the majority of the studies assessing the HPV genomes are based on the DNA-based polymerase chain reaction, and currently, we have seen the emergence of DNA-based *in situ* hybridization (ISH) which has been used in clinical practice in most of the centers worldwide [33]. In the coming years, with refinement and advancement in molecular technology and genomic imprinting, the HPV and its associated inflammatory markers can be identified and extrapolated for future therapeutic intervention.

Epstein Barr Virus (EBV) and the Inflammation

EBV is a known risk factor for nasopharyngeal carcinoma, an important type of head and neck malignancy in certain geographic locations. This NPC is highly prevalent in China, South East Asia, Hong Kong, North Africa, the Arctic regions, and some Mediterranean countries. The EBV may also have interplay roles with other environmental carcinogens such as smoked seafood, salted fish, and pickled vegetables. The accumulation of nitrosamines together with the virus may accelerate the process of carcinogenesis. The mechanisms involved are complex and is not clearly understood. However, recent evidence shows that the epigenetic and genetic events and inflammatory cascades are stimulated and progress in a cohesive manner, which leads to malignant disease development. EBV has been associated with NPC, Burkitt's lymphoma, Hodgkin's disease, and Kaposi's sarcoma.

The most common types of HPV infection that are strongly associated with head and neck cancer is HPV16 and HPV18 [34, 35]. There are more than 170 different types of HPV viruses family that have been identified that able to infect the stratified epithelium of head and neck regions [36]. HPVs are small, circular, non-enveloped, double-stranded DNA viruses that can infect epithelial cells in the upper aerodigestive tract. These viruses can be classified into cutaneous (genital warts) or mucosal types. Mucosal HPV types are mostly found in potentially malignant and cancerous epithelial lesions, leading to their classification as "high-risk HPVs" [36]. Over the last 40 years, the detection of Epstein-Barr virus (EBV) in nasopharyngeal carcinoma (NPC) has evolved from simple serological tests of latent viral infection to highly sensitive measurements of circulating tumor virome [37]. A range of molecular biological methods have now been developed for the detection and genotyping of HPV by polymerase chain reaction (PCR), real-time PCR, *in situ* hybridization, immunohistochemistry, and serum antibody assays at DNA, mRNA, and protein levels [38]. After the infections, EBV resides within B-lymphocytes in a latent phase. The serological markers may present as precursor signals of the actual NPC onset and progression. For instance, anti-IgA antibodies for viral capsid antigen (VCA) and early antigen (EA) have been widely used in the screening of NPC patients.

Transcriptional E6 and E7 activation evidence for viral oncoproteins is seen as a gold standard for clinically relevant HPV, but E6 / E7 mRNA detection requires RNA extraction and PCR amplification is a challenging technique restricted to research labs [39]. Initially, EBV infects a naive B cell where the growth program is implemented by EBV expressing EBNA 1-6, as well as LMP1, LMP2A and LMP2B. The replication of EBV episomes will allow this pattern of expression. Latency III is very immunogenic, and cytotoxic T lymphocytes eliminate cells displaying this pattern. This drives the positive selection of infected B-cells capable of switching to a latency pattern, expressing subdominant immunogenicity only in EBNA1, LMP, and LMP2A [27]. This phenomenon highlights the complexity of the HPV virus mechanism in inducing tumorigenesis. HPV detection is currently emerging as a valid biomarker for discerning the presence and progression of the disease, covering all aspects of patient care, from early detection of cancer to more precise tumor staging to the selection of patients most likely to benefit from specific treatments to tumor surveillance post-treatment [39].

In 2014, prophylactic HPV vaccines were introduced in order to accelerate a decrease in the prevalence of HPV, but the population level in the oral cavity and oropharyngeal subsites was unknown [40]. In the majority of HNSCC samples especially for nasopharyngeal carcinoma, the EBV-positive methods with PCR are used because of the presence of B-lymphocytes in the tumor [41]. Nowadays, most head and neck surgical oncology centers used EBV DNA as a diagnostic marker at the very first patient's clinical presentation. It is an easy and effective diagnostic tool as the cost is inexpensive and the procedure is non-invasive [37]. Fig. (**3**) showed neck metastases in NPC patient.

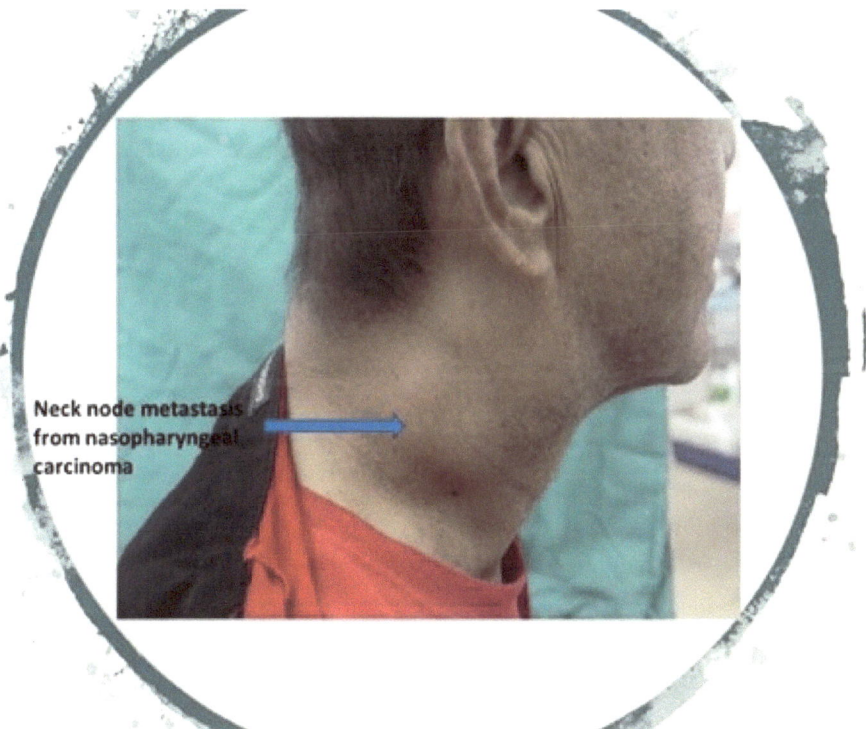

Fig. (**3**))
Nasopharyngeal carcinoma patient with neck nodes metastases.

Dietary Factors and the Risk of Head and Neck Malignancy

In many epidemiological studies, the inverse association of fruit and vegetable consumption with HNC has been reported. The recent World Cancer Research Fund report summarised that the evidence was sufficiently strong to support a causal relationship with non-starchy vegetables, fruits, and carotenoid-containing foods with a decreased HNC risk [42]. The majority of studies highlight that consumption of vegetables and fruit is associated with a reduced risk of head and neck malignancy and the processed meat carries a high risk of getting head and neck cancer. This especially true for the greenery vegetables like cauliflower, broccoli, and cabbage which are high in antioxidant properties and varied color fruits with a high content of tocopherol, phenols, and beta carotenoids [43, 44]. Bauman *et al.* investigate the potential chemopreventative roles of cruciferous vegetables activity against the oral cavity cancers which might reduce the incidence and the tumor size with convincing results [43, 44]. Sulforaphane found in the cruciferous vegetables has shown great antitumor activity and is capable of significantly inhibiting the spread, viability, migration, malignancy and epithelial-to-mesenchymal transition of cancer cells.

Bradshaw *et al.* in their study reported that the consumption of lean protein, in addition to fruit and vegetables (Fig. 4), was associated with a decreased risk of head and neck cancer [45]. On the other end, processed meat, very oily food, high-fat food, and sweet eating were associated with increased risk of head and neck cancer [45]. Health dietary habits should be complemented with regular exercise, which has a positive impact on reducing the risk of head and neck cancer.

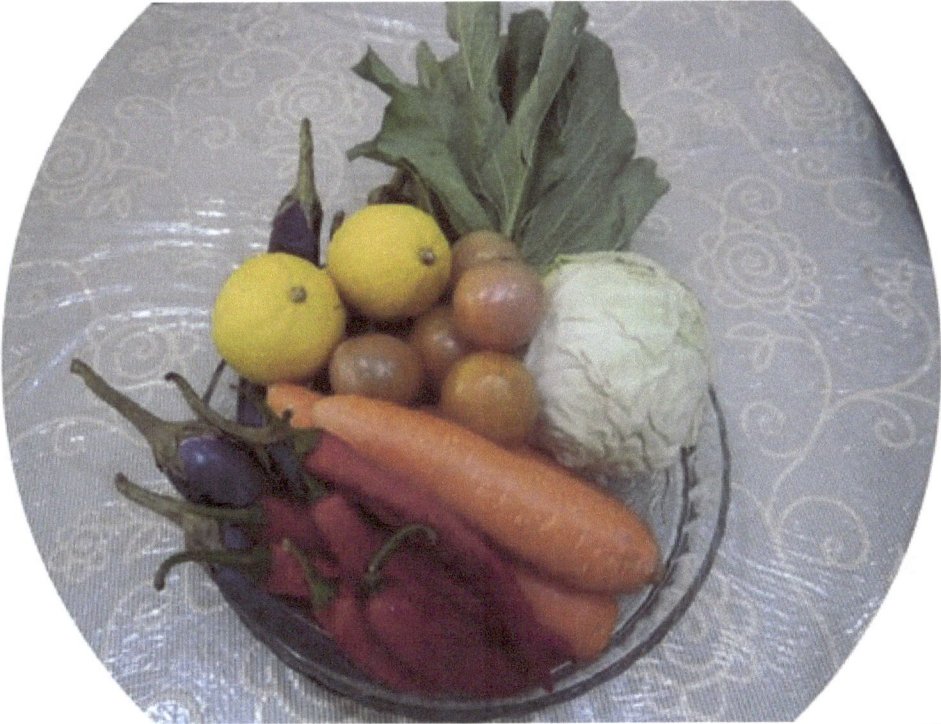

Fig. **(4))**

Vegetables have protective effects against cancer.

Excessive intake of high-fat meat, fried food, sugary foods, and sweets can be observed in patients who are overweight. The overweight patients are prone to have multiple comorbidities including head and neck cancers. This may suggest the possible carcinogenic role of fatty and oily foods.

Some dietary supplements may enhance and regulate the pro-inflammatory cytokines in head and neck cancer patients [46]. The Mediterranean diet is characterized by some common features such as frequent intakes of diversified fruit and vegetables, cereals, fish and seafood, main seasoning fat olive oil, moderate intake of alcohol, and relatively low intake of and dairy products and meat. The Mediterranean diet has been shown to decrease the risk of OPSCC [47]. In younger subjects, in those with a higher level of education, and ex-smokers, the favorable effect of the Mediterranean diet was stronger, although it was also observed in selected patient groups.

Olive oil is largely consumed by the local population in the Mediterranean countries and is the main source of monounsaturated fat. Due to its antioxidant properties attributable both to oleic acid itself and to the presence of other nutrients, such as vitamin E and polyphenols, olive oil has been shown to have a favorable influence on various neoplasms, including OPSCC cancer [47]. Bravi *et al.* in their study provide further evidence on the role of diet on OPSCC cancer risk. They documented that a beneficial effect of vegetables and fruits, whereas a diet high in red meat, eggs, dairy products, potatoes, and sweets raised the risk of cancer of OPSCC [48].

Inverse associations with vegetable protein and fat, polyunsaturated fatty acids, and various antioxidant vitamins have been consistently identified, while direct associations with animal protein and fat, saturated fatty acids, cholesterol, and retinol have been observed [48]. The modifiable risk factors for HNC include an intake of fish and shellfish, a primary source of long-chain omega-3 polyunsaturated fatty acids. The omega-3 fatty acids have been documented to possess anti-inflammatory effects, with the ability to halt tumor development and formation [49].

These long-chain omega-3 fatty acids which are significantly found in fish have been shown to lessen the cancer risk through numerous mechanisms including suppressing the mutations, reducing inflammation markers, inhibiting cell growth as well as enhancing apoptosis [49]. On the contrary high intake of salted fish and preserved vegetables have been linked to the risk of NPC. Salted fish dietary consumption is the most recognized risk factor for NPC, especially in the Guangdong region of South China. Further studies have consistently showed this positive association in Chinese, Thais, Vietnamese, Singaporean, and Indonesian. Early exposure to salted fish during childhood weaning periods in combinations with genetic and familial inheritance plays a crucial role. The pickled vegetables and Cantonese salted fish contain the nitrosamine which is carcinogenic. These foods are categorized in group 1of carcinogenic classification by the International Agency for Cancer Research (IARC) [50]. Importantly, the levels of nitrosamines produced are depending on the types and process of fermentation involved in preparing these salted fish and pickled vegetables.

Genetic and Familial Inheritance in Head and Neck Malignancy

The majority of human malignancy has some genetic abnormality inclusive of head and neck malignancy. The aberrations in genetic profiles of head and neck malignancy are strongly associated with other co-factors which made this malignancy is unique. Evidence of genetic involvement in this malignancy can be seen in various tumor such as nasopharyngeal carcinoma, oral cavity carcinoma, and thyroid carcinoma (Fig. 5). For instance, the ethnic Chinese or Cantonese and their subsequent generations who migrate to America will have similar risk factors of developing NPC with comparison to the natives Cantonese or Chinese in China. This highlights the inheritance pattern that cannot be escaped by related family members, it will exist for generations to come. Other malignancies such as lymphoma (Fig. 6), laryngeal carcinoma and salivary glands carcinoma (Fig. 7) also harbor multiple significant genetic alterations. Hypermethylation of tumor suppressor genes is strongly linked to the development of salivary gland carcinomas. Recent evidence shows that other co-factors like HPV, smoking, and alcohol may act together in producing methylated genes. Thus, combinations of several factors like environmental exposures, dietary habits with the addition of genetic derangement are necessary in promoting carcinogenesis.

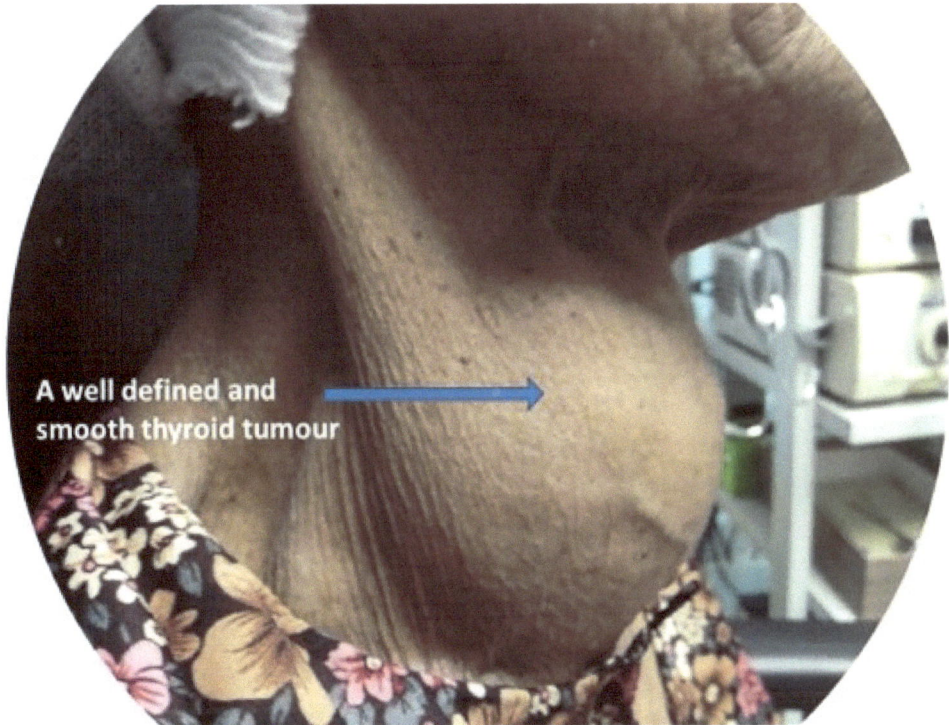

Fig. (5))
Huge goiter in an elderly female with minimal compressive symptoms.

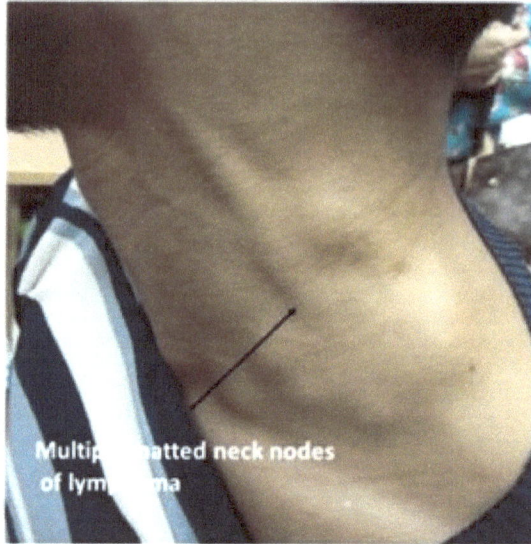

Fig. (6))
Multiple matted left cervical nodes in a young lymphoma patient.

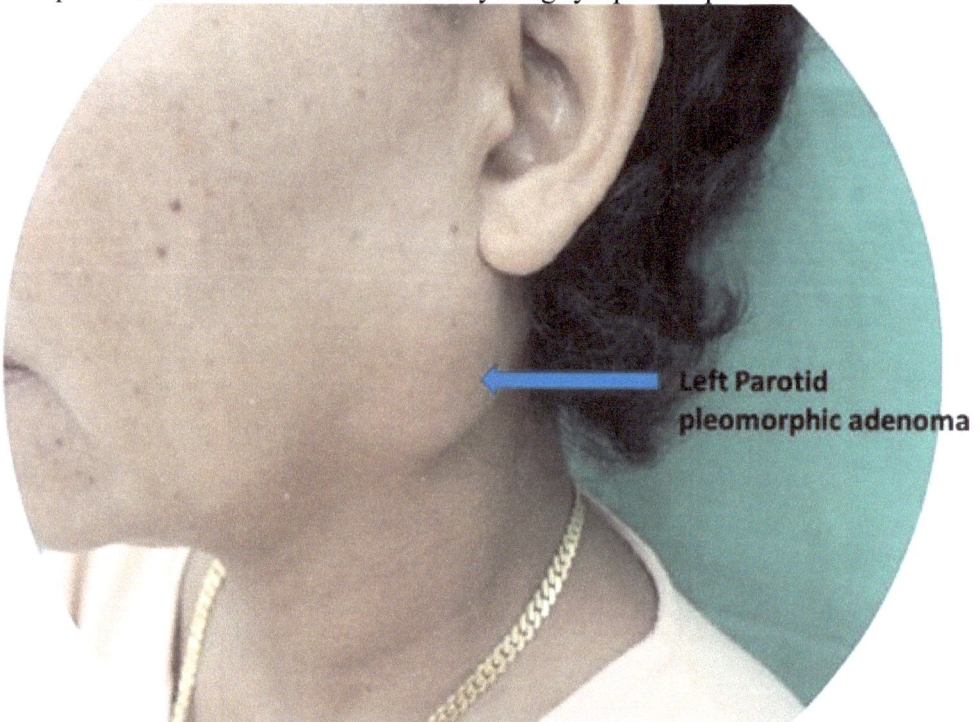

Fig. (7))
Pleomorphic adenoma of left parotid gland.

Chemical Carcinogen and Risk of Inflammation

Environmental factors play a dominant role in the risk of carcinogenesis. Previous literature has documented many types of chemical and industrial carcinogens that are associated with human malignancy. Exposure to chemical materials such as soft leather, crepe rubber, leather, dyeing agents, selected glue type, chlorinated solvents, and flour dust was associated with elevated risks of HNSCC [51, 52]. Exposures to asbestos, formaldehyde, coal acid dust, and acid mists are known to be occupational risk factors for laryngeal cancer and hypopharyngeal cancer [53]. Furthermore, the risk of laryngeal cancer was associated with exposure to polycyclic aromatic hydrocarbons, engine exhaust, textile dust, and working in the rubber industry. Exposure at work is probably an independent risk factor for laryngeal cancer, as defined by occupational categories and title, which warrant more studies [54].

Exposures to asbestos and polycyclic aromatic hydrocarbons were found to be related to an increased risk of oral and pharyngeal cancers [55]. Hypopharyngeal cancer is associated with exposure to organic solvents like petroleum-based products and tetrahydrofuran. The mechanisms involved may be through modulation of chronic inflammation and these agents able to augment the carcinogen absorption into the mucosa of the upper aerodigestive tract [56, 57]. Wood dust exposure on the other hand has been linked to the development of sinonasal carcinoma. Interestingly, the character of the wood also determines the specific malignancy type as softwood is linked to adenocarcinoma whereas hardwood is associated with adenocystic carcinoma. Different molecular events incite by inflammatory substances and molecules could explain this critical difference in the tumor pathology.

Radiation exposure has been associated with several human solid malignancies. In the head and neck region, thyroid carcinoma is linked to radiation exposure. History of radiations in the last 10 -20 years placed a person at 2-3 times increase risk of thyroid malignancy. Other malignancy that is associated with radiation exposure includes salivary glands and sinonasal cavity carcinoma. Avoiding certain identified carcinogens, lifestyle changes and certain vaccinations may reduce the risk of these cancers. Numerous efforts like early screening program, early diagnostic procedures, and early treatment are ongoing to help prevent and delay the development and progression of head and neck cancer globally [58].

THE INTERACTION OF RISK FACTORS IN PROMOTING INFLAMMATION AND CARCINOGENESIS

Smoking, Alcohol, and Oncogenic Viruses

While human genetic variation was linked with the development of NPC, it is evident that lifestyle and dietary differences, together with environmental factors, are likely to increase the risk of this malignancy and cause the unique distribution of NPC. EBV infection, chemical carcinogens, and genetic aberrations may play a significant role in the development of NPCs through a complex of mechanisms and intricate interactions that exist within an ecosystem. The combinations of these factors promote carcinogenesis in NPC [59]. Cigarette smoking and alcohol consumption further causes genetic changes that culminate towards the pathogenesis of head and neck malignancy. Critically history of consumption of alcohol and tobacco smoking is a prognostic factor for overall survival rates of patients with oral cavity, oropharyngeal and laryngeal carcinoma [60]. It has been shown that patients who smoke and drink alcohol are at greater risk to be affected by HPV-related malignancy. However, there was no strong evidence that the stage of HPV or tumor altered the smoking association with survival [61]. Du *et al.* on other hand, reported that the site and stage of tumor, as well as smoking and HPV status, are significant factors in predicting the survivals of head and neck cancer patients [62]. Smoking eliminates the positive impact of HPV on head and neck cancer survival. Non-smoking HPV-positive oropharyngeal cancer patients show 100 percent 10-year OS [63]. Smoking was a major environmental factor, related to increased levels of HPV antibodies [64].

Recently, HPV has been shown to be an important etiologic agent in head and neck carcinomas, particularly in the oropharynx and nasal cancers. Patients with poor PS and a primary 18-positive HPV genotype tumor in sites other than the oropharynx may have a poor prognosis [65]. The oropharynx is exposed to carcinogenic alcohol whereas the nasal cavity is exposed to carcinogens from cigarettes. Certain reports suggest a fairly high exposure of nitrosamines from the cigarette, especially those who smoke more than 20 cigarettes per day is a significant risk of sinonasal cancers as these carcinogens can directly be deposited onto the nasal cavity and nasopharyngeal tissue mucosa [59, 66, 67].

Smoked Fish, Genetic and EBV

Many dietary ingredients have been suggested to be associated with the development of NPC, especially N-nitroso compounds. Epidemiological studies have shown that ingestion of Cantonese-style salted fish is a well-proven risk factor for NPC in Southern China [68, 69]. Canton style herbal tea and cigarette smoking consumption were in positive association with high EBV antibodies observe in patients with NPC [70, 71]. Volatile nitrosamines are known to be present in foods from NPC-high risk areas and are considered to be the etiological factors for NPC. The total volatile nitrosamines were estimated to be in the range of 0.028 to 4.54 mg/kg in Chinese salted fish. Nitrosamine contains in tobacco is equally carcinogenic by causing chronic inflammation and DNA damages [72]. The population who consumed salted fish and smokes cigarettes will have a high level of nitrosamines in their blood. These will also depend on the individual genetic metabolism of nitrosamines.

Interestingly, the boat people of Hong Kong who consumed salted fish as a major food source during the weaning age are observed the highest incidence of NPC [59]. Other food types have also been implicated in NPC development. For instance, the consumption of rancid butter which contains butyrates has also been linked to the development of NPC in certain North African regions. Altogether, these studies show that the incidence of NPC may be increased by the frequent consumption of salted fish and tobacco products, croton oil, or rancid butters which contains nitrosamines, phorbols, and butyrates, respectively.

Obesity

It is well recognized that human cancer development is associated with chronic inflammation, and reactive oxygen species (ROS) released by inflammatory cells may result in DNA damage. Inflammation related to obesity is initially caused by excess nutrients and is located primarily in special adipose tissues [73]. The excess nutrients cause immune alteration, macrophages recruitment, and upregulate the inflammatory cytokines [73, 74]. It has also been reported that spontaneous generation of the ROS and hydrogen peroxide, in tumor tissue was associated with the clinical stage of head and neck squamous cell carcinoma patients. ROS can mediate the cell death pathway and modulate mitochondrial dysfunction [75]. ROS, particularly superoxide and hydrogen peroxides can lead to the activation of NF-κB and AP-1 transcription factors, which play a role in cell proliferation, differentiation, and morphogenesis of cells [19]. Apart from ROS-dependent inflammasome activation, ROS are critical to macrophage phagocytic activity. Specific inflammatory agonists utilize ROS as part of their signaling cascades [76].

Human Papilloma Virus HPV and Inflammations

Several studies have found that patients with HPV-positive tumors are less likely to smoke and consume alcohol compared to patients with HPV-negative tumors. These subsets of patients have a better prognosis. They commonly belong to younger male patients and comes from a higher socioeconomic status. HPV causes oncoprotein expression as well as alterations and mutations in the tumor suppressor genes that subsequently lead to carcinogenesis [31, 77].

D'Souza *et al.* found that exposure to HPV increased the association with oropharyngeal cancer regardless of tobacco and alcohol use [78]. The HPV has been documented to responsible for half of the oropharyngeal cancer cases and the incidence continues to rise [79, 80]. One such exposure that has been linked to HPV infection in the literature is high-risk sexual behavior, particularly oral sex [31]. Patients engaging in high-risk oral sex behaviors are more readily exposed to HPV, which could lead to an increase in malignancy of head and neck subsites [81]. Importantly there are strong geographical differences in the incidence of HPV-positive oropharyngeal cancer. Development of head and neck malignancy appears to differ in relation to individual lifestyle habits, dietary factors, area of residence, and other factors in addition to the presence or absence of HPV.

Masaand *et al.* demonstrated that the effects of heavy smoking and drinking in individuals with HPV16 infection significantly increased the risk of head and neck cancer [33]. This is due to the interactions of the carcinogenic stimuli and alterations in genetic pathways. Robust data indicate that cigarette smoking may modify the clinical behavior of HPV-positive cancers and adversely affecting the prognosis of these neoplasms [15]. However, the incidence of HNC has been increasing worldwide despite a decline in tobacco use that has been attributed to the growing prevalence of oncogenic strains of HPV. This is especially seen in the older male population [12].

PATHOGENESIS OF INFLAMMATION AND OVERALL EFFECTS ON THE HEAD AND NECK MALIGNANCY

Chronic inflammation caused by continuous exposure to chemical carcinogens has been linked to carcinogenesis. Multiple factors and changes occur in an inflammatory cascade that becomes the initial insult responsible for the formation of malignant mass. Numerous cytokines, peptides, immune modulators markers, macrophages are recruited and produced in an intricate inflammation ecosystem.

For instance, the inflammatory enzyme cyclooxygenase 2 (COX2) and the COX2-derived prostaglandin E2 (PGE2) pathway play a key role in promoting the multistep development of cancer, from initiation to metastasis. Significant alterations in the tissue's mucosal and vascularization are induced by potent carcinogenic stimuli. Chronic chemical exposure such as arsenic promotes COX2 expression, which is predominantly expressed in the majority of cancer [81]. Chronic arsenic exposure and other carcinogenic substance cause molecular changes to the cancer stem cells (CSCs). Emerging evidence indicate the central role of CSCs at the top of the cellular hierarchy in tumor initiation, progression, therapeutic resistance, and metastasis. Many more cellular markers, humoral factors, and protein elements induced by dietary habits, tobacco, and alcohol, the oncogenic viruses that are involved in the chronic inflammation phase that underlies the pathogenesis of the majority of head and neck malignancy.

In addition, several studies have suggested that the action of alcohol in head and neck malignancy pathogenesis is mediated by its well-established carcinogen, acetaldehyde. Others have argued that alcohol can directly have adverse effects, either by enhancing the cellular uptake and potency of carcinogens or by inducing hypomethylation of the DNA. The alcohol, cigarette smoking, and HPV infections cause significant genetic and alterations in the epigenetic that underlies the head and neck malignancy [82].

Numerous studies reported that HPV positive head and neck malignancy is diagnosed at more advanced stages than HPV negative head and neck cancers. These subsets of patients, however, have better survival despite being diagnosed with a late-stage tumor. This may have an association with different inflammatory markers that take roles in the pathogenesis of HPV-related malignancy. The overall survival of these patients is better and they have a lower recurrence risk than HPV-negative tumors.

Imperatively, clinicians should consider HPV status and positivity and the extent of disease associated with these tumors in order to strategize a relevant treatment approach based on each patient's tumor characteristics [82, 83]. More studies in the future are needed in order to discover the novel inflammatory markers that can be used for the theranostic approach for head and neck oncology patients.

CONCLUSION

Inflammation and malignancy are inseparable. They are intricately related to each other. The majority of head and neck malignancy is attributed to chronic inflammation, which is induced by, for instance, cigarette, alcohol, viruses, chemicals, dietary products, or radiation. These inciting agents stimulate and secrete critical substances and molecules, which trigger inflammation cascades and induce complex changes within the tissues that eventually lead to malignant mass formation. Combatting head and neck malignancy is feasible since the risk factors and their molecular mechanism can be identified and modulated accordingly. This strategy appears as an effective treatment approach as the tumor can be prevented before it is occurring and progressing. The continuous effort from the scientific community is very crucial in order to maintain future research that will contribute to the discovery of potent diagnostic and therapeutic markers.

CONSENT FOR PUBLICATION

Not applicable.

CONFLICT OF INTEREST

The author confirmed that this chapter's contents have no conflict of interest.

ACKNOWLEDGEMENTS

Declared none.

REFERENCES

[1]   Hakenewerth AM, Millikan RC, Rusyn I, *et al.* Joint effects of alcohol consumption and polymorphisms in alcohol and oxidative stress metabolism genes on risk of head and neck cancer. Cancer Epidemiol Biomarkers Prev 2011; 20(11): 2438-49.[http://dx.doi.org/10.1158/1055-9965.EPI-11-0649]   [PMID: 21940907]

[2]   Giraldi L, Leoncini E, Pastorino R, *et al.* Alcohol and cigarette consumption predict mortality in patients with head and neck cancer: a pooled analysis within the International Head and Neck Cancer Epidemiology (INHANCE) Consortium. Ann Oncol 2017; 28(11): 2843-51.[http://dx.doi.org/10.1093/annonc/mdx486] [PMID: 28945835]

[3]   Priante AV, Castilho EC, Kowalski LP. Second primary tumors in patients with head and neck cancer. Curr Oncol Rep 2011; 13(2): 132-7.[http://dx.doi.org/10.1007/s11912-010-0147-7] [PMID: 21234721]

[4]   Bunbanjerdsuk S, Vorasan N, Saethang T, *et al.* Oncoproteomic and gene expression analyses identify prognostic biomarkers for second primary malignancy in patients with head and neck squamous cell

carcinoma. Mod Pathol 2019; 32(7): 943-56.[http://dx.doi.org/10.1038/s41379-019-0211-2] [PMID: 30737471]

[5]   Tolisano AM, Klem C, Lustik MB, Sniezek JC, Golden JB. Effect of a second primary thyroid carcinoma on patients with head and neck squamous cell carcinoma. Head Neck 2016; 38 (Suppl. 1): E890-4.[http://dx.doi.org/10.1002/hed.24121] [PMID: 25965105]

[6]   Chan JY, Gooi Z, Mydlarz WK, Agrawal N. Risk of thyroid malignancy following an index head and neck squamous cell carcinoma: A population-based study. Ear Nose Throat J 2016; 95(12): E7-E11.[PMID: 27929600]

[7]   Demoor-Goldschmidt C, de Vathaire F. Review of risk factors of secondary cancers among cancer survivors. Br J Radiol 2019; 92(1093): 20180390.[http://dx.doi.org/10.1259/bjr.20180390] [PMID: 30102558]

[8]   Shiga K, Tateda M, Katagiri K, et al. Distinct features of second primary malignancies in head and neck cancer patients in Japan. Tohoku J Exp Med 2011; 225(1): 5-12.[http://dx.doi.org/10.1620/tjem.225.5] [PMID: 21817851]

[9]   Lee DH, Roh JL, Baek S, et al. Second cancer incidence, risk factor, and specific mortality in head and neck squamous cell carcinoma. Otolaryngol Head Neck Surg 2013; 149(4): 579-86.[http://dx.doi.org/10.1177/0194599813496373] [PMID: 23820107]

[10]   Atienza JA, Dasanu CA. Incidence of second primary malignancies in patients with treated head and neck cancer: a comprehensive review of literature. Curr Med Res Opin 2012; 28(12): 1899-909.[http://dx.doi.org/10.1185/03007995.2012.746218] [PMID: 23121148]

[11]   Marur S, Forastiere AA. Head and neck squamous cell carcinoma: update on epidemiology, diagnosis, and treatment. Mayo Clin Proc 2016; 91(3): 386-96.[http://dx.doi.org/10.1016/j.mayocp.2015.12.017] [PMID: 26944243]

[12]   Tsai SC, Huang JY, Lin C, Liaw YP, Lin FC. The association between human papillomavirus infection and head and neck cancer: A population-based cohort study. Medicine (Baltimore) 2019; 98(7): e14436.[http://dx.doi.org/10.1097/MD.0000000000014436] [PMID: 30762752]

[13]   Gillison ML, Chaturvedi AK, Anderson WF, Fakhry C. Epidemiology of human papillomavirus-positive head and neck squamous cell carcinoma. J Clin Oncol 2015; 33(29): 3235-42.[http://dx.doi.org/10.1200/JCO.2015.61.6995] [PMID: 26351338]

[14]   Kim Y, Joo YH, Kim MS, Lee YS. Prevalence of high-risk human papillomavirus and its genotype distribution in head and neck squamous cell carcinomas. J Pathol Transl Med 2020; 54(5): 411-8.[http://dx.doi.org/10.4132/jptm.2020.06.22] [PMID: 32683856]

[15]   Aguayo F, Muñoz JP, Perez-Dominguez F, et al. High-risk human papillomavirus and tobacco smoke interactions in epithelial carcinogenesis. Cancers (Basel) 2020; 12(8): 2201.[http://dx.doi.org/10.3390/cancers12082201] [PMID: 32781676]

[16]   Aldalwg MAH, Brestovac B. Human papillomavirus associated cancers of the head and neck: an australian perspective. Head Neck Pathol 2017; 11(3): 377-84.[http://dx.doi.org/10.1007/s12105-017-0780-7] [PMID: 28176136]

[17]   Hirth J. Disparities in HPV vaccination rates and HPV prevalence in the United States: a review of the literature. Hum Vaccin Immunother 2019; 15(1): 146-55.[http://dx.doi.org/10.1080/21645515.2018.1512453] [PMID: 30148974]

[18]   Marur S, D'Souza G, Westra WH, Forastiere AA. HPV-associated head and neck cancer: a virus-related cancer epidemic. Lancet Oncol 2010; 11(8): 781-9.[http://dx.doi.org/10.1016/S1470-2045(10)70017-6] [PMID: 20451455]

[19]   Ochieng J, Nangami GN, Ogunkua O. The impact of low-dose carcinogens and environmental disruptors on tissue invasion and metastasis. Carcinogenesis 2015; 36(Suppl 1): S128-59.[http://dx.doi.org/10.1093/carcin/bgv034]

[20]   Berthiller J, Straif K, Agudo A, et al. Low frequency of cigarette smoking and the risk of head and neck cancer in the INHANCE consortium pooled analysis. Int J Epidemiol 2016; 45(3): 835-45.[http://dx.doi.org/10.1093/ije/dyv146] [PMID: 26228584]

[21]   Khariwala SS, Ma B, Ruszczak C, et al. High level of tobacco carcinogen-derived dna damage in oral cells is an independent predictor of oral/head and neck cancer risk in smokers. Cancer Prev Res (Phila) 2017; 10(9): 507-13.[http://dx.doi.org/10.1158/1940-6207.CAPR-17-0140] [PMID: 28679497]

[22]   Jethwa AR, Khariwala SS. Tobacco-related carcinogenesis in head and neck cancer. Cancer Metastasis Rev 2017; 36(3): 411-23.[http://dx.doi.org/10.1007/s10555-017-9689-6] [PMID: 28801840]

[23]   Sawabe M, Ito H, Oze I, et al. Heterogeneous impact of alcohol consumption according to treatment method on survival in head and neck cancer: A prospective study. Cancer Sci 2017; 108(1): 91-

100.[http://dx.doi.org/10.1111/cas.13115] [PMID: 27801961]

[24] Huang CC, Hsiao JR, Lee WT, *et al.* Investigating the Association between Alcohol and Risk of Head and Neck Cancer in Taiwan. Sci Rep 2017; 7(1): 9701.[http://dx.doi.org/10.1038/s41598-017-08802-4] [PMID: 28851901]

[25] Wang HJ, Zakhari S, Jung MK. Alcohol, inflammation, and gut-liver-brain interactions in tissue damage and disease development. World J Gastroenterol 2010; 16(11): 1304-13.[http://dx.doi.org/10.3748/wjg.v16.i11.1304] [PMID: 20238396]

[26] Gingerich MA, Smith JD, Michmerhuizen NL, *et al.* Comprehensive review of genetic factors contributing to head and neck squamous cell carcinoma development in low-risk, nontraditional patients. Head Neck 2018; 40(5): 943-54.[http://dx.doi.org/10.1002/hed.25057] [PMID: 29427520]

[27] Mesri EA, Feitelson MA, Munger K. Human viral oncogenesis: a cancer hallmarks analysis. Cell Host Microbe 2014; 15(3): 266-82.[http://dx.doi.org/10.1016/j.chom.2014.02.011] [PMID: 24629334]

[28] Cole L, Polfus L, Peters ES. Examining the incidence of human papillomavirus-associated head and neck cancers by race and ethnicity in the U.S., 1995-2005. PLoS One 2012; 7(3): e32657.[http://dx.doi.org/10.1371/journal.pone.0032657] [PMID: 22448226]

[29] Mourad M, Jetmore T, Jategaonkar AA, Moubayed S, Moshier E, Urken ML. Epidemiological trends of head and neck cancer in the United States: A seer population study. J Oral Maxillofac Surg 2017; 75(12): 2562-72.[http://dx.doi.org/10.1016/j.joms.2017.05.008] [PMID: 28618252]

[30] Bishop JA, Ma XJ, Wang H, *et al.* Detection of transcriptionally active high-risk HPV in patients with head and neck squamous cell carcinoma as visualized by a novel E6/E7 mRNA *in situ* hybridization method. Am J Surg Pathol 2012; 36(12): 1874-82.[http://dx.doi.org/10.1097/PAS.0b013e318265fb2b] [PMID: 23060353]

[31] Boscolo-Rizzo P, Del Mistro A, Bussu F, *et al.* New insights into human papillomavirus-associated head and neck squamous cell carcinoma. Acta Otorhinolaryngol Ital 2013; 33(2): 77-87.[PMID: 23853396]

[32] Tumban E. A current update on human papillomavirus-associated head and neck cancers. Viruses 2019; 11(10): 922.[http://dx.doi.org/10.3390/v11100922] [PMID: 31600915]

[33] Masand RP, El-Mofty SK, Ma XJ, Luo Y, Flanagan JJ, Lewis JS, Jr. Adenosquamous carcinoma of the head and neck: relationship to human papillomavirus and review of the literature. Head Neck Pathol 2011; 5(2): 108-16.[http://dx.doi.org/10.1007/s12105-011-0245-3] [PMID: 21305368]

[34] Bukhari N, Joseph JP, Hussain SS, *et al.* Prevalence of human papilloma virus sub genotypes following head and neck squamous cell carcinomas in asian continent, a systematic review article. Asian Pac J Cancer Prev 2019; 20(11): 3269-77.[http://dx.doi.org/10.31557/APJCP.2019.20.11.3269] [PMID: 31759348]

[35] Lechien JR, Descamps G, Seminerio I, *et al.* HPV involvement in the tumor microenvironment and immune treatment in head and neck squamous cell carcinomas. Cancers (Basel) 2020; 12(5): 1060.[http://dx.doi.org/10.3390/cancers12051060] [PMID: 32344813]

[36] Sabatini ME, Chiocca S. Human papillomavirus as a driver of head and neck cancers. Br J Cancer 2020; 122(3): 306-14.[http://dx.doi.org/10.1038/s41416-019-0602-7] [PMID: 31708575]

[37] Li YQ, Khin NS, Chua MLK. The evolution of epstein-barr virus detection in nasopharyngeal carcinoma. Cancer Biol Med 2018; 15(1): 1-5.[http://dx.doi.org/10.20892/j.issn.2095-3941.2017.0176] [PMID: 29545963]

[38] Rapado-González Ó, Martínez-Reglero C, Salgado-Barreira Á, *et al.* Association of salivary human papillomavirus infection and oral and oropharyngeal cancer: a meta-analysis. J Clin Med 2020; 9(5): 1305.[http://dx.doi.org/10.3390/jcm9051305] [PMID: 32370055]

[39] Economopoulou P, de Bree R, Kotsantis I, Psyrri A. Diagnostic tumor markers in head and neck squamous cell carcinoma (HNSCC) in the clinical setting. Front Oncol 2019; 9: 827.[http://dx.doi.org/10.3389/fonc.2019.00827] [PMID: 31555588]

[40] Menezes FDS, Latorre MDRDO, Conceição GMS, Curado MP, Antunes JLF, Toporcov TN. The emerging risk of oropharyngeal and oral cavity cancer in HPV-related subsites in young people in Brazil. PLoS One 2020; 15(5): e0232871.[http://dx.doi.org/10.1371/journal.pone.0232871] [PMID: 32407339]

[41] Turunen A, Rautava J, Grénman R, Syrjänen K, Syrjänen S. Epstein-Barr virus (EBV)-encoded small RNAs (EBERs) associated with poor prognosis of head and neck carcinomas. Oncotarget 2017; 8(16): 27328-38.[http://dx.doi.org/10.18632/oncotarget.16033] [PMID: 28423694]

[42] Chuang SC, Jenab M, Heck JE, *et al.* Diet and the risk of head and neck cancer: a pooled analysis in the INHANCE consortium. Cancer Causes Control 2012; 23(1): 69-88.[http://dx.doi.org/10.1007/s10552-011-9857-x] [PMID: 22037906]

[43] Bauman JE, Zang Y, Sen M, *et al.* Prevention of carcinogen-induced oral cancer by sulforaphane. Cancer Prev Res (Phila) 2016; 9(7): 547-57.[http://dx.doi.org/10.1158/1940-6207.CAPR-15-0290] [PMID:

27339168]

[44] Russo M, Spagnuolo C, Russo GL, *et al.* Nrf2 targeting by sulforaphane: A potential therapy for cancer treatment. Crit Rev Food Sci Nutr 2018; 58(8): 1391-405.[http://dx.doi.org/10.1080/10408398.2016.1259983] [PMID: 28001083]

[45] Bradshaw PT, Siega-Riz AM, Campbell M, Weissler MC, Funkhouser WK, Olshan AF. Associations between dietary patterns and head and neck cancer: the Carolina head and neck cancer epidemiology study. Am J Epidemiol 2012; 175(12): 1225-33.[http://dx.doi.org/10.1093/aje/kwr468] [PMID: 22575416]

[46] Solís-Martínez O, Plasa-Carvalho V, Phillips-Sixtos G, *et al.* Effect of eicosapentaenoic acid on body composition and inflammation markers in patients with head and neck squamous cell cancer from a public hospital in Mexico. Nutr Cancer 2018; 70(4): 663-70.[http://dx.doi.org/10.1080/01635581.2018.1460678] [PMID: 29697274]

[47] Filomeno M, Bosetti C, Garavello W, *et al.* The role of a Mediterranean diet on the risk of oral and pharyngeal cancer. Br J Cancer 2014; 111(5): 981-6.[http://dx.doi.org/10.1038/bjc.2014.329] [PMID: 24937666]

[48] Bravi F, Bosetti C, Filomeno M, *et al.* Foods, nutrients and the risk of oral and pharyngeal cancer. Br J Cancer 2013; 109(11): 2904-10.[http://dx.doi.org/10.1038/bjc.2013.667] [PMID: 24149181]

[49] McClain KM, Bradshaw PT, Khankari NK, Gammon MD, Olshan AF. Fish/shellfish intake and the risk of head and neck cancer. Eur J Cancer Prev 2019; 28(2): 102-8.[http://dx.doi.org/10.1097/CEJ.0000000000000431] [PMID: 29406335]

[50] Lau HY, Leung CM, Chan YH, *et al.* Secular trends of salted fish consumption and nasopharyngeal carcinoma: a multi-jurisdiction ecological study in 8 regions from 3 continents. BMC Cancer 2013; 13: 298.[http://dx.doi.org/10.1186/1471-2407-13-298] [PMID: 23782497]

[51] Carton M, Menvielle G, Cyr D, *et al.* Icare Study GroupOccupational exposure to flour dust and the risk of head and neck cancer. Am J Ind Med 2018; 61(10): 869-73.[http://dx.doi.org/10.1002/ajim.22899] [PMID: 30124232]

[52] Carton M, Barul C, Menvielle G, *et al.* ICARE Study GroupOccupational exposure to solvents and risk of head and neck cancer in women: a population-based case-control study in France. BMJ Open 2017; 7(1): e012833.[http://dx.doi.org/10.1136/bmjopen-2016-012833] [PMID: 28069619]

[53] Laforest L, Luce D, Goldberg P, *et al.* Laryngeal and hypopharyngeal cancers and occupational exposure to formaldehyde and various dusts: a case-control study in France. Occup Environ Med 2000; 57(11): 767-73.[http://dx.doi.org/10.1136/oem.57.11.767] [PMID: 11024201]

[54] Bayer O, Cámara R, Zeissig SR, *et al.* Occupation and cancer of the larynx: a systematic review and meta-analysis. Eur Arch Otorhinolaryngol 2016; 273(1): 9-20.[http://dx.doi.org/10.1007/s00405-014-3321-y] [PMID: 25311307]

[55] Radoï L, Sylla F, Matrat M, *et al.* ICARE study groupHead and neck cancer and occupational exposure to leather dust: results from the ICARE study, a French case-control study. Environ Health 2019; 18(1): 27.[http://dx.doi.org/10.1186/s12940-019-0469-3] [PMID: 30922305]

[56] Barul C, Carton M, Radoï L, *et al.* ICARE study groupOccupational exposure to petroleum-based and oxygenated solvents and hypopharyngeal and laryngeal cancer in France: the ICARE study. BMC Cancer 2018; 18(1): 388.[http://dx.doi.org/10.1186/s12885-018-4324-7] [PMID: 29621977]

[57] Barul C, Carton M, Radoï L, *et al.* ICARE study groupOccupational exposure to petroleum-based and oxygenated solvents and oral and oropharyngeal cancer risk in men: A population-based case-control study in France. Cancer Epidemiol 2019; 59: 22-8.[http://dx.doi.org/10.1016/j.canep.2019.01.005] [PMID: 30658217]

[58] Alfouzan AF. Head and neck cancer pathology: Old world *versus* new world disease. Niger J Clin Pract 2019; 22(1): 1-8.[http://dx.doi.org/10.4103/njcp.njcp_310_18] [PMID: 30666013]

[59] Fang CY, Huang SY, Wu CC, *et al.* The synergistic effect of chemical carcinogens enhances Epstein-Barr virus reactivation and tumor progression of nasopharyngeal carcinoma cells. PLoS One 2012; 7(9): e44810.[http://dx.doi.org/10.1371/journal.pone.0044810] [PMID: 23024765]

[60] Lazim, Norhafiza & Abdullah, BaharudinCancer biomarkers: strategies for early diagnosis. Cancer Biology and Dietary Factors 2018; 3(1): 208-32.

[61] Beynon RA, Lang S, Schimansky S, *et al.* Tobacco smoking and alcohol drinking at diagnosis of head and neck cancer and all-cause mortality: Results from head and neck 5000, a prospective observational cohort of people with head and neck cancer. Int J Cancer 2018; 143(5): 1114-27.[http://dx.doi.org/10.1002/ijc.31416] [PMID: 29607493]

[62] Du E, Mazul AL, Farquhar D, *et al.* Long-term survival in head and neck cancer: impact of site, stage, smoking, and human papillomavirus status. Laryngoscope 2019; 129(11): 2506-

13.[http://dx.doi.org/10.1002/lary.27807] [PMID: 30637762]

[63] Hoffmann M, Quabius ES, Tribius S, *et al.* Influence of HPV-status on survival of patients with tonsillar carcinomas (TSCC) treated by CO_2-laser surgery plus risk adapted therapy - A 10 year retrospective single centre study. Cancer Lett 2018; 413: 59-68.[http://dx.doi.org/10.1016/j.canlet.2017.10.045] [PMID: 29100961]

[64] He YQ, Xue WQ, Xu FH, *et al.* The relationship between environmental factors and the profile of epstein-barr virus antibodies in the lytic and latent infection periods in healthy populations from endemic and non-endemic nasopharyngeal carcinoma areas in China. EBioMedicine 2018; 30: 184-91.[http://dx.doi.org/10.1016/j.ebiom.2018.02.019] [PMID: 29606628]

[65] Yoo SH, Ock CY, Keam B, *et al.* Poor prognostic factors in human papillomavirus-positive head and neck cancer: who might not be candidates for de-escalation treatment? Korean J Intern Med (Korean Assoc Intern Med) 2019; 34(6): 1313-23.[http://dx.doi.org/10.3904/kjim.2017.397] [PMID: 30428646]

[66] Talmi YP, Wolf M, Horowitz Z, Bedrin L, Kronenberg J, Pfeffer MR. Smoking-induced squamous-cell cancer of the nose. Arch Environ Health 2002; 57(5): 422-4.[http://dx.doi.org/10.1080/00039890209601431] [PMID: 12641183]

[67] Hsu WL, Chien YC, Huang YT, *et al.* GEV-NPC Study GroupCigarette smoking increases the risk of nasopharyngeal carcinoma through the elevated level of IgA antibody against Epstein-Barr virus capsid antigen: A mediation analysis. Cancer Med 2020; 9(5): 1867-76.[http://dx.doi.org/10.1002/cam4.2832] [PMID: 31925935]

[68] Barrett D, Ploner A, Chang ET, *et al.* Past and recent salted fish and preserved food intakes are weakly associated with nasopharyngeal carcinoma risk in adults in Southern China. J Nutr 2019; 149(9): 1596-605.[http://dx.doi.org/10.1093/jn/nxz095] [PMID: 31127847]

[69] Jia WH, Luo XY, Feng BJ, *et al.* Traditional Cantonese diet and nasopharyngeal carcinoma risk: a large-scale case-control study in Guangdong, China. BMC Cancer 2010; 10: 446.[http://dx.doi.org/10.1186/1471-2407-10-446] [PMID: 20727127]

[70] Zhou T, Yang DW, He YQ, *et al.* Associations between environmental factors and serological Epstein-Barr virus antibodies in patients with nasopharyngeal carcinoma in South China. Cancer Med 2019; 8(10): 4852-66.[http://dx.doi.org/10.1002/cam4.2348] [PMID: 31241250]

[71] Yang QY, He YQ, Xue WQ, *et al.* Association between serum cotinine level and serological markers of epstein-barr virus in healthy subjects in South China where nasopharyngeal carcinoma is endemic. Front Oncol 2019; 9: 865.[http://dx.doi.org/10.3389/fonc.2019.00865] [PMID: 31572673]

[72] Yong SK, Ha TC, Yeo MC, Gaborieau V, McKay JD, Wee J. Associations of lifestyle and diet with the risk of nasopharyngeal carcinoma in Singapore: a case-control study. Chin J Cancer 2017; 36(1): 3.[http://dx.doi.org/10.1186/s40880-016-0174-3] [PMID: 28063457]

[73] Wagner M, Samdal Steinskog ES, Wiig H. Adipose tissue macrophages: the inflammatory link between obesity and cancer? Expert Opin Ther Targets 2015; 19(4): 527-38.[http://dx.doi.org/10.1517/14728222.2014.991311] [PMID: 25474374]

[74] Sun S, Ji Y, Kersten S, Qi L. Mechanisms of inflammatory responses in obese adipose tissue. Annu Rev Nutr 2012; 32: 261-86.[http://dx.doi.org/10.1146/annurev-nutr-071811-150623] [PMID: 22404118]

[75] Hsieh YT, Chen YF, Lin SC, Chang KW, Li WC. Targeting cellular metabolism modulates head and neck oncogenesis. Int J Mol Sci 2019; 20(16): 3960.[http://dx.doi.org/10.3390/ijms20163960] [PMID: 31416244]

[76] Forrester SJ, Kikuchi DS, Hernandes MS, Xu Q, Griendling KK. Reactive oxygen species in metabolic and inflammatory signaling. Circ Res 2018; 122(6): 877-902.[http://dx.doi.org/10.1161/CIRCRESAHA.117.311401] [PMID: 29700084]

[77] Wittekindt C, Wagner S, Sharma SJ. HPV - A different view on Head and Neck Cancer. HPV – Das andere Kopf-Hals-Karzinom. Laryngorhinootologie. 2018; 97(S 01): S48-S113.

[78] Desouza G, Kreimer AR, Viscidi R, *et al.* Case control study of human papillomavirus and oropharyngeal cancer. N Eng J Med 2007; 10; 356(19): 1944-56

[79] Reuschenbach M, Wagner S, Würdemann N, *et al.* Humane papillomviren bei plattenepithelkarzinomen der kopf- und halsregion : relevanz für prognose, therapie und prophylaxe. HNO 2016; 64(7): 450-9.[http://dx.doi.org/10.1007/s00106-016-0123-0] [PMID: 26864190]

[80] Zaravinos A. An updated overview of HPV-associated head and neck carcinomas. Oncotarget 2014; 5(12): 3956-69.[http://dx.doi.org/10.18632/oncotarget.1934] [PMID: 24970795]

[81] Ooki A, Begum A, Marchionni L, *et al.* Arsenic promotes the COX2/PGE2-SOX2 axis to increase the malignant stemness properties of urothelial cells. Int J Cancer 2018; 143(1): 113-

26.[http://dx.doi.org/10.1002/ijc.31290] [PMID: 29396848]

[82]   Saad MA, Kuo SZ, Rahimy E, *et al.* Alcohol-dysregulated miR-30a and miR-934 in head and neck squamous cell carcinoma. Mol Cancer 2015; 14: 181.[http://dx.doi.org/10.1186/s12943-015-0452-8] [PMID: 26472042]

[83]   Božinović K, Sabol I, Rakušić Z, *et al.* HPV-driven oropharyngeal squamous cell cancer in Croatia - Demography and survival. PLoS One 2019; 14(2): e0211577.[http://dx.doi.org/10.1371/journal.pone.0211577] [PMID: 30707715]

The Diagnostic Tools for Head and Neck Cancer

Giacomo Spinato[1, 2, *], Paolo Boscolo Rizzo[1], Marco Salvatore[3], Simonetta Ausoni[4], Samuele Frasconi[1], Giuseppe Azzarello[5], Carlo Cavaliere[3], Liberatore Tramontano[3], Maria Cristina Da Mosto[1]

[1] Depatment of Neurosciences, Section of Otolaryngology and Regional Centre for Head and Neck Cancer, University of Padova, Treviso, Italy

[2] Department of Surgery, Oncology and Gastroenterology, Section of Oncology and Immunology, University of Padova, Treviso, Italy

[3] Scientific Institute for Research, Hospitalization and Healthcare - IRCCS - SDN, Naples, Italy

[4] Department of Biomedical Sciences, University of Padua, Padua, Italy

[5] Oncology and Hematology Department, ULSS 3 Serenissima, Mirano Hospital, Venice, Italy

Abstract

Diagnosis plays a key role in overall patient assessment and accurate staging of the malignancy. Diagnosis is the starting point to choose treatment strategies for the disease, as well as the basis upon which therapy success, prognosis and the patient's quality of life will vary. Considering a high level of clinical suspicion of any mucosal alteration or laterocervical swelling is important until medical examinations provide evidence of the contrary. Diagnosis investigation continues with the search, among data collected on the patient's history, of objective signs on which clinical suspicions will focus through further medical and instrumental examinations. Imaging techniques that can be used are ultrasound scan, computerised tomography, magnetic resonance and, in the most complex cases, positron emission computerised tomography. Ultrasonography is the most commonly used imaging technique for head and neck mass, especially for the assessment of lymph nodes, thyroid glands and salivary glands. Magnetic resonance is also considered an important examination in the diagnosis of head and neck tumours, especially for lesions involving the oral cavity, oropharynx, nasopharynx and larynx. Computerised tomography (CT) scan is especially useful when assessing the skull base involvement and the morphology of laryngeal malignancies, for example when the tumour extends over the perichondrium of cartilage structures, as well as when assessing function, *i.e.* evaluating the degree of chordal motility. In head and neck cancers (HNC), predictive factors namely biological characteristics that can be used to predict tumor response to a specific treatment, are currently remarkably lacking. Conversely, some bio-molecular parameters are recognized as prognostic factors of the disease, since they indicate tumor characteristics that inform about cancer outcome,

independently of treatment the patients will undergo. The most prominent prognostic factor for head and neck cancers is viral etiology, specifically HPV-mediated disease for oropharyngeal carcinomas and EBV-mediated disease for nasopharyngeal carcinoma.

Keywords: Biomarkers, Diagnostic tool, Head and neck cancer, Investigation, Imaging, TNM classification.

---

* **Corresponding author Giacomo Spinato:** Department of Neurosciences, Section of Otolaryngology and Regional Centre for Head and Neck Cancer, University of Padova, Treviso, Italy; Tel: +39 0422322324; and Department of Surgery, Oncology and Gastro-enterology, Section of Oncology and Immunology, University of Padova, Treviso, Italy; E-mail: spin.giacomo@gmail.com

INTRODUCTION TO DIAGNOSTIC INVESTIGATIONS IN HEAD AND NECK CANCER

Head and neck cancers may, due to the onset and evolution of the disease and variability of its histology, present in either full-blown or subtler forms. Diagnosis plays a key role in overall patient assessment and accurate staging of the malignancy. Diagnosis is the starting point to choose treatment strategies for the disease, as well as the basis upon which therapy success, prognosis and the patient's quality of life will vary. Approximately half of all head and neck cancers are diagnosed when the disease is at an advanced stage, most likely because the patient tends to see a specialist only when the disease is full-blown because earlier symptoms are often vague or neglectable [1, 2]. Diagnostic errors occur when, in light of one or more patient-reported symptoms, the physician diagnoses the wrong disease or when examinations and tests that are necessary for a correct diagnosis are not performed on the patient.

THE ANAMNESIS ROLE IN THE DIAGNOSIS

The first step to avoid errors in diagnosis is to proceed with an adequate investigation of the patient's history, especially with the aim of building, from the very beginning, a trust relationship between the patient and physician that will last throughout the diagnosis and treatment pathway [3‑5]. When investigating the patient's history, in addition to examining the patient's familiarity in relation to head and neck cancers, another important aspect is to investigate their lifestyle and habits to identify risk factors associated with this type of malignancies, especially tobacco and alcohol abuse and, more recently, promiscuous sexual habits [6‑9].

In addition to lifestyle factors, investigating the patient's profession is also fundamental at this stage, given the known correlation between prolonged exposure to toxic/irritating agents such as heavy metals or wood dust and the onset of upper aerodigestive tract tumours [10]. Agents that are irritating for the mucosa of the upper aerodigestive tracts produce a chronic mucosal phlogosis and can lead to metaplastic or dysplastic phenomena. Factors favouring the onset of chronic mucosal phlogosis in the upper aerodigestive tracts may include gastroesophageal reflux disease, a diet low in antioxidants - especially group A and E vitamins - and viral aetiologic agents, which should be investigated by testing malignant cells for EBV or HPV DNA in patients with nasopharyngeal or oropharyngeal carcinoma respectively [11, 12].

In the case of tumours of the thyroid and salivary glands, investigating any previous exposure to radiation therapy, especially during paediatric age, or high accidental exposure to radiation, as occurred in the past in the Chernobyl disaster, is essential.

Finally, the patient's history investigation should focus on any patient comorbidities, organ failures, home-delivered therapies and allergies that may impact treatment decisions once the precise clinical staging is complete [13‑15].

CLINICAL ASSESSMENT IN HEAD AND NECK CANCER

The analysis and accurate interpretation of reported symptoms and clinical signs is of extreme importance in the setting of head and neck cancers, because the signs and symptoms that may present based on the site of disease onset may vary and differ [16, 17].

Often, during the initial stage of the disease, symptoms might be silent or vague; often, head and neck cancer patients are socially marginalised or live in poor social conditions and thus do not see a specialist until symptoms are full-blown and the disease is already at an advanced stage [18]. Symptoms at onset may be local and most frequently include, based on their site, sore throat, the feeling of a lump, hoarseness, unilateral nasal bleeding and reported symptoms at onset such as ear pain and headache. The most typical symptoms of a malignant evolution in the upper aerodigestive tracts are odynophagia, increasingly severe dysphagia [19], "hot potato" voice, salivary pooling, dyspnea (initially upon exertion), cacosmia, bleeding in the mouth, weight loss. Symptom evolution and the relatively rapid increase in severity are an index for mass growth speed evaluation and, indirectly, tumour malignancy [20, 21].

A typical feature of tumours of the nasopharynx [22] is that the patient reports a generally unilateral feeling of ear fullness associated with the onset of otitis media with effusion after a generally short period of time - a typical onset manifestation in this tumour type. Regarding salivary glands, a setting in which tumours are more frequently benign, the generally slow growth of a lump, alternated with periods of regression (as typically occurs with *cystadenoma lymphomatosum*), is observed in the tail of the parotid gland near the angle of the mandible relative to the superficial parotid gland, or in the mouth and pharynx in some cases of deep parotid lobe cancer, where malignancies may resemble a peritonsillar abscess without signs of acute phlogosis. In case of submandibular and sublingual glands, a level I laterocervical swelling, or lump in the floor of the oral cavity, may be identified. This leads to associated symptoms such as limited tongue motility and trismus with infiltrations in the pterygoid muscles and masticator space, resulting in the patient having difficulties to eat [23, 24].

Regarding parotid masses, odynophagia, ulcers of the skin overlying the glands and even a reduction or deficit of hemiface motility due to more or less direct involvement of the facial nerve may subsequently appear. The degree of involvement of the facial nerve may be evaluated according to the House-Brackmann scale [25], which includes six different grades based on the residual function of mimic muscles or of the *orbicularis oculi* muscle.

The scheme in Table 1 summarises symptoms and tumour position based on the evolution of the malignancy [26-30].

The patient will present to a specialist evaluation in light of the described symptoms and clinical condition [32]. When investigating the patient's history [33], the age may lead to consider certain tumour types. In clinical practice, suspicion of oropharyngeal or nasopharyngeal malignant [34], or more commonly benign tumours in isolated laterocervical swellings originating from the branchial arches or residue of the thyroglossal tract tends to be more frequent in younger than in older patients. Considering with a high level of clinical suspicion, any mucosal alteration or laterocervical swelling is anyway important until medical examinations provide evidence of the contrary. The patient's history needs to take into account familiarity with malignant diseases, the type of dietary habits, daily or accidental exposure to risk factors in the workplace, any predisposing comorbidities, the patient's lifestyle and sexual habits; all the information collected on such aspects shall then be considered when choosing the therapy.

A critical assessment of data collected on the patient's history should be accompanied by a detailed analysis of the timing of the onset and evolution of symptoms and clinical signs mentioned in Table 1 [35-38].

Table 1 **Onset and evolution symptoms in relation to the tumour site [1, 31].**

Anatomical Site	Signs and Symptoms at Onset	Advanced Signs and Symptoms
Nasopharynx	Posterior rhinorrhea, unilateral fullness, cough with haemoptysis	Headache, relapsing posterior epistaxis, cacosmia, unilateral ear pain, symptoms relating to the local invasion of adjacent tissues and skull base
Nasal fossae and paranasal sinuses	Anteroposterior rhinorrhea, cough with haemoptysis, epistaxis, or symptoms of obstructive sinusitis, including facial pain and congestion, sudden onset of nasal obstruction	Complete nasal obstruction, significant relapsing epistaxis, anosmia, septum or cutaneous ulcers, symptoms relating to the local invasion of adjacent tissues, swelling or a mass in the hard palate, upper gum, gingivobuccal sulcus, or cheek. Loose teeth, anesthesia of the skin of the cheek, upper lip, diplopia, and proptosis, trismus, anesthesia in the distribution of the fifth cranial nerve or paralysis of the third, fourth, or sixth cranial nerves

Oral cavity	Feeling of a lump in the mouth	Relapsing bleeding in the mouth, dysphagia, trismus, symptoms relating to the local invasion of adjacent tissues
Oropharynx	Feeling of a lump in the mouth	Relapsing bleeding in the mouth, dysphagia, swallowing dysfunction, nasal regurgitation and aspiration, unilateral ear pain, symptoms relating to the local invasion of adjacent tissues
Hypopharynx	Feeling of a lump in the mouth	Relapsing bleeding in the mouth, dysphagia, hoarseness, dyspnea, nasal regurgitation and aspiration. Symptoms relating to the local invasion of adjacent tissues
Supraglottic larynx	Hoarseness	Relapsing bleeding in the mouth, hoarseness, aphonia, dysphagia, dyspnea. Symptoms relating to the local invasion of adjacent tissues
Glottic larynx	Hoarseness, dyshonia	Relapsing bleeding in the mouth, hoarseness, aphonia, dysphagia, dyspnea. Symptoms relating to the local invasion of adjacent tissues
Hypoglottic larynx	Hoarseness	Relapsing bleeding in the mouth, hoarseness, aphonia, dysphagia, dyspnea. Symptoms relating to the local invasion of adjacent tissues
Cervical esophagus	Dysphagia	Relapsing bleeding in the mouth, hoarseness, dysphagia, dyspnea, nasal regurgitation and aspiration. Symptoms relating to the local invasion of adjacent tissues
Salivary glands	Asymptomatic mass	Dry mouth, V and VII cranial nerve deficit, trismus, dysphagia. Ear pain, symptoms relating to the local invasion of adjacent tissues

CLINICAL EXAMINATION IN HEAD AND NECK CANCER

Diagnosis investigation continues with the search, among data collected on the patient's history, of objective signs which clinical suspicions will focus on through further medical examinations. The first diagnostic approach consists of an accurate examination of the patient. A general inspection of the patient may confirm part of the information gained from data on the patient's history, such as their nutritional state, smoke or alcohol abuse and willingness to collaborate;

all such information is essential for subsequent therapy planning [39-41].

Ear, nose and throat examination should, first of all, include the observation of face, scalp and neck skin; furthermore, the presence of any suspicious swollen, ulcerating or dyschromic lesions or facial asymmetries should be assessed [42]. In case of clinical signs, further information may be suggested by an accurate superficial and deep palpation to assess lesion texture, fixity and tenderness, together with the presence of pus from superinfection or cutaneous ulceration. Palpation of parotid swelling and any way of the main salivary glands should always be performed using two hands and should be associated to the inspection of the type of sputum produced by salivary ducts in order to differentiate diagnosis from purely infectious diseases.

Neck palpation extends to the region behind the preauricular area and all the way to the supraclavear area, assessing evident laterocervical swellings and identifying any suspicious lymph node beds that deserve more in-depth diagnostic evaluation [43, 44]. Lymph node characteristics worthy of assessment by means of palpation include, in particular, texture (soft *vs.* hard), size, speed of evolution (higher in more aggressive forms), site (uni- *vs.* bilateral) and tenderness (which is typically absent in suspicious forms [45].

Lymph node beds should be examined at all levels whenever possible. The conventional and international American Head and Neck Society classification involves seven levels, each draining lymph from a specific cutaneous or mucosal anatomical site of the head and neck region; such levels are categorized as follows;

- Level IA (submental level), which includes the area extending from the hyoid bone inferiorly, the midline medially and the lateral margin of the anterior belly of the digastric muscle laterally;
- Level IB (submandibular level), which is comprised within the mandibular branch inferiorly, the anterior belly of the digastric muscle anteriorly and the stylohyoid muscle posteriorly;
- Level II (upper jugular chain level), which is delimited by the cranial base superiorly, the stylohyoid muscle medially, the hyoid bone inferiorly and the posterior margin of the sternocleidomastoid muscle posteriorly; based on the point of emergence of the accessory spinal nerve, a perpendicular line can be traced to divide sublevel II in bed IIA, located anteroinferior to it, and sublevel IIB, which includes lymph nodes located posterosuperior;
- Level III (middle internal jugular chain level), which is included between the hyoid bone superiorly, the belly of the sternocleidomastoid muscle externally and the inferior margin of the cricoid cartilage inferiorly;
- Level IV (deep jugular chain level), which is the most deeply located site in respect of the sternocleidomastoid muscle and is delimited by the posterior margin of its muscular belly posteriorly, by the inferior

margin of the cricoid cartilage superiorly and by the upper margin of the superior clavicle inferiorly;

- Level V (posterior triangle level), which is comprised of the triangle delimited by the posterior margin of the sternocleidomastoid muscle anteriorly, by the lateral margin and belly of the trapezius posterolaterally; a line can be traced perpendicularly to the midline, following the accessory nerve passing through the cricoid cartilage to divide level V into sublevel VA, located superiorly to such line, and sublevel VB, located in the inferior section;
- Level VI (anterior jugular chain level), which is comprised within the hyoid bone superiorly, the carotid artery laterally and the superior margin of the sternal manubrium inferiorly;
- Level VII (superior mediastinal level), which includes the pretracheal, paratracheal and oesophageal folds extending from the level of the superior margin of the sternal manubrium to the innominate artery.

Lymph drainage occurring at each level is summarised below:

- Level IA (submental level) drains the anteroinferior portions of the mouth (lip, gums and tongue) and of the sublingual gland;
- Level IB (submandibular level) drains the mid-level of third middle of buccal structures (lip, palate, dental arch and tongue), of the lateral portion of the mental region and of the submandibular gland;
- Level II (superior jugular chain level) drains lymph coming from nasal cavities, structures belonging to the posterior portion of the oral cavity, the parotid gland, the supraglottic larynx and the pharynx;
- Level III (middle jugular chain level) drains the pharynx and larynx;
- Level IV (inferior jugular chain level) drains lymph circulating in the larynx, thyroid, hypopharynx and cervical oesophagus;
- Level V (posterior triangle level) drains the pharynx, parotid gland and, through the retro-auricular and occipital lymph node beds, the respective areas of the scalp;
- Level VI (anterior jugular chain level) collects lymph coming from the thyroid, muscles of the anterior cervical compartment, larynx and cervical oesophagus;
- Level VII (superior mediastinal level), which includes the pretracheal, paratracheal and oesophageal folds extending from the level of the superior margin of the sternal manubrium to the innominate artery.

During the clinical investigation of the mucosa, all upper aerodigestive tract regions should be inspected with the help of both the simplest tools, such as headlight, cold spatula and nasal speculum and more sophisticated equipment such as white or filtered light optics to identify any suspicious, ulcerating, dyschromic, hyperplastic or neoangiogenic lesions [46, 47]. Ear examination using an otoscope, microscope or endoscope is essential for differential diagnosis of reported ear pain *versus* otodynia, as well as in the evaluation of the skin of the outer ear.

The accurate examination of the oral cavity, which is often underestimated, should involve various areas. To begin with, the condition of the patient's dentition and gum mucosa of both dental arches may provide a significant amount of information on the patient's overall conditions and personal care and hygiene, their lifestyle habits, any mucosal lesions due to poor oral hygiene, chronic trauma caused by sharp teeth or inadequate removable prostheses; moreover, a class II malocclusion and significant development of superior incisors may be a criterion for exclusion from transoral surgery. The accurate description of the dental state may furthermore prevent subsequent medical-legal post-intubation litigations or surgery in case of trauma or chipped teeth. Tongue examination considers aspect, hydration and any morphological or motility asymmetries of the mucosa. The examination of the floor of the oral cavity also includes the assessment of submandibular and sublingual gland excretory ducts. When suspicious lesions are recognized in any site of the oral cavity, accurate palpation follows in order to gain further information on its size and any infiltration of the malignancy. Different from the oral cavity, the oropharynx features sites that cannot be viewed directly, such as the tonsillar crypts or basis of the tongue so, in case of suspicion following an inspection or optic fibre pharyngoscopy, seeking clinical confirmation through deep palpation remains fundamental.

Portions of the head and neck area excluded from direct inspection and anterior rhinoscopy, *i.e.* nasopharynx [48, 49], nasal fossae posteriorly, part of the oropharynx and the area of the hypopharynx and larynx, require second-level tools that enable a full exploration. Based on convenience and clinical experience, either rigid or flexible endoscopic tools can be used. Nowadays, assessment of upper aerodigestive tracts by means of indirect pharyngolaryngoscopy specula is no longer sustainable in oncologic clinical evaluation, as the latter are not precise enough in terms of image resolution and are strictly operator-dependant. In rhinoscopy and endoscopy, suspicious - especially unilateral, ulcerating or bleeding - lesions should be sought.

Regarding the nasopharynx from choanae to the soft palate, obtaining evidence on the palatovelar function in swallowing and phonation, as well as on the patency of tubal ostia is important. Assessment of the hypopharynx and larynx, as well as the oropharynx as a whole, is feasible by means of rigid, angulated optic fibre video laryngoscopy, although the latter is not always accepted by patients with marked emetic reflex in spite of locally applied anaesthesia, which often facilitates evaluation. In the latter cases, a fibroscopy is performed using a flexible endoscope that bypasses the palatoglossal arch causing the emetic reflex.

The hypopharynx is a particular and anatomically complex structure consisting of portions that are clearly visible at endoscopy and expandable regions, such as the pyriform sinuses and retrocricoid region. An important, indirect suspicious clinical clue regarding expandable regions involves salivary pooling or lumen asymmetry when a clear investigation of the mucosa is not possible. The larynx includes subsites that can be more or less visible with laryngoscopy. While lesions of the glottic plane are easily recognisable even at an initial stage because of the early presence of hoarseness, other lesions, such as those in the hypoglottic cone and laryngeal ventricle, have a subtler clinical, symptomatic and laryngoscopic manifestation. Alterations in the motility of the hemilarynx can also be linked to conditions relating to mediastinal diseases. Information that is particularly important to collect when describing the larynx includes the patency of pyriform sinuses - areas from where squamous cell cancers frequently originate - as well as the aspect of motility of the cricoarytenoid units, which typically appear altered in the presence of suspected infiltrating lesions.

While high definition (HD) light optic fibre endoscopies enable a macroscopic view of mucosas, narrow band imaging (NBI) and autofluorescence technologies [50-53] allow, by means of specific filters, to distinguish the pathological lesion, characterised by its typical anarchic hypervascularisation, from the rest of the healthy mucosa, leading to early lesion diagnosis and directing further biopsy investigations. Beyond what is made possible by clinical examinations pertaining to the ENT specialist's competence, using diagnostic radiography is anyway essential to continue the diagnosing pathway - thus the already mentioned importance of a multidisciplinary approach in the treatment of an oncologic disease. As a matter of fact, diagnostic radiography images enable specialists to stage the disease by knowing its actual local and, if applicable, distant depth extension.

IMAGING TOOLS IN HEAD AND NECK

Cross-sectional imaging techniques are ultrasound (US) scan with or without fine-needle aspiration cytology (FNAC), contrast-enhanced computed tomography (CECT), magnetic resonance imaging (MRI) with or without diffusion-weighted (DW) sequences (DW MRI), positron emission tomography (PET)/CT or a combination of these techniques [54].

Each modality has its own strengths and drawbacks and findings provided by the different imaging modalities are usually complementary. The imaging role encompasses for the detection/exclusion of lesion, its characterization in terms of size, extent, regional lymph nodal involvement, perineural or perivascular spread, bone infiltration or long-ranging metastasis. Advanced imaging is also used to address biopsies, to decide and plan tailored treatments, and to assess/follow-up treatment response in head and neck tumors.

According to local (Tumor size and surrounding diffusion - T), regional (involvement of lymph nodes - N) and distant (presence/absence of metastases - M), the union for international cancer control (UICC) has classified head and neck tumors into different stages (TNM classification), determining a specific treatment (surgery and/or chemotherapy and/or radiotherapy) and prognosis. While different histological subtypes and anatomical subsites have different T staging [55], the N parameter is related to the site, number and laterality of the lymph nodes involved by the primary tumour site.

N staging for most tumours (except the nasopharynx and thyroid)

Nx means that the regional lymph nodes cannot be assessed

N0 no node involvement

N1 single ipsilateral lymph node 3 cm or less in greatest diameter

N2a single ipsilateral lymph node between 3 and 6 cm

N2b multiple ipsilateral lymph nodes less than 6 cm

N2c contralateral or bilateral lymph nodes less than 6 cm

N3 any lymph node larger than 6 cm.

N staging of nasopharyngeal tumours (midline nodes are considered ipsilateral)

N0 no node involvement

N1 ipsilateral single lymph node above the supraclavicular fossa, and/or unilateral or bilateral retropharyngeal lymph node(s), 3 cm or less in greatest dimension

N2a ipsilateral single lymph node between 3 to 6 cm

N2b multiple ipsilateral lymph nodes less than 6 cm

N2c contralateral or bilateral lymph node(s) 6 cm in greatest diameter above the supraclavicular fossa

N3a lymph node or nodes larger than 6 cm, unilateral or bilateral

N3b extension to the supraclavicular fossa

N staging for thyroid cancer

N1a level VI (pretracheal, paratracheal, prelaryngeal/Delphian lymph nodes)

N1b unilateral, bilateral or contralateral cervical (level I-V), retropharyngeal or superior mediastinal (level VII) nodes.

Distant metastases represent another crucial prognostic factor conditioning the therapeutical approach, referring to M0 for no distant metastasis and M1 for diffusion to distant organs beyond the regional lymph nodes. Al already mentioned, each imaging modality has intrinsic advantages and weakness in a so complex district as the head and neck region, differently contributing to each of the T, N, and M parameter.

As for the primary tumor assessment (T parameter), MRI, and CT differently contribute to the diagnostic phase, according to the subset and the clinical issue, while US has a limited role and it is performed mainly to evaluate salivary gland tumors, drive biopsies or to characterize/monitoring regional lymph nodal involvement [56]. Thanks to the colour Doppler technique, it enables to assess the way vascularisation behaves in the area, which can be peripheral or, in suspicious cases, intralesional with an increased flow. PET/CT, instead, is commonly prescribed to assess regional nodal infiltration and/or distant metastases in advanced stage head and neck tumors, and it is commonly performed with 18 fluoro-deoxyglucose tracers, which is preferentially transported and trapped into hypermetabolic cancerous or inflamed tissues.

MRI represents the imaging gold standard to characterize nasopharyngeal malignancy because of its superior contrast resolution, mainly for the assessment of adjacent soft tissue invasion (*e.g.*, the pharyngobasilar fascia, sinus of Morgagni, skull base, intracranial involvement, and perineural spread). CT, instead, provides meaningful information regarding possible bony invasion, mainly for sinonasal pathology, and for the planning of open or endoscopic sinus surgery.

Regarding the carcinomas of the oral cavity and oropharynx, the choice of the cross-sectional imaging technique is often tricky, for example, due to dental hardware artifacts, mainly for CT scan, or movement artifacts due to patient swallowing and breathing, mainly for MR acquisition. While according to clinical issue, CT often represents the first step to define possible mandible and maxilla invasion, MR is more informative to establish bone marrow invasion and perineural spread, or to characterize small soft tissue tumors, such as primary tongue tumor's submucosal extension [57‾59].

Finally, considering the primary laryngeal or hypopharyngeal malignancies, CT is generally preferred to assess cartilaginous erosion, almost for the MR longer acquisition time that can be affected by swallowing artifacts [60]. Head and neck oncological lesions can appear as an asymmetry of the aerial lumen, or an asymmetrical thickening of the mucosa, or a soft tissue density mass on CT, that generally show a T2-weighted hyperintense signal and a T1-weighted hypo-isointensity on MR sequences, compared to healthy muscle [61]. If absent procedural contraindications like severe renal failure or previous anaphylactic reaction to contrast media, all the histological subtypes can enhance after contrasted medium injection, according to their vascularity. The more recent introduction of diffusion-weighted sequences (DW-MRI) can help to better identify hypercellular tumors, and mainly to distinguish between a disease relapse from phlogosis/scars caused by post-treatment alterations during the follow-up.

As for bony invasion assessment, imaging findings are often represented by a discontinuity of the normal hyper-attenuating cortical on CT or hypointense signal on MR, that can be paralleled by a medullary alteration, better detected by short tau inversion-recovery (STIR) sequence on MRI or spectral acquisitions on modern CT scan [61]. Regarding perineural diffusion, while CT shows only indirect signs as foramina enlargement or surrounding soft-tissue inhomogeneity, MRI can highlight a thickening of the nerve with a clearer hyperintensity following contrast medium injection [61].

Finally, considering the complementarity of information provided by PET/CT and MRI, several technological efforts have been done to combine these two modalities in a simultaneous PET/MR scanner. This need arises from the evidences of a relatively poor soft-tissue contrast especially when using low-dose PET/CT acquisition protocols or when intravenous contrast material is not injected, and from the additional CT radiation dose administered to the patient, that can have detrimental effects mainly in pediatric patients and in strict longitudinal follow-ups [62].

Despite the initial euphoria generated by the implementation of PET/MRI scanners for clinical use (Fig. 1), scientific data evaluating the clinical usefulness of hybrid PET/MRI systems remain at an early stage, and only very few studies have so far addressed the clinical workflow, feasibility and optimized imaging protocols in the head and neck [63‾69].

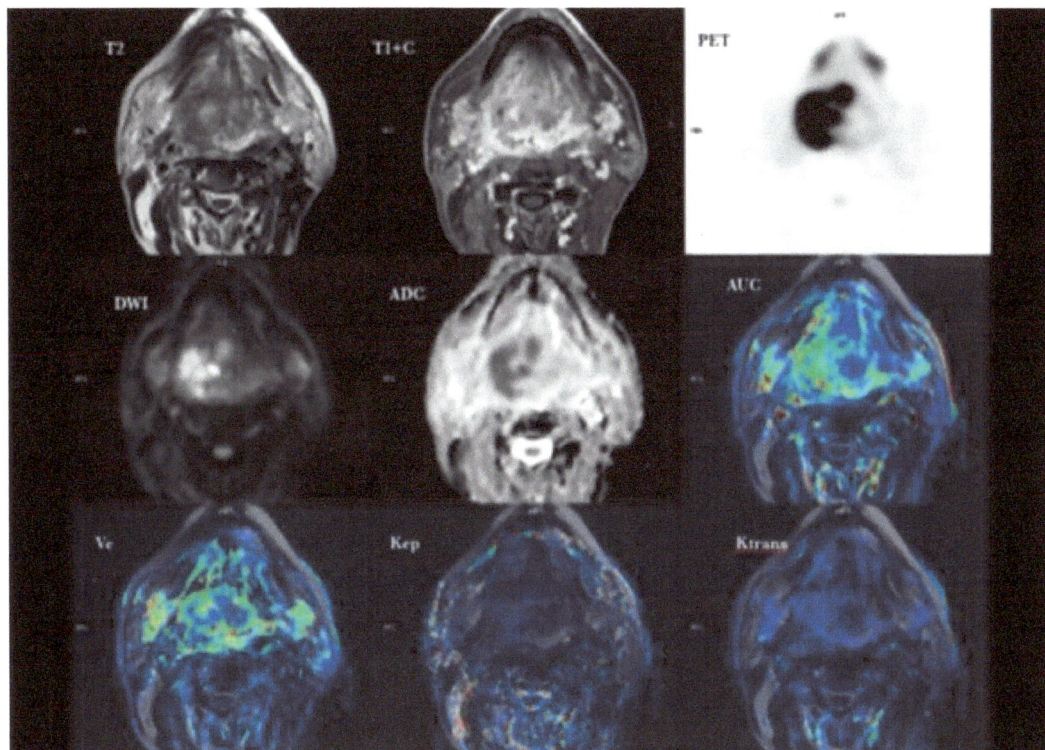

Fig. **(1))**
PET/MRI of tongue tumour.

As for N parameter, detection of nodal metastases occurs in about 50% of patients at diagnosis, deeply affecting prognosis and survival rates in head and neck cancers [70]. Although the need for an accurate imaging method to assess lymph nodes is paramount, both CT and MRI, commonly used to characterize nodal involvement, missed at least an half of occult metastases [71]. This finding is due to the evidence that all currently available diagnostic imaging methods for nodal involvement assessment, rely on size (transversal short axis diameter of more than 1.5 cm for Level II nodes, and more than 1 cm for all other nodes) and morphologic criteria (rounded shape and loss of fatty hilum) [72‑75] and that the identification of lymph node necrosis, the most predictive finding, has a limited role in smaller nodes (< 3cm) [76, 77]. Imaging signs that suggest an extracapsular nodal spread include capsular enhancement and irregularity, and infiltration of adjacent fat or muscle planes [61, 78‑82]. The extracapsular spread is a crucial prognostic factor, considered the increased locoregional failure if treatment consists of only surgery.

Although, hybrid PET/MRI has demonstrated higher accuracy in the assessment of primary tumor (T-staging), no significant added value has been shown for lymph nodes involvement (N-staging) and limited improvement for metastasis detection (M-staging) when compared to PET/CT scan [83, 84]. As for imaging follow-up in head and neck cancer, an effort has been made by the ACR to standardize imaging surveillance and reporting with the introduction in August 2016 of the Neck Imaging Reporting and Data Systems (NI-RADS) [85]. Originally developed for CECT [86], NI-RADS template can be adapted to other cross-sectional imaging techniques [87] categorizing the disease's status from 0 to 4, according to imaging suspicion (0 - incomplete, 1- negative, 2- low suspicion, 3- high suspicion, and 4- definite recurrence). Nevertheless, it has to be taken into account that imaging pattern varies accordingly to the type of treatment received, including edema, inflammation, fibrosis, and others that can render tricky differentiate between tumor recurrence and post-treatment alterations in the early stages [88].

More recently, radiomics technique has been introduced [89⁻91], as an high-throughput extraction approach of quantitative imaging features, able to (I) non-invasively characterize the overall tumor accounting for heterogeneity; (II) produce prognostic and/or predictive biomarker value derived from routine, standard of care imaging data as-is; and (III) allow for a fast, low-cost, and repeatable means for longitudinal monitoring [92⁻94]. This kind of approach can be applied to all cross-sectional imaging techniques to non-invasively disentangle among the heterogeneous composition of head and neck cancers toward a personalized patient's treatment. Several promising applications of radiomics framework have been applied to classify and segment head and neck cancers. For instance, different studies have classified head and neck tumors by human papillomavirus (HPV) status with textural analysis [95⁻98], or segmented in an automatic manner healthy by cancerous tissue [99⁻101].

PREDICTIVE AND PROGNOSTIC BIOMOLECULAR TOOLS FOR HEAD AND NECK CANCER

In head and neck cancers (HNC) predictive factors - namely, biological characteristics that can be used to predict tumor response to a specific treatment - are currently remarkably lacking. Conversely, some bio-molecular parameters are recognized as prognostic factors of the disease, since they indicate tumor characteristics that inform about cancer outcome, independently of treatment the patients will undergo. The most prominent prognostic factor for head and neck cancers is viral etiology, specifically HPV-mediated disease for oropharyngeal carcinomas and EBV-mediated disease for nasopharyngeal carcinoma.

Biomarkers Related to Viral Etiology

High-risk a-human papillomaviruses (HPVs), and in particular HPV type 16, have been etiologically linked to a subgroup of oropharyngeal squamous cell carcinomas (OPSCCs) arising from the epithelium lining the crypt of the palatine and lingual tonsils and are responsible for a substantial fraction of SCCs from unknown primary metastatic to the neck nodes [102]. These HPV-driven SCCs are increasing in many Western countries and are associated with a platform-independent survival benefit compared to non-HPV-driven cases, with several studies reporting a considerably reduced risk of death (up to 80%) and relapse (up to 70%) [103]. Thus, identifying those HPV infections that are the real driving force behind the carcinogenesis process is of paramount importance. Detection of HPV E6/E7 mRNA by polymerase chain reaction (PCR) in frozen samples is considered the gold standard for diagnosis of oncologically-relevant HPV infections but it is often clinically unfeasible. In a clinical setting, HPV-status is primarily assessed using FFPE-based diagnostic tests such as HPV DNA detection (by PCR or *in situ* hybridisation) or immunostaining for cyclin-dependent kinase inhibitor $p16^{INK4a}$, considered a surrogate marker for active HPV involvement in OPSCC tumorigenesis. Unfortunately, both markers lack adequate sensitivity and/or specificity. HPV DNA testing positive to PCR sequencing may be related to transient, non-transforming HPV infection or to laboratory contamination [104]. Additionally, $p16^{INK4a}$ over-expression could be triggered by HPV-independent deregulation of $p16^{INK4a}$/RB signaling pathway with 10 to 20% of $p16^{INK4a}$-positive OPSCC resulting in HPV-DNA/RNA negative [102, 105⁻107].

Furthermore, immunostaining for $p16^{INK4a}$ is unable to discriminate between infections supported by HPV16 and non-HPV16 strains and recent studies have highlighted the negative prognostic role of non-HPV16 strains, especially HPV33 [108]. Finally, fluorescence *in situ* hybridization has acceptable specificity but lacks adequate sensitivity. Consistently, prognostic stratification based on HPV-DNA or $p16^{INK4a}$ immunostaining as standalone tests is disappointing and patients testing $p16^{positive}$/HPV DNA^{negative} have significantly poorer survival compared to double-positive cases [106]. Regrettably, the eighth edition of the AJCC/UICC TNM staging system and most of the ongoing clinical trials exploring treatment de-escalation in patients with OPSCC are classifying patients as harboring and HPV-related cancer on the basis of $p16^{INK4a}$ immunostaining positivity alone [109]. This raises ethical concerns because it would expose a fraction of the patients whose $p16^{INK4a}$ over-expression is triggered by an HPV-independent mechanism to prognostic misclassification and suboptimal treatment. Thus, it is strongly recommended to aim for the positivity to both p16^{INK4a} immunostaining and HPV DNA to define an OPSCC as HPV-driven in order to obtain more accurate prognostic information [110].

The contemporary anatomy-based staging system for nasopharyngeal carcinoma (NPC) is inadequate for predicting prognosis or treatment benefits. Pre-treatment EBV DNA is found in about 95% of patients with NPC in endemic areas. Circulating serum EBV DNA has been established as a robust prognostic biomarker in patients with NPC and has been used for population screening, predicting treatment response for therapeutic adaptation, and disease surveillance, and prognostication [111]. Particularly, high pre-treatment EBV DNA levels, unfavorable EBV DNA response after chemotherapy, midcourse of radiotherapy, or post-treatment are adverse prognosticators for clinical outcomes, including distant relapse and worse survival.

Biomarkers in the Era of Target Therapy and Immune Checkpoint Inhibitors

Among the other biomarkers of head and neck cancers, the most widely studied is the epidermal growth factor receptor (EGFR), whose biological role in these tumors has been established since the late decades of the last century. Aberrant EGFR activity in head and neck cancers is the result of different molecular mechanisms, including overexpression of receptor or ligands, *EGFR* gene amplification, protein mutations/polymorphisms, and transactivation by other tyrosine kinases receptors [112-114]. The direct causative role of EGFR and its pathway in the pathogenesis of head and neck cancers has been proved by *in vitro* studies and in patients and has led to the development of the molecular target therapy with anti-EGFR antibody Cetuximab. This pharmacological approach is currently applied in both curative and palliative settings [115, 116], and more antibodies against EGFR have been tested in controlled clinical trials [117].

Several studies investigated the prognostic value of EGFR in head and neck cancers, while only a limited number of studies explored the predictive role of EGFR in relation to a specific treatment. Overall, results indicate that neither EGFR overexpression nor the gene copy number can be used as predictive or prognostic tools for the treatment with EGFR inhibitors. For other treatments, current evidence supports the predictive and prognostic role of EGFR overexpression (assessed with quantitative assays) only in cases of exclusive radiotherapy, but not in multimodal treatments (surgery and chemoradiotherapy) [118].

Immunotherapy with programmed death 1 (PD-1) and programmed death-ligand 1 (PD-L1) targeted monoclonal antibodies is significantly changing the therapeutic approach and disease prognosis of head and neck cancers. Since 2016, when US Food and Drug Administration granted the approval for the first antiPD-1 immune checkpoint inhibitors nivolumab and pembrolizumab for recurrent head and neck squamous cell carcinoma refractory to platinum-based therapy, a significant number of controlled clinical trials have been produced, and positive results have led to the approval of pembrolizumab as first-line therapy [119]. A critical review of these studies is part of another chapter of this book, however, the role of biomarker testing (PD-L1) in patients with head and neck cancers deserves some comments. Very recent results of the randomized phase III clinical trial Keynote 048 [119] demonstrated a significant increase in overall survival after pembrolizumab monotherapy only in patients with PD-L1 immunohistochemical positivity. Conversely, the combination of pembrolizumab and chemotherapy provided significant benefit regardless of the expression of PD-L1. The best predictive value of the PD-L1 biomarker test was the combined positive score (CPS), which is the number of PD-L1 staining cells (tumor cells plus infiltrating lymphocytes and macrophages) divided by the total number of viable tumor cells, multiplied by 100. Currently, the international consensus documents underline the requirement of a validated immunohistochemical platform with validated PD-L1 antibodies to test the expression of PD-L1 with predictive value (8.9). Predictive CPS values are greater than or equal to 1, obtained with the immunohistochemical technique. Given that clinical responses have also been obtained in patients without significant expression of PD-L1, in the near future the identification of new and alternative biomarkers will be critical to improve the selection of patients with a better chance of responding to the new immune checkpoint inhibitors [120, 121].

Based on clinical objectivity, diagnostic, radiological and biomolecular investigations, a precise staging according to the AJCC TNM clinical criteria [122⁻124] is identified as follows in Table 2.

Table 2 **Exemplified Head and Neck TNM Staging [124].**

Clinical Tumor Classification (cT)		Clinical Nodes Classification (cN)	
Nasopharynx			
T1	Confined to nasopharynx or extension to oropharynx/nasal cavity	N1	Cervical unilateral metastasis/unilateral or bilateral retropharyngeal metastasis 6 cm or smaller above the caudal border of the cricoid cartilage

T2	Extension to parapharyngeal space/soft tissue of medial or lateral pterygoid or prevertebral muscles	N2	Cervical bilateral metastasis 6 cm or smaller above the caudal border of the cricoid cartilage
T3	Bony structures at skull base, cervical vertebra, pterygoid, paranasal sinuses	N3	Cervical unilateral/bilateral metastasis larger than 6 cm or extension below the caudal border of the cricoid cartilage
T4	Intracranial extension, cranial nerves, orbite, hypopharynx, parotid, soft tissue beyond the lateral pterygoid muscle		

Nasal Cavity and Ethmoid Sinus

T1	Restricted to any one subsite	N1	Single ipsilateral node <= 3 cm, without extranodal extension (ENE-)
T2	Extension to two subsites in a single region or adjacent region within the nasoethmoidal complex	N2a	3 – 6 cm single ipsilateral node, ENE-
		N2b	Multiple ipsilateral nodes <= 6 cm, ENE-
		N2c	Bilateral or controlateral nodes <= 6 cm, ENE-
T3	Extension to the medial wall/floor of the orbity/maxillary sinus/palate/cribriform plate	N3a	Node > 6 cm, ENE-
T4a	Extension to anterior orbital contents/nose or cheek skin/minimal extension to anterior cranial fossa/pterygoid plates/sphenoid or frontal sinuses		
T4b	Invasion of orbital apex/dura/brain/middle cranial fossa/nasopharynx/clivus/cranial nerves		

Maxillary Sinus

T1	Restricted to the mucosa of the maxillary sinus		
T2	Extension to bone of the sinus or extension into the hard palate/middle nasal meatus		
T3	Extension to the posterior wall of maxillary sinus/subcutaneous tissues/floor or medial wall of orbit/pterygoid fossa/etmoid sinuses	N3b	Any node with ENE
T4a	Extension to orbital contents/skin of cheek/pterygoid plates/infratemporal fossa/cribriform plate/sphenoid or frontal sinuses		
T4b	Invasion of orbital apex/dura/brain/middle cranial fossa/nasopharynx/clivus/cranial		

	nerves		
Oropharynx (p16+) – HPV Mediated			
T1	<= 2cm	N1	1 or multiple ipsilateral nodes < 6cm
T2	2-4 cm	N2	Controlateral/bilateral nodes < 6cm
T3	> 4cm/extension to lingual surface of epiglottis	N3	1 or multiple nodes > 6cm
T4	extension to larynx/extrinsic muscle of tongue/medial pterygoid/hard palate/mandible		
Oropharynx (p16-)			
T1	<= 2cm	N1	Single ipsilateral node <= 3 cm, ENE-
T2	2-4 cm	N2a	Single ipsilateral node 3-6 cm, ENE-
T3	> 4cm/extension to lingual surface of epiglottis	N2b	Multiple ipsilateral node <= 6 cm, ENE-
T4a	extension to larynx/extrinsic muscle of tongue/medial pterygoid/hard palate/mandible		
T4b	Invasion of pterygoid muscle/pterygoid plates/lateral nasopharynx/skull base/ carotid artery	N3a	Any node > 6cm ENE-
Oral Cavity			
T1	<= 2cm with Deep Of Invasion (DOI)<=5mm	N1	Single ipsilateral node <= 3 cm, ENE-
T2	2-4 cm with DOI <= 10mm	N2a	Single ipsilateral node 3-6 cm, ENE-
T3	> 4cm with DOI <= 10mm	N2b	Multiple ipsilateral node <= 6 cm, ENE-
	or 2-4 cm with DOI > 10mm	N2c	Bilateral/controlateral node <= 6 cm, ENE-
T4a	> 4cm with DOI > 10mm	N3a	Any node > 6cm ENE-
	or invasion of adjacent structures (mandible, maxilla, face skin, maxillary sinus)	N3b	Any node with ENE
Oral Cavity			
T4b	Invasion of masticatory space/pterygoid plates/skull base/internal carotid artery (ICA)	-	-

Hypopharynx		
T1	<= 2cm / limited to one subsite of hypopharynx	
T2	2-4 cm without fixation of hemilarynx / ivasion > 1 hypopharynx subsite or adjacent site	
T3	> 4cm with fixation of hemilarynx / esophageal mucosa extension	
T4a	invasion of thyroid/cricoid/hyoid bone/thyroid gland/esophageal muscle/central compartment soft tissue (with strap muscles and subcutaneous fat)	
T4b	Invasion of prevertebral fascia/carotid artery/mediastinal structures	
Larynx: Supraglottis		
T1	limited to one subsite of supraglottis with normal vocal cord mobility	
T2	ivasion of mucosa of adjacent subsites of glottis/supraglottis/region outside supraglottis (mucosa of ase of tongue, vallecula, medial wall of pyrform sinus without fixation of the larynx	
T3	Limited to larynx with vocal cord fixation / invasion of postcricoid area/preepiglottic space/paraglottic space/inner cortex of thyroid cartilage	
T4a	invasion through the cortex of thyroid cartilage / trachea/deep extrinsic tongue muscles/strap muscles/thyroid/esophagus	
T4b	Invasion of prevertebral spce/carotid artery/mediastinal structures	
Larynx: Glottis	-	-
T1a	limited to one vocal cord	N1	Single ipsilateral node <= 3 cm, ENE-
T1b	Involves both vocal cord	N2a	Single ipsilateral node 3-6 cm, ENE-
T2	extension to supraglottis/subglottis/impaired vocal cord mobility	N2b	Multiple ipsilateral nodes <= 6 cm, ENE-
T3	Limited to larynx with vocal cord fixation / invasion of paraglottic space/inner cortex of thyroid cartilage	N2c	Bilateral or controlateral nodes <= 6 cm, ENE-

T4a	invasion through the cortex of thyroid cartilage / trachea/cricoid/deep extrinsic tongue muscles/strap muscles/thyroid/esophagus	N3a	Node > 6 cm, ENE-
T4b	Invasion of prevertebral spce/carotid artery/mediastinal structures	N3b	Any node with ENE
Larynx: Subglottis		-	-
T1	limited to the subglottis		
T2	ivasion of vocal cord with normal/impaired mobility		
T3	Limited to larynx with vocal cord fixation / invasion of paraglottic space/inner cortex of thyroid cartilage	-	-
T4a	invasion of thyroid cartilage / cricoid/trachea/deep extrinsic tongue muscles/strap muscles/thyroid/esophagus		
T4b	Invasion of prevertebral spce/carotid artery/mediastinal structures		

Clinical Definition of Distant Metastasis (cM)	
M0	No distant metastasis
M1	Distant metastasis

CONCLUSIONS

Performing a correct and in-depth assessment is important in order to reach to an exact tumor diagnosis and staging. To know the correct stage of the disease, it is necessary to follow, thoroughly and precisely, a proper approach to the patient through a clear investigation and assessment composed of detailed medical history, clinical evidence, diagnostic, radiological and biomolecular investigations. The accurate stage of the disease is critical to determine for a multidisciplinary therapeutic choice that is most suitable for the patient, in terms of oncological radicality, improvement of prognosis and quality of life of any head and neck cancer patients.

CONSENT FOR PUBLICATION

Not applicable.

CONFLICT OF INTEREST

The authors confirm that the content of this chapter have no conflict of interest.

ACKNOWLEDGEMENTS

Declared none.

REFERENCES

[1]   Robbins KT, Clayman G, Levine PA, *et al.* American Head and Neck SocietyAmerican Academy of Otolaryngology--Head and Neck SurgeryNeck dissection classification update: revisions proposed by the American Head and Neck Society and the American Academy of Otolaryngology-Head and Neck Surgery. Arch Otolaryngol Head Neck Surg 2002; 128(7): 751-8.[http://dx.doi.org/10.1001/archotol.128.7.751] [PMID: 12117328]

[2]   Beahrs O, Henson DE, Hutter RVP, Kennedy BJ. American Joint Committee on Cancer: manual for staging of cancer (4th ed.), 4th ed.1992.

[3]   Marcy A. List PhD, Chris Ritter-Sterr MS, RN, Shirley BLansky MD A performance status scale for head and neck cancer patients. ACS J 1990.[http://dx.doi.org/10.1002/1097-0142(19900801)66:3564:   AID-CNCR2820660326>3.0.CO;2-D (1990)]

[4]   Cerezo L, Millán I, Torre A, Aragón G, Otero J. Prognostic factors for survival and tumor control in cervical lymph node metastases from head and neck cancer. A multivariate study of 492 cases. Cancer 1992; 69(5): 1224-34.[http://dx.doi.org/10.1002/cncr.2820690526] [PMID: 1739921]

[5]   Deleyiannis FW, Thomas DB, Vaughan TL, Davis S. Alcoholism: independent predictor of survival in patients with head and neck cancer. J Natl Cancer Inst 1996; 88(8): 542-9.[http://dx.doi.org/10.1093/jnci/88.8.542] [PMID: 8606383]

[6]   Amini A, Jasem J, Jones BL, *et al.* Predictors of overall survival in human papillomavirus-associated oropharyngeal cancer using the National Cancer Data Base. Oral Oncol 2016; 56(56): 1-7.[http://dx.doi.org/10.1016/j.oraloncology.2016.02.011] [PMID: 27086480]

[7]   Faye-Lund H, Abdelnoor M. Prognostic factors of survival in a cohort of head and neck cancer patients in Oslo. Eur J Cancer B Oral Oncol 1996; 32B(2): 83-90.[http://dx.doi.org/10.1016/0964-1955(95)00073-9] [PMID: 8736169]

[8]   Von Gunten CF. Palliative Care and Rehabilitation of Cancer Patients Kluwer Academic Publishers 1999.[http://dx.doi.org/10.1007/978-1-4615-5003-7]

[9]   Lee DH, Roh JL, Baek S, *et al.* Second cancer incidence, risk factor, and specific mortality in head and neck squamous cell carcinoma. Otolaryngol Head Neck Surg 2013; 149(4): 579-86.[http://dx.doi.org/10.1177/0194599813496373] [PMID: 23820107]

[10]   Huang SH, Xu W, Waldron J. Refining american joint committtee on cancer/union for international cancer control tnm stage and prognostic groups for human papillomavirus-related oropharyngeal carcinomas. J Clin Oncol 1992; 25: 231-41.

[11]   Daniel GD, Jeremy DR, Samir SK, Ferris RL, Wang MB. The "new" head and neck cancer patient-young, nonsmoker, nondrinker, and HPV positive: evaluation. Otolaryngol Head Neck Surg 2014; 151(3): 375-80.

[12]   Piccirillo JF. Inclusion of comorbidity in a staging system for head and neck cancer. Oncology (Williston Park) 1995; 9(9): 831-6.[PMID: 8562325]

[13]   Urist MM, O'Brien CJ, Soong SJ, Visscher DW, Maddox WA. Squamous cell carcinoma of the buccal mucosa: analysis of prognostic factors. Am J Surg 1987; 154(4): 411-4.[http://dx.doi.org/10.1016/0002-9610(89)90014-7] [PMID: 3661845]

[14]   Medina JE. A rational classification of neck dissections. Otolaryngol Head Neck Surg 1989; 100(3): 169-76.[http://dx.doi.org/10.1177/019459988910000301] [PMID: 2496376]

[15] Pauloski BR, Logemann JA, Colangelo LA, *et al*. Surgical variables affecting speech in treated patients with oral and oropharyngeal cancer. Laryngoscope 1998; 108(6): 908-16.[http://dx.doi.org/10.1097/00005537-199806000-00022] [PMID: 9628509]

[16] Colangelo LA, Logemann JA, Pauloski BR, Pelzer JR, Rademaker AW. T stage and functional outcome in oral and oropharyngeal cancer patients. Head Neck 1996; 18(3): 259-68.[http://dx.doi.org/10.1002/(SICI)1097-0347(199605/06)18:3<259::AID-HED8>3.0.CO;2-Z] [PMID: 8860768]

[17] de Leeuw JRJ, de Graeff A, Ros WJG, Blijham GH, Hordijk GJ, Winnubst JA. Prediction of depressive symptomatology after treatment of head and neck cancer: the influence of pre-treatment physical and depressive symptoms, coping, and social support. Head Neck 2000; 22(8): 799-807.[http://dx.doi.org/10.1002/1097-0347(200012)22:8<799::AID-HED9>3.0.CO;2-E] [PMID: 11084641]

[18] Levendag PC, Teguh DN, Voet P. Dysphagia disorders in patients with cancer of the oropharynx are significantly affected by the radiation dose-effect relationship. Radiother Oncol 2007; 85: 54-73.[http://dx.doi.org/10.1016/j.radonc.2007.07.009] [PMID: 17714815]

[19] Ansarin M, Cattaneo A, De Benedetto L, *et al*. Retrospective analysis of factors influencing oncologic outcome in 590 patients with early-intermediate glottic cancer treated by transoral laser microsurgery. Head Neck 2017; 39(1): 71-81.[http://dx.doi.org/10.1002/hed.24534] [PMID: 27453475]

[20] Richard JM, Sancho-Garnier H, Micheau C, Saravane D, Cachin Y. Prognostic factors in cervical lymph node metastasis in upper respiratory and digestive tract carcinomas: study of 1,713 cases during a 15-year period. Laryngoscope 1987; 97(1): 97-101.[http://dx.doi.org/10.1288/00005537-198701000-00019] [PMID: 3796181]

[21] Chan JKC, Pilch BZ, Kuo TT, Wenig BM, Lee AWM. Tumours of the nasopharynx. In: Eveson BL, JW RP, Sidransky D, eds. World Health Organization classification of tumour, pathology and genetics Eveson BL, JW RP, Sidransky D. 2005815-97.

[22] Kujan O, Glenny AM, Oliver RJ, Thakker N, Sloan P. Screening programmes for the early detection and prevention of oral cancer. Cochrane Database Syst Rev 2006; 3(3): CD004150.[http://dx.doi.org/10.1002/14651858.CD004150.pub2] [PMID: 16856035]

[23] Chu EA, Kim YJ. Laryngeal cancer: diagnosis and preoperative work-up. Otolaryngol Clin North Am 2008; 41(4): 673-95.[http://dx.doi.org/10.1016/j.otc.2008.01.016] [PMID: 18570953]

[24] House JW, Brackmann DE. Facial nerve grading system. Otolaryngol Head Neck Surg 1985; 93(2): 146-7.[http://dx.doi.org/10.1177/019459988509300202] [PMID: 3921901]

[25] Strong EW, Kasdorf H, Henk JM. Squamous cell carcinoma of the head and neck. In: Hermanek P, Gospodarowicz MK, Henson DE, eds. Prognostic factors in cancer, UICC Geneva Hermanek P, Gospodarowicz MK, Henson DE. 199523-7.[http://dx.doi.org/10.1007/978-3-642-79395-0_2]

[26] Elackattu A, Jalisi S. Living with head and neck cancer and coping with dying when treatments fail. Otolaryngol Clin North Am 2009; 42(1): 171-84.[http://dx.doi.org/10.1016/j.otc.2008.09.004] [PMID: 19134499]

[27] Lind SE, DelVecchio Good MJ, Seidel S, Csordas T, Good BJ. Telling the diagnosis of cancer. J Clin Oncol 1989; 7(5): 583-9.[http://dx.doi.org/10.1200/JCO.1989.7.5.583] [PMID: 2709087]

[28] Warnakulasuriya S, Johnson NW, van der Waal I. Nomenclature and classification of potentially malignant disorders of the oral mucosa. J Oral Pathol Med 2007; 36(10): 575-80.[http://dx.doi.org/10.1111/j.1600-0714.2007.00582.x] [PMID: 17944749]

[29] Napier S, Speight P. Natural history of potentially malignant oral lesions and conditions: an overview of the literature. J Oral Pathol Med 2007; 36: 575-80.[PMID: 18154571]

[30] Standring S, Ellis H, Berkovitz BKB. Larynx. In: Standring S, Ellis H, Berkovitz BKB, eds. Gray's anatomy: the anatomical basis of clinical practice (39th ed.) 39th ed.Standring S, Ellis H, Berkovitz BKB. 2005633-46.

[31] Jatin P. Shah, Snehal G Patel, Bhuvanesh Singh Head and Neck Surgery and Oncology 2012.

[32] Bosetti C, Garavello W, Gallus S, La Vecchia C. Effects of smoking cessation on the risk of laryngeal cancer: an overview of published studies. Oral Oncol 2006; 42(9): 866-72.[http://dx.doi.org/10.1016/j.oraloncology.2006.02.008] [PMID: 16931120]

[33] Batsakis JG. The pathology of head and neck tumors: nasal cavity and paranasal sinuses, part 5. Head Neck Surg 1980; 2(5): 410-9.[http://dx.doi.org/10.1002/hed.2890020510] [PMID: 7364592]

[34] Arnold W, Ganzer U. Checkliste Hals-Nasen-Ohren-Heilkunde (4th ed.), 4th ed.2005.

[35] Kachlik D, Baca V, Bozdechova I, Cech P, Musil V. Anatomical terminology and nomenclature: past, present and highlights. Surg Radiol Anat 2008; 30(6): 459-66.[http://dx.doi.org/10.1007/s00276-008-0357-y]

[PMID: 18488135]

[36] Wendell-Smith CP. Fascia: an illustrative problem in international terminology. Surg Radiol Anat 1997; 19(5): 273-7.[http://dx.doi.org/10.1007/BF01637586] [PMID: 9413070]

[37] Funk GF, Karnell LH, Christensen AJ. Long-term health-related quality of life in survivors of head and neck cancer. Arch Otolaryngol Head Neck Surg 2012; 138(2): 123-33.[http://dx.doi.org/10.1001/archoto.2011.234] [PMID: 22248560]

[38] Boenninghaus HG, Lenarz T. Hals-Nasen-Ohrenheilkunde für Medizinstudenten HNO (13th ed.), 13th ed.2007.

[39] Lee KJ, Toh EH. Otolaryngology A surgical notebook 2007.[http://dx.doi.org/10.1055/b-002-72243]

[40] Myers EN. Operative otolaryngology: head and neck surgery (2nd ed.), 2nd ed.2008.

[41] Seiden AM, Tami TA, Pensak ML, Cotton RT, Gluckman JL. Otolaryngology. The Essentials 2001.

[42] Lee A, Foo W, Law S. N-staging of nasopharyngeal carcinoma: discrepancy between UICC/AJCC and Ho systems. Clin Oncol (R Coll Radiol) 1995; 17: 377-81.[PMID: 8814369]

[43] Pugliano FA, Piccirillo JF, Zequeira MR, et al. Clinical-severity staging system for oropharyngeal cancer: five-year survival rates. Arch Otolaryngol Head Neck Surg 1997; 123(10): 1118-24.[http://dx.doi.org/10.1001/archotol.1997.01900100094013] [PMID: 9339990]

[44] Robbins KT, Clayman G, Levine PA. Neck dissection classification update: revisions proposed by the American head and neck society and the American academy of otolaryngology-head and neck surgery. Arch Otolaryngol Head Neck Surg 2002; 128: 751-8.

[45] Schechter GL, Kalafsky JT. Cancer of the hypopharynx and cervical esophagus: management concepts. Oncology (Williston Park) 1988; 2(5): 17-24, 34-35.[PMID: 3079327]

[46] Au JSK, Law CK, Foo W, Lau WH. In-depth evaluation of the AJCC/UICC 1997 staging system of nasopharyngeal carcinoma: prognostic homogeneity and proposed refinements. Int J Radiat Oncol Biol Phys 2003; 56(2): 413-26.[http://dx.doi.org/10.1016/S0360-3016(02)04610-2] [PMID: 12738316]

[47] Low JS, Heng DM, Wee JT. The question of T2a and N3a in the UICC/AJCC (1997) staging system for nasopharyngeal carcinoma. Clin Oncol (R Coll Radiol) 2004; 16(8): 581-3.[http://dx.doi.org/10.1016/j.clon.2004.08.003] [PMID: 15630856]

[48] Roh J-L, Sung MW, Kim KH, et al. Nasopharyngeal carcinoma with skull base invasion: a necessity of staging subdivision. Am J Otolaryngol 2004; 25(1): 26-32.[http://dx.doi.org/10.1016/j.amjoto.2003.09.011] [PMID: 15011203]

[49] Cosway B, Drinnan M, Paleri V. Narrow band imaging for the diagnosis of head and neck squamous cell carcinoma: A systematic review. Head Neck 2016; 38 (Suppl. 1): E2358-67.[http://dx.doi.org/10.1002/hed.24300] [PMID: 26891200]

[50] Piazza C, Del Bon F, Peretti G, Nicolai P. Narrow band imaging in endoscopic evaluation of the larynx. Curr Opin Otolaryngol Head Neck Surg 2012; 20(6): 472-6.[http://dx.doi.org/10.1097/MOO.0b013e32835908ac] [PMID: 23000733]

[51] Watanabe A, Taniguchi M, Tsujie H, Hosokawa M, Fujita M, Sasaki S. The value of narrow band imaging for early detection of laryngeal cancer. Eur Arch Otorhinolaryngol 2009; 266(7): 1017-23.[http://dx.doi.org/10.1007/s00405-008-0835-1] [PMID: 18982341]

[52] Tirelli G, Piovesana M, Bonini P, Gatto A, Azzarello G, Boscolo Nata F. Follow-up of oral and oropharyngeal cancer using narrow-band imaging and high-definition television with rigid endoscope to obtain an early diagnosis of second primary tumors: a prospective study. Eur Arch Otorhinolaryngol 2017; 274(6): 2529-36.[http://dx.doi.org/10.1007/s00405-017-4515-x] [PMID: 28283788]

[53] Bolzoni A, Cappiello J, Piazza C, et al. Diagnostic accuracy of magnetic resonance imaging in the assessment of mandibular involvement in oral-oropharyngeal squamous cell carcinoma: a prospective study. Arch Otolaryngol Head Neck Surg 2004; 130(7): 837-43.[http://dx.doi.org/10.1001/archotol.130.7.837] [PMID: 15262760]

[54] Tshering Vogel DW, Thoeny HC. Cross-sectional imaging in cancers of the head and neck: how we review and report. Cancer Imaging 2016; 16(1): 20.[http://dx.doi.org/10.1186/s40644-016-0075-3] [PMID: 27487932]

[55] Sobin LH, Gospodaroqicz MK, Wittekind C. TNM classification of malignant tumours (7th.), 7th.2009.

[56] Baatenburg de Jong RJ, Rongen RJ, Verwoerd CD, van Overhagen H, Laméris JS, Knegt P. Ultrasound-guided fine-needle aspiration biopsy of neck nodes. Arch Otolaryngol Head Neck Surg 1991; 117(4): 402-4.[http://dx.doi.org/10.1001/archotol.1991.01870160056008] [PMID: 2007009]

[57] Kim SY, Roh JL, Kim JS, *et al.* Utility of FDG PET in patients with squamous cell carcinomas of the oral cavity. Eur J Surg Oncol 2008; 34(2): 208-15.[http://dx.doi.org/10.1016/j.ejso.2007.03.015] [PMID: 17482789]

[58] Ng SH, Yen TC, Chang JT, *et al.* Prospective study of [18F]fluorodeoxyglucose positron emission tomography and computed tomography and magnetic resonance imaging in oral cavity squamous cell carcinoma with palpably negative neck. J Clin Oncol 2006; 24(27): 4371-6.[http://dx.doi.org/10.1200/JCO.2006.05.7349] [PMID: 16983105]

[59] Hsu WC, Loevner LA, Karpati R, *et al.* Accuracy of magnetic resonance imaging in predicting absence of fixation of head and neck cancer to the prevertebral space. Head Neck 2005; 27(2): 95-100.[http://dx.doi.org/10.1002/hed.20128] [PMID: 15627263]

[60] Keberle M, Kenn W, Hahn D. Current concepts in imaging of laryngeal and hypopharyngeal cancer. Eur Radiol 2002; 12(7): 1672-83.[http://dx.doi.org/10.1007/s00330-002-1319-0] [PMID: 12111057]

[61] Abraham J. Imaging for head and neck cancer. Surg Oncol Clin N Am 2015; 24(3): 455-71.[http://dx.doi.org/10.1016/j.soc.2015.03.012] [PMID: 25979394]

[62] Aiello M, Cavaliere C, Marchitelli R, d'Albore A, De Vita E, Salvatore M. Hybrid pet/mri methodology. Int Rev Neurobiol 2018; 141: 97-128.[http://dx.doi.org/10.1016/bs.irn.2018.07.026] [PMID: 30314608]

[63] Boss A, Stegger L, Bisdas S, *et al.* Feasibility of simultaneous PET/MR imaging in the head and upper neck area. Eur Radiol 2011; 21(7): 1439-46.[http://dx.doi.org/10.1007/s00330-011-2072-z] [PMID: 21308378]

[64] Vargas MI, Becker M, Garibotto V, *et al.* Approaches for the optimization of MR protocols in clinical hybrid PET/MRI studies. MAGMA 2013; 26(1): 57-69.[http://dx.doi.org/10.1007/s10334-012-0340-9] [PMID: 23008016]

[65] Varoquaux A, Rager O, Poncet A, *et al.* Detection and quantification of focal uptake in head and neck tumours: (18)F-FDG PET/MR *versus* PET/CT. Eur J Nucl Med Mol Imaging 2014; 41(3): 462-75.[http://dx.doi.org/10.1007/s00259-013-2580-y] [PMID: 24108458]

[66] Becker M, Zaidi H. Imaging in head and neck squamous cell carcinoma: the potential role of PET/MRI. Br J Radiol 2014; 87(1036): 20130677.[http://dx.doi.org/10.1259/bjr.20130677] [PMID: 24649835]

[67] Covello M, Cavaliere C, Aiello M, *et al.* Simultaneous PET/MR head-neck cancer imaging: Preliminary clinical experience and multiparametric evaluation. Eur J Radiol 2015; 84(7): 1269-76.[http://dx.doi.org/10.1016/j.ejrad.2015.04.010] [PMID: 25958189]

[68] Cavaliere C, Romeo V, Aiello M, *et al.* Multiparametric evaluation by simultaneous PET-MRI examination in patients with histologically proven laryngeal cancer. Eur J Radiol 2017; 88: 47-55.[http://dx.doi.org/10.1016/j.ejrad.2016.12.034] [PMID: 28189208]

[69] Monti S, Cavaliere C, Covello M, Nicolai E, Salvatore M, Aiello M. An Evaluation of the Benefits of Simultaneous Acquisition on PET/MR Coregistration in Head/Neck Imaging. J Healthc Eng 2017; 2017: 2634389.[http://dx.doi.org/10.1155/2017/2634389] [PMID: 29065582]

[70] Chong VF, Khoo JB, Fan YF. Imaging of the nasopharynx and skull base. Magn Reson Imaging Clin N Am 2002; 10(4): 547-71.[http://dx.doi.org/10.1016/S1064-9689(02)00010-7] [PMID: 12685495]

[71] Genden EM, Ferlito A, Silver CE, *et al.* Contemporary management of cancer of the oral cavity. Eur Arch Otorhinolaryngol 2010; 267(7): 1001-17.[http://dx.doi.org/10.1007/s00405-010-1206-2] [PMID: 20155361]

[72] Castelijns JA, van den Brekel MW. Detection of lymph node metastases in the neck: radiologic criteria. AJNR Am J Neuroradiol 2001; 22(1): 3-4.[PMID: 11158879]

[73] Williams AD, Cousins C, Soutter WP, *et al.* Detection of pelvic lymph node metastases in gynecologic malignancy: a comparison of CT, MR imaging, and positron emission tomography. AJR Am J Roentgenol 2001; 177(2): 343-8.[http://dx.doi.org/10.2214/ajr.177.2.1770343] [PMID: 11461859]

[74] Heusch P, Sproll C, Buchbender C, *et al.* Diagnostic accuracy of ultrasound, ^{18}F-FDG-PET/CT, and fused ^{18}F-FDG-PET-MR images with DWI for the detection of cervical lymph node metastases of HNSCC. Clin Oral Investig 2014; 18(3): 969-78.[http://dx.doi.org/10.1007/s00784-013-1050-z] [PMID: 23892450]

[75] Torabi M, Aquino SL, Harisinghani MG. Current concepts in lymph node imaging. J Nucl Med 2004; 45(9): 1509-18.[PMID: 15347718]

[76] Som PM. Detection of metastasis in cervical lymph nodes: CT and MR criteria and differential diagnosis. AJR Am J Roentgenol 1992; 158(5): 961-9.[http://dx.doi.org/10.2214/ajr.158.5.1566697] [PMID: 1566697]

[77] van den Brekel MW, Stel HV, Castelijns JA, *et al.* Cervical lymph node metastasis: assessment of radiologic criteria. Radiology 1990; 177(2): 379-84.[http://dx.doi.org/10.1148/radiology.177.2.2217772] [PMID: 2217772]

[78] van den Brekel MW, van der Waal I, Meijer CJ, Freeman JL, Castelijns JA, Snow GB. The incidence of

micrometastases in neck dissection specimens obtained from elective neck dissections. Laryngoscope 1996; 106(8): 987-91.[http://dx.doi.org/10.1097/00005537-199608000-00014] [PMID: 8699914]

[79] Yousem DM, Som PM, Hackney DB, Schwaibold F, Hendrix RA. Central nodal necrosis and extracapsular neoplastic spread in cervical lymph nodes: MR imaging versus CT. Radiology 1992; 182(3): 753-9.[http://dx.doi.org/10.1148/radiology.182.3.1535890] [PMID: 1535890]

[80] Steinkamp HJ, Hosten N, Richter C, Schedel H, Felix R. Enlarged cervical lymph nodes at helical CT. Radiology 1994; 191(3): 795-8.[http://dx.doi.org/10.1148/radiology.191.3.8184067] [PMID: 8184067]

[81] Tartaglione T, Summaria V, Medoro A, Brunetti D, Di Lella GM, Zacchei P. Metastatic lymphadenopathy from ENT carcinoma: role of diagnostic imaging. Rays 2000; 25(4): 429-46.[PMID: 11367912]

[82] Hudgins PA, Kingdom TT, Weissler MC, Mukherji SK. Selective neck dissection: CT and MR imaging findings. AJNR Am J Neuroradiol 2005; 26(5): 1174-7.[PMID: 15891180]

[83] Buchbender C, Heusner TA, Lauenstein TC, Bockisch A, Antoch G. Oncologic PET/MRI, part 1: tumors of the brain, head and neck, chest, abdomen, and pelvis. J Nucl Med 2012; 53(6): 928-38.[http://dx.doi.org/10.2967/jnumed.112.105338] [PMID: 22582048]

[84] Kim SG, Friedman K, Patel S, Hagiwara M. Potential role of pet/mri for imaging metastatic lymph nodes in head and neck cancer. Am J Roentgenol 2016; 207(2): 248-56.[http://dx.doi.org/10.2214/AJR.16.16265] [PMID: 27163282]

[85] Aiken AH, Rath TJ, Anzai Y, et al. ACR Neck Imaging Reporting and Data Systems (NI-RADS): A White Paper of the ACR NI-RADS Committee. J Am Coll Radiol 2018; 15(8): 1097-108.[http://dx.doi.org/10.1016/j.jacr.2018.05.006] [PMID: 29983244]

[86] Aiken AH, Farley A, Baugnon KL. Implementation of a novel surveillance template for head and neck cancer: Neck Imaging Reporting and Data System (NI-RADS). J Am Coll Radiol 2016; 13: 743-746 e741.

[87] Krieger DA, Hudgins PA, Nayak GK, et al. Initial performance of NI- RADS to predict residual or recurrent head and neck squamous cell carcinoma. Am J Neuroradiol 2017; 38(6): 1193-9.[http://dx.doi.org/10.3174/ajnr.A5157] [PMID: 28364010]

[88] Hermans R. Posttreatment imaging in head and neck cancer. Eur J Radiol 2008; 66(3): 501-11.[http://dx.doi.org/10.1016/j.ejrad.2008.01.021] [PMID: 18328660]

[89] Zanfardino M, Franzese M, Pane K, et al. Bringing radiomics into a multi-omics framework for a comprehensive genotype-phenotype characterization of oncological diseases. J Transl Med 2019; 17(1): 337.[http://dx.doi.org/10.1186/s12967-019-2073-2] [PMID: 31590671]

[90] Aiello M, Cavaliere C, D'Albore A, Salvatore M. The challenges of diagnostic imaging in the era of big data. J Clin Med 2019; 8(3): E316.[http://dx.doi.org/10.3390/jcm8030316] [PMID: 30845692]

[91] Incoronato M, Aiello M, Infante T, et al. Radiogenomic analysis of oncological data: a technical survey. Int J Mol Sci 2017; 18(4): E805.[http://dx.doi.org/10.3390/ijms18040805] [PMID: 28417933]

[92] Gillies RJ, Kinahan PE, Hricak H. Radiomics: images are more than pictures, they are data. Radiology 2016; 278(2): 563-77.[http://dx.doi.org/10.1148/radiol.2015151169] [PMID: 26579733]

[93] Kumar V, Gu Y, Basu S, et al. Radiomics: the process and the challenges. Magn Reson Imaging 2012; 30(9): 1234-48.[http://dx.doi.org/10.1016/j.mri.2012.06.010] [PMID: 22898692]

[94] Wong AJ, Kanwar A, Mohamed AS, Fuller CD. Radiomics in head and neck cancer: from exploration to application. Transl Cancer Res 2016; 5(4): 371-82.[http://dx.doi.org/10.21037/tcr.2016.07.18] [PMID: 30627523]

[95] Buch K, Fujita A, Li B, Kawashima Y, Qureshi MM, Sakai O. Using texture analysis to determine human papillomavirus status of oropharyngeal squamous cell carcinomas on CT. AJNR Am J Neuroradiol 2015; 36(7): 1343-8.[http://dx.doi.org/10.3174/ajnr.A4285] [PMID: 25836725]

[96] Fujita A, Buch K, Li B, Kawashima Y, Qureshi MM, Sakai O. Difference between HPV-positive and HPV-negative non-oropharyngeal head and neck cancer: texture analysis features on CT. J Comput Assist Tomogr 2016; 40(1): 43-7.[http://dx.doi.org/10.1097/RCT.0000000000000320] [PMID: 26466116]

[97] Vallieres M, Kumar A, Sultanem K. FDG-PET image-derived features can determine HPV status in head-and-neck cancer. Int J Radiat Oncol Biol Phys 2013; 87: S467.[http://dx.doi.org/10.1016/j.ijrobp.2013.06.1236]

[98] Fruehwald-Pallamar J, Czerny C, Holzer-Fruehwald L, et al. Texture-based and diffusion-weighted discrimination of parotid gland lesions on MR images at 3.0 Tesla. NMR Biomed 2013; 26(11): 1372-9.[http://dx.doi.org/10.1002/nbm.2962] [PMID: 23703801]

[99] Yang X, Wu N, Cheng G, et al. Automated segmentation of the parotid gland based on atlas registration and machine learning: a longitudinal MRI study in head-and-neck radiation therapy. Int J Radiat Oncol Biol Phys

2014; 90(5): 1225-33.[http://dx.doi.org/10.1016/j.ijrobp.2014.08.350] [PMID: 25442347]

[100] Park M, Kim J, Choi YS, *et al.* Application of dynamic contrast-enhanced mri parameters for differentiating squamous cell carcinoma and malignant lymphoma of the oropharynx. Am J Roentgenol 2016; 206(2): 401-7.[http://dx.doi.org/10.2214/AJR.15.14550] [PMID: 26797371]

[101] Fruehwald-Pallamar J, Hesselink JR, Mafee MF, Holzer-Fruehwald L, Czerny C, Mayerhoefer ME. Texture-based analysis of 100 mr examinations of head and neck tumors - is it possible to discriminate between benign and malignant masses in a multicenter trial? RoFo Fortschr Geb Rontgenstr Nuklearmed 2016; 188(2): 195-202.[PMID: 26422418]

[102] Schroeder L, Boscolo-Rizzo P, Dal Cin E. Human papillomavirus as prognostic marker with rising prevalence in neck squamous cell carcinoma of unknown primary: A retrospective multicentre study. Eur J Cancer Oxf Engl 2017; 74: 73-81.[http://dx.doi.org/10.1016/j.ejca.2016.12.020]

[103] O'Rorke MA, Ellison MV, Murray LJ, Moran M, James J, Anderson LA. Human papillomavirus related head and neck cancer survival: a systematic review and meta-analysis. Oral Oncol 2012; 48(12): 1191-201.[http://dx.doi.org/10.1016/j.oraloncology.2012.06.019] [PMID: 22841677]

[104] Boscolo-Rizzo P, Pawlita M, Holzinger D. From HPV-positive towards HPV-driven oropharyngeal squamous cell carcinomas. Cancer Treat Rev 2016; 42: 24-9.[http://dx.doi.org/10.1016/j.ctrv.2015.10.009] [PMID: 26547133]

[105] Rietbergen MM, Snijders PJ, Beekzada D, Braakhuis BJ, Brink A, Heideman DA. Molecular characterization of p16-immunopositive but HPV DNA-negative oropharyngeal carcinomas 2014; 134: 2366-72.[http://dx.doi.org/10.1002/ijc.28580]

[106] Nauta IH, Rietbergen MM, van Bokhoven AAJD, *et al.* Evaluation of the eighth TNM classification on p16-positive oropharyngeal squamous cell carcinomas in the Netherlands and the importance of additional HPV DNA testing. Ann Oncol 2018; 29(5): 1273-9.[http://dx.doi.org/10.1093/annonc/mdy060] [PMID: 29438466]

[107] Spinato G, Stellin M, Azzarello G, *et al.* Multicenter research into the quality of life of patients with advanced oropharyngeal carcinoma with long-term survival associated with human papilloma virus. Oncol Lett 2017; 14(1): 185-93.[http://dx.doi.org/10.3892/ol.2017.6152] [PMID: 28693152]

[108] Chatfield-Reed K, Gui S, O'Neill WQ, Teknos TN, Pan Q. HPV33+ HNSCC is associated with poor prognosis and has unique genomic and immunologic landscapes. Oral Oncol 2020; 100: 104488.[http://dx.doi.org/10.1016/j.oraloncology.2019.104488] [PMID: 31835137]

[109] Boscolo-Rizzo P, Dietz A. The AJCC/UICC eighth edition for staging head and neck cancers: Is it wise to de-escalate treatment regimens in p16-positive oropharyngeal cancer patients? Int J Cancer 2017; 141: 1490-.[http://dx.doi.org/10.1002/ijc.30837]

[110] Mena M, Taberna M, Tous S, *et al.* Double positivity for HPV-DNA/p16^{ink4a} is the biomarker with strongest diagnostic accuracy and prognostic value for human papillomavirus related oropharyngeal cancer patients. Oral Oncol 2018; 78: 137-44.[http://dx.doi.org/10.1016/j.oraloncology.2018.01.010] [PMID: 29496041]

[111] Chen Y-P, Chan ATC, Le Q-T, Blanchard P, Sun Y, Ma J. Nasopharyngeal carcinoma. Lancet 2019; 394(10192): 64-80.[http://dx.doi.org/10.1016/S0140-6736(19)30956-0] [PMID: 31178151]

[112] Maxwell SA, Sacks PG, Gutterman JU, Gallick GE. Epidermal growth factor receptor protein-tyrosine kinase activity in human cell lines established from squamous carcinomas of the head and neck. Cancer Res 1989; 49(5): 1130-7.[PMID: 2783883]

[113] Kearsley JH, Furlong KL, Cooke RA, Waters MJ, Waters MJ. An immunohistochemical assessment of cellular proliferation markers in head and neck squamous cell cancers. Br J Cancer 1990; 61(6): 821-7.[http://dx.doi.org/10.1038/bjc.1990.184] [PMID: 2372483]

[114] Ishitoya J, Toriyama M, Oguchi N, *et al.* Gene amplification and overexpression of EGF receptor in squamous cell carcinomas of the head and neck. Br J Cancer 1989; 59(4): 559-62.[http://dx.doi.org/10.1038/bjc.1989.113] [PMID: 2713242]

[115] Bonner JA, Raisch KP, Trummell HQ, *et al.* Enhanced apoptosis with combination C225/radiation treatment serves as the impetus for clinical investigation in head and neck cancers. J Clin Oncol 2000; 18(21) (Suppl.): 47S-53S.[PMID: 11060327]

[116] Vermorken JB, Mesia R, Rivera F, *et al.* Platinum-based chemotherapy plus cetuximab in head and neck cancer. N Engl J Med 2008; 359(11): 1116-27.[http://dx.doi.org/10.1056/NEJMoa0802656] [PMID: 18784101]

[117] Zibelman M, Mehra R. Overview of current treatment and investigational targeted therapies for locally advanced squamous cell carcinoma of the head and neck. Am J Clin Oncol 2016; 39(4): 396-406.[http://dx.doi.org/10.1097/COC.0000000000000283] [PMID: 26967327]

[118] Bossi P, Resteghini C, Paielli N, Licitra L, Pilotti S, Perrone F. Prognostic and predictive value of EGFR in head and neck squamous cell carcinoma. Oncotarget 2016; 7(45): 74362-79.[http://dx.doi.org/10.18632/oncotarget.11413] [PMID: 27556186]

[119] Rischin D, Harrington KJ, Greil R, Soulieres D, Tahara M, de Catro G. protocol-specified final analysis of the phase 3 keynote-048 trial of pembrolizumab as first line therapy for recurrent/metastatic head and neck squamous cell carcinoma. J Clin Oncol 2019; 37(15): 6000-0.[http://dx.doi.org/10.1200/JCO.2019.37.15_suppl.6000]

[120] Cohen EEW, Bell RB, Bifulco CB, et al. The Society for Immunotherapy of Cancer consensus statement on immunotherapy for the treatment of squamous cell carcinoma of the head and neck (HNSCC). J Immunother Cancer 2019; 7(1): 184.[http://dx.doi.org/10.1186/s40425-019-0662-5] [PMID: 31307547]

[121] Ancevski Hunter K, Socinski MA, Villaruz LC. PD-L1 testing in guiding patient selection for PD-1/PD-L1 inhibitor therapy in lung cancer. Mol Diagn Ther 2018; 22(1): 1-10.[http://dx.doi.org/10.1007/s40291-017-0308-6] [PMID: 29119407]

[122] Lee AWM, Au JS, Teo PM, et al. Staging of nasopharyngeal carcinoma: suggestions for improving the current UICC/AJCC Staging System. Clin Oncol (R Coll Radiol) 2004; 16(4): 269-76.[http://dx.doi.org/10.1016/j.clon.2004.01.008] [PMID: 15214651]

[123] Liu MZ, Tang LL, Zong JF. Evaluation of the sixth edition of AJCC Staging System for nasopharyngeal carcinoma and proposed improvement. Int J Radiat Oncol Biol Phys 2008; 70(4): 1115-23.

[124] AJCC cancer staging manual8th Edition 2016.

The Emergence of New Inflammatory Markers of Head and Neck Cancer and their Potentials

Norhafiza Mat Lazim[1], *, Baharudin Abdullah[1]

[1] Department of Otorhinolaryngology-Head and Neck Surgery, School of Medical Sciences, Universiti Sains Malaysia, Health Campus 16150, Kubang Kerian, Kelantan, Malaysia

Abstract

Inflammation plays a critical role in the process of carcinogenesis as well as in modulating treatment effects of many therapeutic agents for head and neck malignancy. Current research indicates that a myriad of new diagnostic tools and treatment modality works in harmony in producing a desired effective cancer treatment regime. Imperatively, multiple inflammatory markers have surged in the genomic and molecular ecospheres as highly potential agents that can be used in screening, diagnosis, treatment as well as follow up of head and neck cancer patients. These markers include arrays of cytokines, peptides, macrophages, acute phase proteins, growth factors, and many more. The tumor microenvironment is a complex ecosystem and has an intricate relationship with its surrounding biosphere. The multiple interactions within the molecules in the cancer microenvironment play significant roles in mediating and promoting carcinogenesis as well as mitigating the treatment response. These complex ecosystems are also responsible for the occurrence of metastatic diseases, recurrences, and residual diseases. This chapter highlights some of the critical inflammatory markers that can be potentially used as a potent theranostic approach for head and neck tumors in the near future.

Keywords: Carcinogenesis, Chemokines, Head and neck malignancy, Immunomodulation, Inflammatory cascades, Inflammation ecosystem, Tumor microenvironment.

* **Corresponding author Norhafiza Mat Lazim:** Department of Otorhinolaryngology-Head and Neck Surgery, School of Medical Sciences, Universiti Sains Malaysia, Health Campus 16150, Kubang Kerian, Kelantan, Malaysia; Tel: +60199442664; E-mail: norhafiza@usm.my

INTRODUCTION

Head and neck squamous cell carcinoma (HNSCC) is known to be aggressive, with a high incidence of local recurrence and distant metastases despite multimodality treatment. This may be attributed to the heterogeneity of the populated tumor cells as wells as tumor and patient's biology. Patients who are exposed to inflammatory agents such as alcohol, smoke, viruses, environmental

chemical agents, and selected dietary factors are at greater risk of developing HNSCC. Selective groups of HNSCC are resistant to treatment and prone to develop metastatic disease. They are known to have aggressive natures and a tendency to recur. Clinical presentation of each type of HNSCC varies and depends on the primary anatomic locations and organ involvement. The majority of the patients are in the middle and older age group, with a smaller percentage of the pediatric patient population, who are at increased risk of developing HNSCC. Assessment of HNSCC requires a multi-step process and numerous procedures, and the involvement of a dedicated team is a pre-requisite for optimal treatment planning and execution.

Importantly, the risk factors of HNSCC are strongly related to inflammation. For instance, viruses, dietary factors, and environmental carcinogens always cause acute inflammation as an initial insult, which then progresses to chronic inflammation. This later will be followed by the development and promotion of carcinogenesis. Multiple factors and molecules are involved in the process of carcinogenesis originating from the initial inflammation insult. The interaction between these factors in the tumor microenvironment is responsible for the progression of carcinoma. Several excellent reviews have discussed the probable role of cell and molecular inflammation in cancer growth. Most studies reported consistent associations between chronic inflammatory conditions and inflammatory-inducing risk factors, such as alcohol and tobacco consumption, the oncogenic viruses (EBV and HPV), wood dust exposure, in carcinogenesis of head and neck malignancy [1ˉ3].

The process of carcinogenesis is complex and involves multifactorial tissue elements. It is an intricate process, which commonly involves a primary insult, mitigated by factors that can further promote carcinoma development. Peyton Rous was the first to identify that cancers arise from "neoplastic substrate states" induced by viral or chemical carcinogens that trigger somatic changes. These somatic changes are critical insult points in cancer progression. They can be induced by carcinogenic stimuli like chemical carcinogens, nitrosamines in the preserved vegetables and salted fish, acetaldehyde from alcohol, and many chemical components in tobacco, aflatoxins, aromatic amines, and other genotoxic compounds [4]. The steps of initiation and promotion are crucial in carcinogenesis and are both modulated by multiple factors. Significant DNA changes occur during the initial stage, and they are mostly permanent. Chronic exposure to inflammation-induced factors serves as the second stage *i.e.* the promotion. This multistep process of carcinogenesis is very complex and requires intricate genomic changes and chronic exposure of the mucosa of head and neck cancer subsites [5]. It is crucial to understand the true process of carcinogenesis involving the inciting agents that illicit inflammatory cascades.

Other tissue factors are also equally crucial in the development of carcinoma and mitigating carcinogenesis. This can involve vascularization, genetic aberrations, and other deranged physiological processes in a specific microenvironment. Indeed, inflammation is a mechanism that facilitates many forms of cancer. It is suspected to influence the development and progression of cancer through many etiological pathways. These include increased levels of DNA adduction, mutations of oncogenes and tumor suppressor genes, increased vascularization, aberrant anti-apoptotic signaling, and immune evasion [1, 6, 7]. DNA methylation especially hypermethylation, has been known to cause certain HNSCC such as oral cavity carcinoma and salivary glands carcinomas. The process of angiogenesis is paramount as most of the tumoral mass displays various patterns of vascularization. This angiogenic pattern is responsible for tumor characteristics and the true biology of the HNSCC. Several of these processes may interact with each other in producing harmful effects that lead to carcinogenesis and malignant mass formation.

INFLAMMATION AS A PRIMARY CAUSE OF CANCER PROGRESSION

Although cancer is multifactorial in origin, various epidemiological and experimental studies suggest that chronic inflammation has an important role in all stages of cancer, from initiation to progression and even survival of the patient. Inflammatory products like cytokines, chemokines, leucocytes, prostaglandins, cyclooxygenase, reactive oxygen, and nitrogen species are all involved in the development of carcinomas. The other equally important elements are the aberrant genetic factors and processes such as metalloproteinase that able to induce genetic and epigenetic changes in normal cells and damaging their DNA. They can also inhibit their repair, modify transcription factors, suppress apoptosis, and induce angiogenesis, resulting in carcinogenesis. All these markers play a vital role not only in promoting cancers but also in diagnosis, assessment, treatment, and post-treatment surveillance. Thus, these inflammatory mediators have a potential role to become cancer biomarkers for all stages of cancer as many of them can be measured in a cost-effective manner [8]. These biomarkers may emerge as potential therapeutic agents in combatting head and neck malignancy from the very beginning.

The role of inflammation in cancer is indisputable. To illustrate this strong relationship further, the recent literature has highlighted many chronic inflammation reactions as the primary causes of the majority of solid and epithelial malignancies in humankind globally. Numerous writers have reported that many studies highlight the strong association of inflammation with chronic diseases. Accumulating data indicates that chronic inflammation is a precursor to tumor formation such as gastric carcinoma, hepatocellular carcinoma, colonic carcinoma, cervical cancer, and so forth [9⁻11]. Myriads of molecules and markers have been identified that able to promote cascades of an event, which eventually lead to cancer development. Gastritis *i.e.*, inflammation of the lining of the stomach, is the initial insult that eventually leads to gastric cancer. The persistence of chronic active infection in gastric mucosa, together with the presence of *H. pylori* infection, stimulates the initial phase of invasive gastric carcinoma [10]. Lung cancer has been strongly related to cigarette smokers, which results in numerous molecular changes and inflammation that lead to malignancy [12]. Similarly, patient with inflammatory bowel disease has a higher incidence of colorectal carcinoma [13, 14]. Indeed, this cancer-related chronic inflammation plays critical key roles in various aspects of tumor growth, including the proliferation of malignant cells, cell transformation and survival, the progression of invasion, systemic metastases, and tumor response to the drugs.

Increased development of pro-inflammatory mediators, such as cytokines, chemokines, and reactive oxygen intermediates, are the molecular mechanisms by which chronic inflammation drives cancer initiation and promotion. Other factors and components, such as increased oncogene expression, cyclo-oxygenases, matrix metalloproteinase (MMPs), and pro-inflammatory transcription factors, are responsible for tumor progression and response to treatment [15]. These inflammatory-associated molecules are activated by a variety of environmental and carcinogenic stimuli, including the virus, tobacco and alcohol consumption, chemical reagents, and so forth. Of note, all of these in combination are thought to drive the majority of human solid malignancies.

Although inflammation promotes the development of cancer, microenvironmental tumor components such as tumor and stromal cell, inflammatory and immune cells infiltrate produce many stimulative pro-inflammatory molecules that play important roles in tumor initiation, promotion, and progression [16]. Recent studies have shown that cancer-related inflammation results from contact between the host and tumor cells to create a reciprocal interplay that often leads to structural changes, immune suppression, evasion, and malignant progression [17]. Overexpression and abnormal activation of these pro-inflammatory mediators further promote tumor promotion and progression. It is this complex interaction that exists within a tissue biosphere that needs to be comprehensively studied by scientists and clinicians in order to discover novel markers.

Additionally, Tumor-infiltrating lymphocytes (TILs) may also be involved in carcinogenesis. TILs are thought to function in both promoting tumor growth and changes of treatment response to for instance chemotherapy due to its anti-tumor immunity effects. The lymphocytes count in relation to the neutrophil count has also been investigated and shoed to have prognostic significance [18]. This inflammatory marker, neutrophil-lymphocyte ratio (NLR) has been reported to have a strong association with recurrence and survival in HPV-positive cancers [19⁻21]. Importantly, organ transplantation often raises both local and systemic levels of inflammation and is associated with elevated rates of malignancies. Inflammatory markers, such as interleukin-6 (IL-6), tumor necrosis factor and C-reactive protein (CRP), have been shown to increase tissue damage and active disease and influence surgical outcomes [22, 23]. Both cancer risk and plasma levels of inflammatory markers increase with age. Importantly, the levels of circulating inflammatory markers are associated with an increased risk of cancer [22]. This critical finding mandates further intense research as it has a significant impact on the armamentarium of head and neck oncology management.

Some of the head and neck malignancies that are highly related to inflammation include oral cavity carcinoma, nasopharyngeal carcinoma, buccal carcinoma, and thyroid tumors (Figs. 1⁻4).

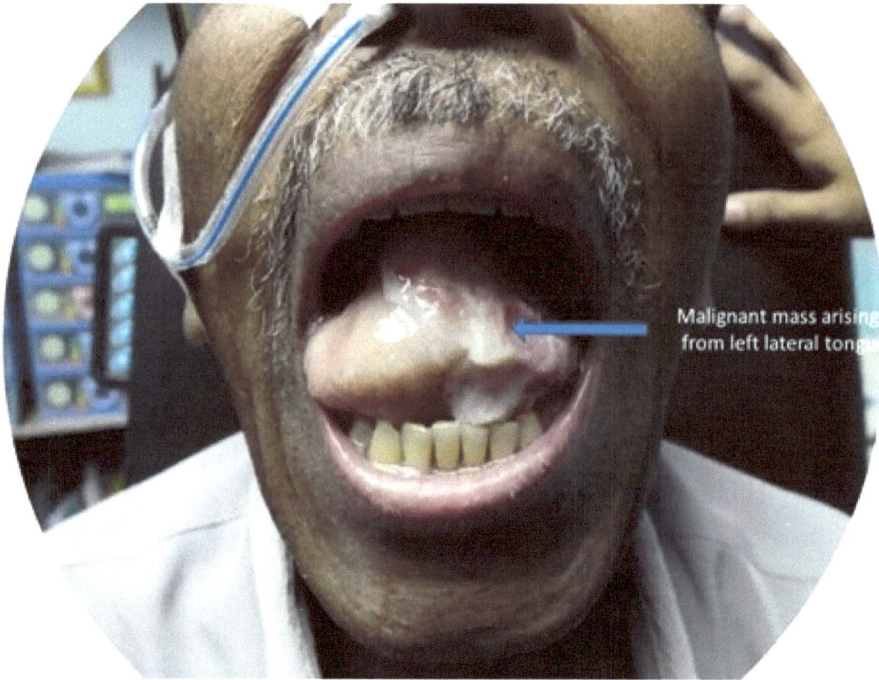

Fig. (1))

Carcinoma of left lateral border of the tongue.

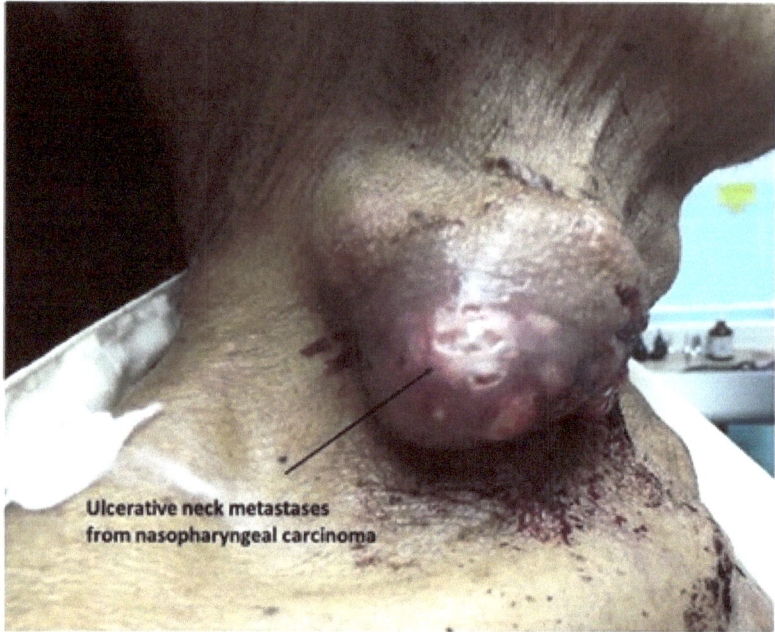

Fig. (2))

Nasopharyngeal carcinoma patient with neck node metastases. The malignant tumor has breached the skin.

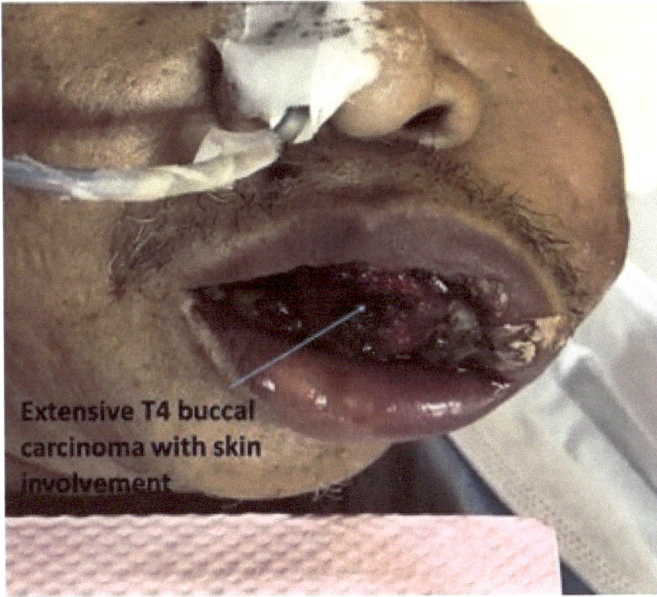

Fig. (3))
Oral cavity carcinoma ie extensive T4 buccal carcinoma.

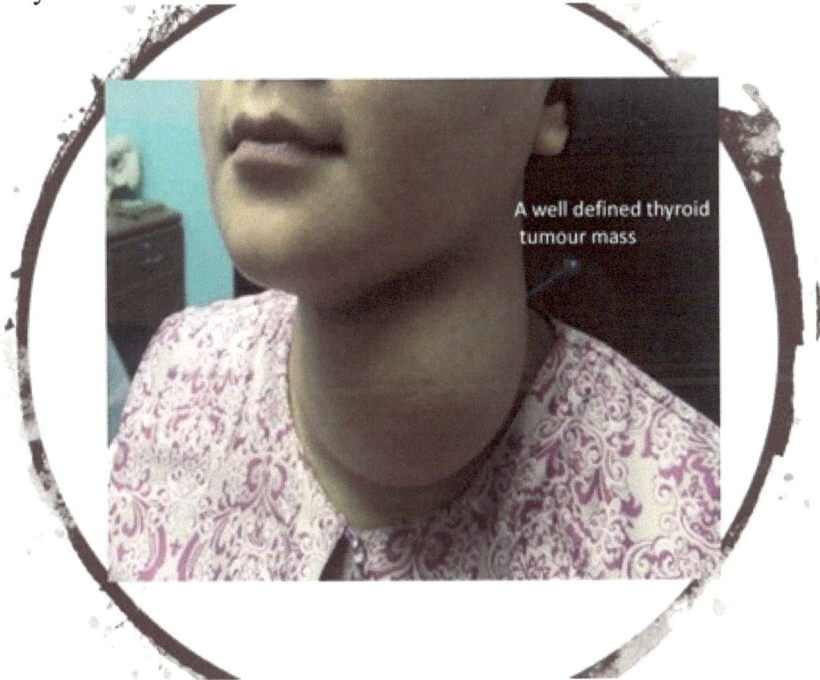

Fig. (4))
Multinodular goiter in a young lady.

EPIDEMIOLOGY OF HEAD AND NECK TUMOUR AND INFLAMMATION DRIVEN CAUSES

According to the WHO cancer statistics, the incidence of head and neck cancer showed an increase in trends, in the majority of the continents especially in the area where the living status is suboptimal. At certain geographic locations, more patients have been diagnosed annually with head and neck cancers includes pediatric malignancies. There have been many identifiable risk factors that have been and are currently being investigated and linked to the carcinogenesis of head and neck malignancy. Oral cavity carcinoma is highly prevalent in India and is strongly related to betel nut chewing and reversed smoking. On the other hand, nasopharyngeal carcinoma is known to be prominent in the South East Asia region, china, Taiwan, Hong Kong, and Japan. This different geographic location reflects different inflammatory agents that may have involved in this malignancy.

Chronic diseases, obesity, alcohol, tobacco, radiation, environmental contaminants, and high-calorie diets have been reported as significant risk factors for the most common forms of cancer including head and neck malignancy [24, 25]. Most of these risk factors are related to cancer progression *via* inflammation. Imperatively, acute inflammation mediates host protection against infections, long-term chronic inflammation can predispose the host to various chronic diseases, including cancers [26]. In the head and neck region, chronic infection with EBV is well known with nasopharyngeal carcinoma whereas chronic infection of human papilloma virus is associated with laryngeal and oropharyngeal tumors [27]. Smoke inhalants, wood dust, smoked seafood, salty fish, and pickled vegetables can all induced malignancy like sinonasal carcinoma and NPC through the chronic inflammation process. The many interactions that exist between the molecules and tissue vasculature in the specific tissue microenvironment driven a lethal pathogenic cascade that eventually leads to the formation of a tumor.

It is crucial to understand the process of inflammation. Inflammation can be divided into two stages, acute and chronic inflammation. Acute inflammation is a part of the innate immunity of immune cells, which lasts for a short period. There are multiple markers involved in this phase that primarily act to initiate tissue healing and repair. However, if the inflammation continues, the second stage of inflammation called chronic inflammation persists. This chronic inflammation underlies the pathogenesis of multiple chronic diseases and cancer *via* alteration of various signaling pathways and inflammatory cascades [28, 29]. Chronic inflammation triggers multiple critical events and produces changes that take place in the tissue with subsequent recruitment of particles and molecules which causes angiogenesis, granulation tissues, and scarring. Angiogenesis is an important element in tumor survivals. It also plays role in diagnostic as well as therapeutic for head and neck malignancies.

INFLAMMATION AS A POTENT RISK FACTOR FOR HEAD AND NECK MALIGNANCY

Clinical and epidemiological studies have shown a significant correlation between chronic infection, inflammation, and cancer. This correlation initially proposed by Rudolf Virchow when he observed an increased number of leukocytes were present in tumor tissues and indicated that tumors could be related to chronic inflammation [30]. Thereafter, a surge of literature focusing on inflammation and cancer took place and extensive research also starts expanding globally. Scientists, physicians, clinicians, epidemiologist, pathologist embarks on mutual collaborative works and studies in gathering information in order to get the data on the nature of solid malignancies in humans.

Numerous molecules that play a critical role in inflammation have been identified in the last two decades of intensive research. These include tumor necrosis factor (TNF), interleukin-chemokines, cyclooxygenases, matrix metalloproteases (MMP), a vascular endothelial growth factor that play major roles in carcinogenesis either in tumor progression or mediate treatment effects [26, 31⁻35]. As aforementioned, malignancy of the head and neck is associated with multiple environmental factors, dietary habits, smoking and alcohol, workplace hazards, chemical, and radiation exposures as well as viruses. Chronic inflammation due to these inciting agents is thought to encourage carcinogenesis and can predispose individuals to particular types of malignancy. Non-infectious chronic inflammation is also associated with several types of cancers including head and neck carcinoma [22]. This portrays numerous factors in the tissue ecosystem that trigger the inflammation cascade responsible for cancer development.

Thus far, we have seen that cancer is one of the main diseases caused by chronic inflammation. In 2009, Colotta *et al*. suggested cancer-related inflammation as the seventh mark of cancer [36]. This is a pertinent discovery that alters the focus of the study in the pathogenesis of head and neck malignancy. Both the internal and external pathways link cancer and inflammation. The oncogenes control the inflammatory microenvironment, while the inflammatory microenvironment facilitates the progression of cancer [28, 37]. The tumor microenvironment comprises a milieu of factors, protease, extracellular matrix, and proteins that are involved in a complex ecosystem to maintain and generate cancer stem cells [37, 38]. Many of these tumor microenvironment constituents play significant roles in head and neck malignancy, for instance in oral squamous cell carcinoma [39]. These carcinogenic stimuli and inflammatory inciting agents influence the level and the mode of actions of the TME elements in the carcinogenesis. Inflammatory stimuli may include bacterial infection *H. pylori* in gastric cancer and tobacco in lung cancer [26]. During the initiation stage, the addition of genetic changes is necessary for tumor formation to occur and progress. The carcinogenic stimuli initiate the mucosa changes but only with persistent mutational changes that will allow carcinogenesis to develop.

Promotion and progression of tumors rely on signals that derive from non-mutant cells in the microenvironment of the tumor. The microenvironment of the tumor consists not only of tumor cells but also of stromal cells, cells of the innate immune system, neutrophils, mast cells, myeloid-derived suppressor cells, macrophages, dendritic cells, lymphocytes, and so forth. This microenvironment can either facilitate tumor progression or become a potential barrier for tumor proliferation through a complex system of immune system interaction, angiogenic proliferation, and growth factors stimulations [40]. It can also be used in the development of anti-cancer therapy [41]. These cell types secrete cytokines, growth factors, proteases, and many more factors that can act in an autocrine or paracrine manner. During the carcinogenesis process, dampening effects of anti-tumor activity take place, and activated proinflammatory events and cascade occurs that lead to the formation of tumor, vascularization, and metastases [30].

Infectious organisms cause inflammation by activating receptors cell and interfering with the composition of wall components and nucleic acids. The mucosal breach facilitates the entry of the organism. Sometimes the architecture of the mucosa itself, like the tonsillar region which has multiple crypts is an ideal place for an oncogenic particle like the viruses to reside. The HPV positive oropharyngeal carcinoma is exclusively in reference to the tonsillar carcinoma, which has different presentations, treatment approach, and prognostication [42⁻44].

However, insufficient eradication of pathogens or persistent infection with prolonged inflammatory signaling and malfunctions in anti-inflammatory pathways and cascades can all contribute to chronic inflammation with the eventual development of malignancy [45]. Arrays of chemical carcinogens, nitrosamines, aflatoxins, tobacco, and alcohol also incite similar inflammation trends. By understanding this complex interaction and pathogenesis that exist between the carcinogenic stimuli and inflammatory changes, it will lead to new insights into cancer and inflammatory diseases and transcend common perspectives on cancer and inflammation [46, 47]. Tumor-associated macrophages and their mediators influence key elements in the multi-step phase of invasion and metastases [48]. Some reports stated that a higher number of TAM is associated with poor prognosis for example in oral cavity cancer and nasopharyngeal carcinoma [49⁻52]. TAM also has cute roles in angiogenesis, invasion, immune evasion, and tumor metastatic potential [53, 54].

Important activation of inflammatory mediators like interleukin and signaling pathways in the buccal epithelium was observed in subjects who burned smoky coal relative to smokeless coal [55]. TAM, lymphocytes, c-reactive proteins, and cyclo-oxygenase also have critical roles in the promotion of oral tumor carcinogenesis [56]. These inflammatory mediators also are a potential marker for the diagnosis and prognosis of oral cavity carcinoma. In order to identify the malignant transformation of neoplasms and to expose the functional mechanism that allows cancer cells to progress, the detailed cancer characteristics of cancer cells and their microenvironment need to be intensely investigated [46].

SIGNIFICANT INFLAMMATORY MARKERS IN HEAD AND NECK CANCER

There are six groups of an inflammation-related biomarker that have been identified which includes cytokines or chemokines, immune-related factors, acute phase proteins, reactive oxygen and nitrogen species, prostaglandins and cyclooxygenase-related factors, and mediators such as transcription and growth factors [1]. These biomarkers have numerous significant roles in carcinogenesis and malignancy development. Other markers that are associated with immune evasion have also been identified and are responsible for the immune escape mechanism for cell proliferation, invasion, and metastasize. These markers include macrophages, NLR, cytokines, growth factors, and TAMs.

Some of these markers can be used to give a clinical prediction of tumor behavior, response to treatment, and development of recurrence. Certain markers have been used to assess the risk of lymph node metastases in papillary thyroid carcinoma. Selected cytokines have been associated with the growth and development of human gastric carcinoma, colorectal cancer, and esophageal cancer [29]. Studies are also looking at the roles of cytokines in the prediction of head and neck cancer regional spread, for instance, cytokines produce due to radiation therapy [57, 58]. Cytokines that are present in saliva have been reported to be different between pre- and post-treatment which can be used to monitor treatment response [59, 60].

Clinical trials evaluating systemic inflammatory response in cancer patients for prognostication is escalating. The neutrophil-to-lymphocyte ratio (NLR) is one of the main biomarkers of systemic inflammation and has been associated with increased tumor burden and disease spread as well as monitor treatment response to immune-targeted therapy [61⁻63]. NLR is elevated in patients with laryngeal squamous cell carcinoma relative to those with benign and precancerous lesions. NLR is also an independent indicator of decreased overall survival in most epithelial cancers [64].

Tumor Microenvironment and Inflammatory Markers

In normal tissue, the cellular microenvironment is capable of suppressing malignant cell development. However, tumor-stromal interactions that modulate the microenvironment are more permissive to malignant cell proliferation and increase cell motility and adherence. This tumorigenic process includes angiogenesis, lymphangiogenesis, and multiple inflammation cascades that able to be amplified with the presence of growth factors, cytokines, proteases, and so forth. In addition, the composition and function of the basement membrane are generally altered in cancer, along with changes in growth factor expression, recruitment of inflammatory cytokines, and increased fibroblast proliferation, all of which lead to the metastatic spread of tumor cells. It is indeed to manage head and neck malignancy as in the majority of cases, treatment response is poor due to aggressive tumor and issues of chemo-radioresistance and cancer-prone to recurs. This will impair the patient's survival and quality of life [65].

Of note, the tumor microenvironment is capable of influencing malignant cell growth by releasing ECM proteins, growth factors, and cytokine. Critically, tumors themselves secrete growth factors and proteases that are capable of altering their local microenvironment, promoting the interaction among the tumor cell themselves, and facilitate immune surveillance [66, 67]. This is a crucial relationship in the carcinogenesis events as these markers become disproportionately unbalanced, altering the cellular process within the ecosystem. Most current data support the notion that acute inflammation caused by tumor-infiltration of host leukocytes does not have natural immune-protective mechanisms that contribute to the eradication of cancer and antitumor immunity. Instead, overly and excessively developed pro-inflammatory mediators are thought to contribute to tumor promotion and progression.

In the microenvironment of the tumor, there is a delicate balance between antitumor immunity and tumor-originated proinflammatory activity, which weakens antitumor immunity that will allow the tumor to expand rapidly [45]. A summary of some of the critical markers is listed in Table 1.

Table 1 **Selected classes of inflammatory markers and their roles in head and neck malignancy.**

Groups of Inflammatory Biomarkers	Cancer Sites	Roles of Specific Markers
Peptide	HNSCC (Wright *et al.*, 2016) [31] HNSCC (Yoshitake *et al.*, 2015) [32]	• Tumor targeting peptides for to improve imaging sensitivity (angiogenic cyclic RGD peptide cilengitide) • 12 amino acid peptide HN1 may have relation to HPV positive HNSCC • Cancer vaccine therapy (Multiple tumor antigens TAA derived peptide)
Chemokines	Adenoid Cystic carcinoma of Salivary gland (Muller *et al.*, 2016) [33] HNSCC (Muller *et al.*, 2016) HNSCC (Wolff *et al.*, 2011) [34] HNSCC (Antonio LP *et al.*, 2015) [35]	• Chemokine receptors as indicative of metastases. (CXCR4) • May suppress apoptosis induced by chemotherapy agent of tumor load • Lymph nodes metastases (CCR7) • B Cell Lymphoma (CXCR5) • Chemotherapy Resistance • High CXCR4 expression increased risk of nodal invasion (high CXCR4 expression) • Low risk of local and distant recurrence (low CXCL12 expression)
Macrophages	OCSCC (Evrard *et al.*, 2019) [36] HNSCC + OCSCC (Kumar *et al.*, 2019) [37]	• TAMS indicate poor prognosis • correlate with increased lymph node metastasis, extracapsular extension, and advanced stage
CRP proteins	OCSCC (Katano *et al.*,2017; Chen IH *et al.*, 2014, Chen HH *et al.*, 2013) [22, 23, 38]	• Prognostic Markers • Lymph node metastasis • Recurrence • Clinical tumor status • Extracapsular (ECS) lymph nodes spread
Interleukins	HNSCC (Choudhary *et al.*, 2016) [25] HNSCC (Aderhold *et al.*, 2014) [39] HNSCC (von Biberstein *et al.*, 1996) [40]	• Tumor stage (IL6 elevation • indicate high tumor stage • Lymph nodes positivity • Chemoradiotherapy resistance • Tumor Metastases and progression • IL 4 as a potential screening marker • unrestricted growth and metastasis of (Increased IL-1 index)
VEGF	HNSCC (Aderhold	• Tumor node metastases TNM staging

	et al., 2014) [39]	

The findings of the Illyasoya *et al*. studies indicate that;

1. CRP levels are a more consistent measure of cancer risk than IL-6;
2. The correlation between cancer incidence and inflammatory markers may be site-specific;
3. An increased level of inflammatory markers displays a greater correlation with the risk of cancer death compared to the risk of cancer incidence [22].

This indicates that inflammatory markers can be used to delineate the primary tumor of origins as well as giving the prognostication for that specific cancer. Importantly, other critical mechanisms by which inflammation can lead to carcinogenesis includes (Table 2):

Table 2 **Selected classes of inflammatory markers and their roles in head and neck malignancy.**

S. No.	Mechanisms of Inflammation that Lead to Cancer Development
1.	Apoptosis resistance
2.	Tumor neovascularization
3.	Invasion of tumor-related basement membrane
4.	Formation of reactive oxygen and nitrogen species
5.	Induction of genomic instability
6.	Alteration of genetic events
7.	Altered gene expression
8.	Increase the proliferation of damage-initiated cells [16]

The genetic changes in combination with the inflammation agents thus is a serious condition that can alter the process of carcinogenesis and giving the different behavior of each type of cancer. Many of the proinflammatory mediators transform the angiogenic switches mainly mediated by the growth factors, thus inducing inflammatory angiogenesis and tumor cell-stromal contact. This would end with angiogenesis, metastases, and invasion of the tumor. In addition, cellular microRNAs are emerging as a possible link between inflammation and cancer [16]. Tumor-associated macrophages (TAMs) are a significant component of inflammatory infiltrates in neoplastic tissues and are produced from monocytes. TAMs have a dual function in neoplasms and contain a variety of potent angiogenic and lymphangiogenic growth factors, cytokines, and proteases which are mediators that promote the progression of malignant tissue formation [68].

Chemokines and Cytokines

Systemic cytokine concentrations have been associated with both cancer risk and cancer progression. There are nearly hundreds of cytokines identified which possessed multiple pivotal functions in the head and neck cancer ecosystem. For example, circulating IL-6 was associated with lung and colorectal cancer [1]. Importantly, a number of chemokines and cytokines with their receptors have been shown to be strongly related to squamous cell carcinoma of the head and neck which can, for example, encourage chemotherapy resistance or use as a clinical indicator of disease progression [69, 70]. The chemoradiation resistance is responsible for disease progression and recurrence in the majority of head and neck malignancy.

Cytokines are central to vast networks that include both synergistic and antagonistic interactions. They have both negative and positive regulatory effects on different target cells. The macrophages and T lymphocytes are the primary producers of cytokines that may have primarily pro-inflammatory activity. Such examples include IL-1α, IL-1β, IL-2, IL-6, Il-8, IL-12, TNF-α, IFN-γ or anti-inflammatory properties such as IL-4, IL-5, IL-10, TGF-β) [1]. Some of this cytokine has been shown to be promising markers for monitoring disease progression, risk of recurrence and metastases, and in optimizing surgical therapy of HNSCC. For example, IFN-γ has been shown to be a promising marker for predicting neck metastases in HNSCC, sensitivity to chemotherapy as well as serves as a reference for selecting types of required neck dissections [71]. Mburu *et al.* demonstrate that up-regulation of NF-κB in HNSCC patients correlates with lower patient survival because of metastatic disease. Of note, certain cytokines also able to stratify cancer according to their aggressiveness [72]. With the advent of research in the future, more true roles of these cytokines can be identified and refined in order to optimize HNSCC management.

Chemokine molecules are a superfamily, functioning mainly as chemo-attractors and activators of particular forms of leukocytes [71]. During both acute and chronic inflammatory processes, the cytokines are involved in the recruitment of leukocytes *via* increased expression of cell adhesion molecules and chemo-attraction [1, 71]. Measuring cytokines as an indicator of inflammatory status in a population-based study is an area of great promise, but it poses many challenges due to the biochemistry of molecules, especially their short half-life [1].

Immune-Related Effectors

Leukocytes are an important part of the innate, as well as the adaptive immune system, which include granulocytes, monocytes, macrophages, dendritic cells, lymphocytes that may have immunostimulatory or immunosuppressive roles. In general, many mechanisms can be activated in cancer patients in order to inhibit the successful adaptive immune response which can prevent the destruction of the tumor by immune cells. Leukocytes also facilitate the release of cytokines and growth factors that promote tumor growth. Above all, the actions of the immune system contribute to a shift in the blood leukocyte profile, which acts as a marker for the systemic inflammatory response [1].

At this juncture, different measures of leukocyte count, such as WBC count, platelet to lymphocyte ratio (PLR), and neutrophil to lymphocyte ratio (NLR) were correlated with an increased risk of many forms of cancer, including breast cancer, colorectal cancer, and tumor progression [1]. Additionally, these markers also can be potentially used for prognostication, monitoring treatment responses, and predict the recurrence risk. for instance, reports show that elevated CRP in nasopharyngeal carcinoma patients who had chemoradiation indicates they have a poor prognosis [73]. Numerous inflammatory markers have been identified to have clinical utility in current practice in terms of predicting the treatment outcomes of HNSCC patients.

Acute Phase Protein

CRP is an acute-phase protein present in the blood that is synthesized in the liver in response to inflammation. Physiologically, the protein stimulates the complement system. When triggered, the complement system helps remove the wounded or dead cells from the tissues. CRP has been associated with systemic levels of inflammation in multiple inflammatory disorders as well as chronic diseases such as cardiovascular disease and type II diabetes [1]. Katanano *et al.* reported that a high pre-treatment level of CRP is a critical prognostic factor for esophageal cancer, hepatocellular carcinoma, renal cell carcinoma, non-small cell lung carcinoma, and prostate carcinoma [74].

In oral cavity carcinoma, CRP has also been shown to confer prognostication. Additionally, CRP has been reported to have a significant association with lymph node metastases and recurrence [75]. Chen *et al.* also stated that elevated serum CRP is correlated with advanced tumor status, skin invasion, and bone invasion and that there are important associations between CRP, DFS, and OS levels [75]. Some studies also investigating the role of CRP in relation to the lymph node metastases and recurrence of head and neck squamous cell carcinoma [76]. Reports from the SCC oral cavity research indicated a link between CRP level and poor prognosis, pathological tumor status, nodal status, and extracapsular lymph node spread [75].

Role of STAT3 in HNSCC Cancer Patients

Various cancer cell growth factors, including IL-6 and EGF, can activate STAT3. Constitutively active STAT3 has been documented for multiple myeloma, chronic lymphocytic leukemia, gastric cancer, lung cancer, and laryngeal carcinoma [26]. For instance, IL6/STAT 3 offer as a potential target for HNSCC. Curcumin has been shown to mediate its anti-tumor effects by inhibiting a variety of signaling pathways including IL-6/STAT3 pathways. Targeting the pathway of IL-6/STAT3 head and neck cancer seems very exciting that can potentially lead to the discovery of a novel marker [77].

Role of COX2 in HNSCC Cancer Patients

Cyclooxygenase has emerged as another significant mediator of inflammation. Overexpression of COX2 has been demonstrated in patients with different forms of cancer. Its overexpression has been associated with low survival in prostate cancer, with a high risk of recurrence, shorter survival in patients with lung cancer, development of oral cancer, and esophageal cancer. The COX overexpression has been linked to poor prognosis of breast cancer, promoting angiogenesis in Hodgkin's lymphoma, and shorten the progression-free survival in multiple myeloma patients [26].

Role of TNF in HNSCC Cancer Patients

One of the first mentions of a potential function for TNF was a decade ago, during the initial study, based on the molecular cancer network. TNF was found to be elevated in lung cancer. ovarian cancer and lymphoma and may serve beneficial functions as inflammatory markers [26, 78, 79]. More recent studies reported that TNF can be used as an index of prognostication and indicate the risk of malignant transformation in oral cavity cancer [80]. The TNF is also reported to have effects in antiapoptotic signaling pathways and is the candidate for developing potent anti-cancer therapy [81]. It has also been assessed to have critical in cancer cachexia that significantly impairs the patient's head and neck quality of life [82].

Role of VEGF in HNSCC Cancer Patients

For tumor progression, angiogenesis is a necessary process and is driven by molecular interactions between cancer cells and neighboring endothelial vascular cells. Vascular endothelial growth factors and their respective receptors on endothelial cells are the primary mediators of angiogenesis. VEGF is another cytokine that plays a key role in the spread of endothelial cells and angiogenesis. The expression of VEGF has been associated with metastases, poor prognosis, and relapse of multiple cancers including papillary thyroid carcinoma, nasopharyngeal carcinoma, and melanoma [26]. The VEGF expression is related to advanced tumor and poor survival rates of a patient who had oral cavity carcinoma and laryngeal carcinoma [83⁻86].

VEGF may also play roles in mediating the radioresistance in head and neck cancer which responsible for poor treatment outcomes [87]. Clinical trials are conducted for the efficacy of anti-angiogenic agents combined with chemoradiation therapy in head and neck cancer that show positive response by increasing the response rate [88, 89]. Currently, there are a number of U.S. Food and Drug Administration clinically approved anti-angiogenic agents that have been used in clinical practice.

INFLAMMATION AS AN ANTI-CANCER THERAPEUTIC OPPORTUNITY

We have discussed many significant inflammatory markers that can be potentially used in the near future, to combat head and neck malignancy. The aforementioned markers can be developed as an effective agent for:

1. Screening of at-risk patient populations
2. Early diagnosis of head and neck cancer
3. Stratify patient prognosis
4. Treatment outcomes monitoring
5. Reduce the chemoradioresistance
6. Escalate treatment response with minimal treatment-related side effects

Many reported studies have highlighted the potential roles of these inflammatory markers that signify the elements of the inflammation ecosystem that functions in a cohesive manner [90].

Inflammation plays a crucial role in cancer development, making it an ideal therapeutic focus. Several biomarkers have been identified as a useful marker for the management of head and neck cancer [91]. We can foresee that in coming decades that more therapeutics drugs will be made available with more potency and fewer morbidities. These potential drugs or agents can be used as effective chemoprevention regimes. This has been partly proved by the emergence of, for instance, angiogenic inhibitors, immune checkpoint blockade, nanotag probes, and so forth. The newer therapeutic agents can be complemented with recent advancement in technology such as artificial intelligence, in order to escalate therapeutic response and lessening the treatment-related morbidities.

The deeper comprehension of the molecular changes that occur in the microenvironment of the tumor and their significance during tumor growth, recurrence and metastasis will pave the way for optimum strategies that target particular cytokines, growth factors, immune cells, macrophages, and proteases in achieving the objectives as highlighted above. Several phases I and phase II trials are currently investigating the safety and efficacy of these interventions in various malignancies. Developing these highly potential markers and make them available for early usage in clinical practice is not an easy task. This requires multi-team effort and commitment from all health professionals involved, whether it be the surgeon, physician, scientist, researcher, technologist, and so forth.

CONCLUSION

A true understanding of inflammatory markers and their numerous roles is a pre-requisite for clinicians, scientists, and other health-related professionals. By knowing their roles and interactions that exist between molecules in the delicate tumor microenvironment, scientists will be able to embark on a well-defined path for a novel discovery of agents, molecules, and substances that can be used as a treatment hybrid for diagnostic and therapeutic markers in the near future. Cancer is a complex disease, yet robust data is accumulating and have shed light on the carcinogenesis of most human malignancies including head and neck malignancy. These available data can be used to move forward in the management armamentarium of head and neck cancers globally. Funded research and clinical trials will allow these potential identifiable markers to be fully used in clinical practices at a very short time.

CONSENT FOR PUBLICATION

Not applicable.

CONFLICT OF INTEREST

The author declares no conflict of interest, financial or otherwise.

ACKNOWLEDGEMENTS

Declared none.

REFERENCES

[1] Brenner DR, Scherer D, Muir K. A review of the application of inflammatory biomarkers in epidemiologic cancer research. Cancer Epidemiol Biomarkers Prev 2014; 23(9): 1729-51.[http://dx.doi.org/10.1158/1055-9965.EPI-14-0064]

[2] Domingo-Vidal M, Whitaker-Menezes D, Martos-Rus C, et al. Cigarette smoke induces metabolic reprogramming of the tumor stroma in head and neck squamous cell carcinoma. Mol Cancer Res 2019; 17(9): 1893-909.[http://dx.doi.org/10.1158/1541-7786.MCR-18-1191] [PMID: 31239287]

[3] Konings H, Stappers S, Geens M, et al. A literature review of the potential diagnostic biomarkers of head and neck neoplasms. Front Oncol 2020; 10: 1020.[http://dx.doi.org/10.3389/fonc.2020.01020] [PMID: 32670885]

[4] Hartwig A, Arand M, Epe B, et al. Mode of action-based risk assessment of genotoxic carcinogens. Arch Toxicol 2020; 94(6): 1787-877.[http://dx.doi.org/10.1007/s00204-020-02733-2] [PMID: 32542409]

[5] Coussens LM, Werb Z. Inflammation and cancer. Nature 2002; 420(6917): 860-7.[http://dx.doi.org/10.1038/nature01322] [PMID: 12490959]

[6] Leemans CR, Snijders PJF, Brakenhoff RH. The molecular landscape of head and neck cancer. Nat Rev Cancer 2018; 18(5): 269-82.[http://dx.doi.org/10.1038/nrc.2018.11] [PMID: 29497144]

[7] Saada-Bouzid E, Peyrade F, Guigay J. Molecular genetics of head and neck squamous cell carcinoma. Curr Opin Oncol 2019; 31(3): 131-7.[http://dx.doi.org/10.1097/CCO.0000000000000536] [PMID: 30893149]

[8] Chaunhan R, Trivedi V. Inflammatory markers in Cancers: Potential resources. Front Biosci 2020; 12: 1-24.[http://dx.doi.org/10.2741/s537]

[9] Refolo MG, Messa C, Guerra V, Carr BI, D'Alessandro R. Inflammatory Mechanisms of HCC Development. Cancers (Basel) 2020; 12(3): 641.[http://dx.doi.org/10.3390/cancers12030641] [PMID: 32164265]

[10] Wessler S, Krisch LM, Elmer DP, Aberger F. From inflammation to gastric cancer - the importance of Hedgehog/GLI signaling in *Helicobacter pylori*-induced chronic inflammatory and neoplastic diseases. Cell Commun Signal 2017; 15(1): 15.[http://dx.doi.org/10.1186/s12964-017-0171-4] [PMID: 28427431]

[11] Fernandes JV, DE Medeiros Fernandes TA, DE Azevedo JC, et al. Link between chronic inflammation and human papillomavirus-induced carcinogenesis (Review). Oncol Lett 2015; 9(3): 1015-26.[http://dx.doi.org/10.3892/ol.2015.2884] [PMID: 25663851]

[12] Gomes M, Teixeira AL, Coelho A, Araújo A, Medeiros R. The role of inflammation in lung cancer. Adv Exp Med Biol 2014; 816: 1-23.[http://dx.doi.org/10.1007/978-3-0348-0837-8_1] [PMID: 24818717]

[13] Gupta SC, Kunnumakkara AB, Aggarwal S, Aggarwal BB. Inflammation, a double-edge sword for cancer and other age-related diseases. Front Immunol 2018; 9: 2160.[http://dx.doi.org/10.3389/fimmu.2018.02160] [PMID: 30319623]

[14] Long AG, Lundsmith ET, Hamilton KE. Inflammation and colorectal cancer. Curr Colorectal Cancer Rep 2017; 13(4): 341-51.[http://dx.doi.org/10.1007/s11888-017-0373-6] [PMID: 29129972]

[15] Sethi G, Shanmugam MK, Ramachandran L, Kumar AP, Tergaonkar V. Multifaceted link between cancer and inflammation. Biosci Rep 2012; 32(1): 1-15.[http://dx.doi.org/10.1042/BSR20100136] [PMID: 21981137]

[16] Kundu JK, Surh YJ. Inflammation: gearing the journey to cancer. Mutat Res 2008; 659(1-2): 15-30.[http://dx.doi.org/10.1016/j.mrrev.2008.03.002] [PMID: 18485806]

[17] Charles KA, Harris BD, Haddad CR, et al. Systemic inflammation is an independent predictive marker of clinical outcomes in mucosal squamous cell carcinoma of the head and neck in oropharyngeal and non-oropharyngeal patients. BMC Cancer 2016; 16: 124.[http://dx.doi.org/10.1186/s12885-016-2089-4] [PMID: 26892430]

[18] Wu F, Wu LL, Zhu LX. Neutrophil to lymphocyte ratio in peripheral blood: a novel independent prognostic factor in patients with head and neck squamous cell carcinoma. Zhonghua Zhong Liu Za Zhi 2017; 39(1): 29-32.[http://dx.doi.org/10.3760/cma.j.issn.0253-3766.2017.01.006] [PMID: 28104030]

[19] Rosculet N, Zhou XC, Ha P, et al. Neutrophil-to-lymphocyte ratio: Prognostic indicator for head and neck squamous cell carcinoma. Head Neck 2017; 39(4): 662-7.[http://dx.doi.org/10.1002/hed.24658] [PMID: 28075517]

[20] Bojaxhiu B, Templeton AJ, Elicin O, et al. Relation of baseline neutrophil-to-lymphocyte ratio to survival and toxicity in head and neck cancer patients treated with (chemo-) radiation. Radiat Oncol 2018; 13(1): 216.[http://dx.doi.org/10.1186/s13014-018-1159-y] [PMID: 30400969]

[21] Tham T, Wotman M, Chung C, *et al.* Systemic immune response in squamous cell carcinoma of the head and neck: a comparative concordance index analysis. Eur Arch Otorhinolaryngol 2019; 276(10): 2913-22.[http://dx.doi.org/10.1007/s00405-019-05554-x] [PMID: 31312922]

[22] Il'yasova D, Colbert LH, Harris TB, *et al.* Circulating levels of inflammatory markers and cancer risk in the health aging and body composition cohort. Cancer Epidemiol Biomarkers Prev 2005; 14(10): 2413-8.

[23] Lassig AAD, Lindgren BR, Itabiyi R, Joseph AM, Gupta K. Excessive inflammation portends complications: Wound cytokines and head and neck surgery outcomes. Laryngoscope 2019; 129(7): E238-46.[http://dx.doi.org/10.1002/lary.27796] [PMID: 30628094]

[24] Ng SP, Pollard C, III, Kamal M, *et al.* Risk of second primary malignancies in head and neck cancer patients treated with definitive radiotherapy. NPJ Precis Oncol 2019; 3: 22.[http://dx.doi.org/10.1038/s41698-019-0097-y] [PMID: 31583278]

[25] Zamani SA, McClain KM, Graubard BI, *et al.* Dietary polyunsaturated fat intake in relation to head and neck, esophageal, and gastric cancer incidence in the national institutes of health-aarp diet and health study. Am J Epidemiol 2020; 189(10): 1096-113.[http://dx.doi.org/10.1093/aje/kwaa024] [PMID: 32141493]

[26] Aggarwal BB, Vijayalekshmi RV, Sung B. Targeting inflammatory pathways for prevention and therapy of cancer: short-term friend, long-term foe. Clin Cancer Res 2009; 15(2): 425-30.[http://dx.doi.org/10.1158/1078-0432.CCR-08-0149] [PMID: 19147746]

[27] Mat Lazim N, Abdullah B. Risk Factors and etiopathogenesis of NPC. In: Abdullah B, Balasubramaniam A, Mat Lazim N, eds. An Evidence-Based Approach to the Management of Nasopharyngeal Cancer: From Basic Sciences to Clinical Presentation and Treatment Abdullah B, Balasubramaniam A, Mat Lazim N. 202011-30. https://www.elsevier.com/books-and-journals[http://dx.doi.org/10.1016/B978-0-12-814403-9.00002-1]

[28] Kunnumakkara AB, Sailo BL, Banik K, *et al.* Chronic diseases, inflammation, and spices: how are they linked? J Transl Med 2018; 16(1): 14.[http://dx.doi.org/10.1186/s12967-018-1381-2] [PMID: 29370858]

[29] Aggarwal BB, Gehlot P. Inflammation and cancer: how friendly is the relationship for cancer patients? Curr Opin Pharmacol 2009; 9(4): 351-69.[http://dx.doi.org/10.1016/j.coph.2009.06.020]

[30] Bollrath J, Greten FR. IKK/NF-kappaB and STAT3 pathways: central signalling hubs in inflammation-mediated tumour promotion and metastasis. EMBO Rep 2009; 10(12): 1314-9.[http://dx.doi.org/10.1038/embor.2009.243] [PMID: 19893576]

[31] Wolff HA, Rolke D, Rave-Fränk M, *et al.* Analysis of chemokine and chemokine receptor expression in squamous cell carcinoma of the head and neck (SCCHN) cell lines. Radiat Environ Biophys 2011; 50(1): 145-54.[http://dx.doi.org/10.1007/s00411-010-0341-x] [PMID: 21085979]

[32] Gkouveris I, Nikitakis NG, Aseervatham J, Rao N, Ogbureke KUE. Matrix metalloproteinases in head and neck cancer: current perspectives. Metalloproteinases Med 2017; 4: 47-61.[http://dx.doi.org/10.2147/MNM.S105770]

[33] Hauff SJ, Raju SC, Orosco RK, *et al.* Matrix-metalloproteinases in head and neck carcinoma-cancer genome atlas analysis and fluorescence imaging in mice. Otolaryngol Head Neck Surg 2014; 151(4): 612-8.[http://dx.doi.org/10.1177/0194599814545083] [PMID: 25091190]

[34] Peltanova B, Raudenska M, Masarik M. Effect of tumor microenvironment on pathogenesis of the head and neck squamous cell carcinoma: a systematic review. Mol Cancer 2019; 18(1): 63.[http://dx.doi.org/10.1186/s12943-019-0983-5] [PMID: 30927923]

[35] Haibe Y, Kreidieh M, El Hajj H, *et al.* Resistance mechanisms to anti-angiogenic therapies in cancer. Front Oncol 2020; 10: 221.[http://dx.doi.org/10.3389/fonc.2020.00221] [PMID: 32175278]

[36] Colotta F, Allavena P, Sica A, Garlanda C, Mantovani A. Cancer-related inflammation, the seventh hallmark of cancer: links to genetic instability. Carcinogenesis 2009; 30(7): 1073-81.[http://dx.doi.org/10.1093/carcin/bgp127] [PMID: 19468060]

[37] Zheng J, Gao P. Toward normalization of the tumor microenvironment for cancer therapy. Integr Cancer Ther 2019; 18: 1534735419862352.[http://dx.doi.org/10.1177/1534735419862352] [PMID: 31282197]

[38] Laplane L, Duluc D, Bikfalvi A, Larmonier N, Pradeu T. Beyond the tumour microenvironment. Int J Cancer 2019; 145(10): 2611-8.[http://dx.doi.org/10.1002/ijc.32343] [PMID: 30989643]

[39] Salo T, Vered M, Bello IO, *et al.* Insights into the role of components of the tumor microenvironment in oral carcinoma call for new therapeutic approaches. Exp Cell Res 2014; 325(2): 58-64.[http://dx.doi.org/10.1016/j.yexcr.2013.12.029] [PMID: 24462456]

[40] Anari F, Ramamurthy C, Zibelman M. Impact of tumor microenvironment composition on therapeutic responses and clinical outcomes in cancer. Future Oncol 2018; 14(14): 1409-21.[http://dx.doi.org/10.2217/fon-2017-0585] [PMID: 29848096]

[41] Chen Q, Liu G, Liu S, *et al.* Remodeling the tumor microenvironment with emerging nanotherapeutics.

Trends Pharmacol Sci 2018; 39(1): 59-74.[http://dx.doi.org/10.1016/j.tips.2017.10.009] [PMID: 29153879]

[42] Kim KY, Lewis JS, Jr, Chen Z. Current status of clinical testing for human papillomavirus in oropharyngeal squamous cell carcinoma. J Pathol Clin Res 2018; 4(4): 213-26.[http://dx.doi.org/10.1002/cjp2.111] [PMID: 30058293]

[43] Nguyen B, Meehan K, Pereira MR, et al. A comparative study of extracellular vesicle-associated and cell-free DNA and RNA for HPV detection in oropharyngeal squamous cell carcinoma. Sci Rep 2020; 10(1): 6083.[http://dx.doi.org/10.1038/s41598-020-63180-8] [PMID: 32269293]

[44] Damerla RR, Lee NY, You D. Detection of early human papillomavirus-associated cancers by liquid biopsy. JCO Precis Oncol 2019; 3. [http://dx.doi.org/10.1200/PO.18.00276]

[45] Lin WW, Karin M. A cytokine-mediated link between innate immunity, inflammation, and cancer. J Clin Invest 2007; 117(5): 1175-83.[http://dx.doi.org/10.1172/JCI31537] [PMID: 17476347]

[46] Mierke CT. The fundamental role of mechanical properties in the progression of cancer disease and inflammation. Rep Prog Phys 2014; 77(7): 076602.[http://dx.doi.org/10.1088/0034-4885/77/7/076602] [PMID: 25006689]

[47] Plzák J, Bouček J, Bandúrová V, et al. The head and neck squamous cell carcinoma microenvironment as a potential target for cancer therapy. Cancers (Basel) 2019; 11(4): 440.[http://dx.doi.org/10.3390/cancers11040440] [PMID: 30925774]

[48] Solinas G, Marchesi F, Garlanda C, Mantovani A, Allavena P. Inflammation-mediated promotion of invasion and metastasis. Cancer Metastasis Rev 2010; 29(2): 243-8.[http://dx.doi.org/10.1007/s10555-010-9227-2] [PMID: 20414701]

[49] Evrard D, Szturz P, Tijeras-Raballand A, et al. Macrophages in the microenvironment of head and neck cancer: potential targets for cancer therapy. Oral Oncol 2019; 88: 29-38.[http://dx.doi.org/10.1016/j.oraloncology.2018.10.040] [PMID: 30616794]

[50] Ooft ML, van Ipenburg JA, Sanders ME, et al. Prognostic role of tumour-associated macrophages and regulatory T cells in EBV-positive and EBV-negative nasopharyngeal carcinoma. J Clin Pathol 2018; 71(3): 267-74.[http://dx.doi.org/10.1136/jclinpath-2017-204664] [PMID: 28877959]

[51] Kumar AT, Knops A, Swendseid B, et al. Prognostic significance of tumor-associated macrophage content in head and neck squamous cell carcinoma: a meta-analysis. Front Oncol 2019; 9: 656.[http://dx.doi.org/10.3389/fonc.2019.00656] [PMID: 31396482]

[52] Li B, Ren M, Zhou X, Han Q, Cheng L. Targeting tumor-associated macrophages in head and neck squamous cell carcinoma. Oral Oncol 2020; 106: 104723.[http://dx.doi.org/10.1016/j.oraloncology.2020.104723] [PMID: 32315971]

[53] Zhou K, Cheng T, Zhan J, et al. Targeting tumor-associated macrophages in the tumor microenvironment. Oncol Lett 2020; 20(5): 234.[http://dx.doi.org/10.3892/ol.2020.12097] [PMID: 32968456]

[54] Wu K, Lin K, Li X, et al. Redefining Tumor-Associated Macrophage Subpopulations and Functions in the Tumor Microenvironment. Front Immunol 2020; 11: 1731.[http://dx.doi.org/10.3389/fimmu.2020.01731] [PMID: 32849616]

[55] Wang TW, Vermeulen RC, Hu W, et al. Gene-expression profiling of buccal epithelium among non-smoking women exposed to household air pollution from smoky coal. Carcinogenesis 2015; 36(12): 1494-501.[http://dx.doi.org/10.1093/carcin/bgv150] [PMID: 26468118]

[56] Tampa M, Mitran MI, Mitran CI, et al. Mediators of Inflammation - A Potential Source of Biomarkers in Oral Squamous Cell Carcinoma. J Immunol Res 2018; 2018: 1061780.[http://dx.doi.org/10.1155/2018/1061780] [PMID: 30539028]

[57] Bussu F, Graziani C, Gallus R, et al. IFN-γ and other serum cytokines in head and neck squamous cell carcinomas. Acta Otorhinolaryngol Ital 2018; 38(2): 94-102.[http://dx.doi.org/10.14639/0392-100X-1530] [PMID: 29967556]

[58] Berggren KL, Restrepo Cruz S, Hixon MD, et al. MAPKAPK2 (MK2) inhibition mediates radiation-induced inflammatory cytokine production and tumor growth in head and neck squamous cell carcinoma. Oncogene 2019; 38(48): 7329-41.[http://dx.doi.org/10.1038/s41388-019-0945-9] [PMID: 31417185]

[59] Russo N, Bellile E, Murdoch-Kinch CA, et al. Cytokines in saliva increase in head and neck cancer patients after treatment. Oral Surg Oral Med Oral Pathol Oral Radiol 2016; 122(4): 483-90.[http://dx.doi.org/10.1016/j.oooo.2016.05.020] [PMID: 27554375]

[60] Druzgal CH, Chen Z, Yeh NT, et al. A pilot study of longitudinal serum cytokine and angiogenesis factor levels as markers of therapeutic response and survival in patients with head and neck squamous cell carcinoma. Head Neck 2005; 27(9): 771-84.[http://dx.doi.org/10.1002/hed.20246] [PMID: 15920746]

[61] Ueda T, Chikuie N, Takumida M, et al. Baseline neutrophil-to-lymphocyte ratio (NLR) is associated with

clinical outcome in recurrent or metastatic head and neck cancer patients treated with nivolumab. Acta Otolaryngol 2020; 140(2): 181-7.[http://dx.doi.org/10.1080/00016489.2019.1699250] [PMID: 31825711]

[62]   Sacdalan DB, Lucero JA, Sacdalan DL. Prognostic utility of baseline neutrophil-to-lymphocyte ratio in patients receiving immune checkpoint inhibitors: a review and meta-analysis. OncoTargets Ther 2018; 11: 955-65.[http://dx.doi.org/10.2147/OTT.S153290] [PMID: 29503570]

[63]   Mascarella MA, Mannard E, Silva SD, Zeitouni A. Neutrophil-to-lymphocyte ratio in head and neck cancer prognosis: A systematic review and meta-analysis. Head Neck 2018; 40(5): 1091-100.[http://dx.doi.org/10.1002/hed.25075] [PMID: 29356179]

[64]   Cho JK, Kim MW, Choi IS, et al. Optimal cutoff of pretreatment neutrophil-to-lymphocyte ratio in head and neck cancer patients: a meta-analysis and validation study. BMC Cancer 2018; 18(1): 969.[http://dx.doi.org/10.1186/s12885-018-4876-6] [PMID: 30309318]

[65]   Alsahafi E, Begg K, Amelio I, et al. Clinical update on head and neck cancer: molecular biology and ongoing challenges. Cell Death Dis 2019; 10(8): 540.[http://dx.doi.org/10.1038/s41419-019-1769-9] [PMID: 31308358]

[66]   Finger EC, Giaccia AJ. Hypoxia, inflammation, and the tumor microenvironment in metastatic disease. Cancer Metastasis Rev 2010; 29(2): 285-93.[http://dx.doi.org/10.1007/s10555-010-9224-5] [PMID: 20393783]

[67]   Chen SMY, Krinsky AL, Woolaver RA, Wang X, Chen Z, Wang JH. Tumor immune microenvironment in head and neck cancers. Mol Carcinog 2020; 59(7): 766-74.[http://dx.doi.org/10.1002/mc.23162] [PMID: 32017286]

[68]   Gupta SC, Tyagi AK, Deshmukh-Taskar P, Hinojosa M, Prasad S, Aggarwal BB. Downregulation of tumor necrosis factor and other proinflammatory biomarkers by polyphenols. Arch Biochem Biophys 2014; 559: 91-9.[http://dx.doi.org/10.1016/j.abb.2014.06.006] [PMID: 24946050]

[69]   Mat Lazim N. Cancer biomarkers: strategies for early diagnosis. Functional Foods and Cancer: Cancer Biology and Dietary Factors 2017; 3: 315-27. https://www.elsevier.com/books-and-journals

[70]   Shkeir O, Athanassiou-Papaefthymiou M, Lapadatescu M, et al. In vitro cytokine release profile: predictive value for metastatic potential in head and neck squamous cell carcinomas. Head Neck 2013; 35(11): 1542-50.[http://dx.doi.org/10.1002/hed.23191] [PMID: 23322448]

[71]   Chi LM, Lee CW, Chang KP, et al. Enhanced interferon signaling pathway in oral cancer revealed by quantitative proteome analysis of microdissected specimens using 16O/18O labeling and integrated two-dimensional LC-ESI-MALDI tandem MS. Mol Cell Proteomics 2009; 8(7): 1453-74.[http://dx.doi.org/10.1074/mcp.M800460-MCP200] [PMID: 19297561]

[72]   Mburu YK, Egloff AM, Walker WH, et al. Chemokine receptor 7 (CCR7) gene expression is regulated by NF-κB and activator protein 1 (AP1) in metastatic squamous cell carcinoma of head and neck (SCCHN). J Biol Chem 2012; 287(5): 3581-90.[http://dx.doi.org/10.1074/jbc.M111.294876] [PMID: 22158872]

[73]   Balasubramaniam A, Mat Lazim N. Nasopharyngeal Carcinoma screening and prevention programme. In: Abdullah B, Balasubramaniam A, Mat Lazim N, eds. An Evidence-Based Approach to the Management of Nasopharyngeal Cancer: From Basic Sciences to Clinical Presentation and Treatment Abdullah B, Balasubramaniam A, Mat Lazim N. 202011-30. https://www.elsevier.com/books-and-journals[http://dx.doi.org/10.1016/B978-0-12-814403-9.00012-4]

[74]   Katano A, Takahashi W, Yamashita H, et al. The impact of elevated C-reactive protein level on the prognosis for oro-hypopharynx cancer patients treated with radiotherapy. Sci Rep 2017; 7(1): 17805.[http://dx.doi.org/10.1038/s41598-017-18233-w] [PMID: 29259311]

[75]   Chen IH, Liao CT, Wang HM, Huang JJ, Kang CJ, Huang SF. Using SCC antigen and CRP levels as prognostic biomarkers in recurrent oral cavity squamous cell carcinoma. PLoS One 2014; 9(7): e103265.[http://dx.doi.org/10.1371/journal.pone.0103265] [PMID: 25061977]

[76]   Kruse AL, Luebbers HT, Grätz KW. C-reactive protein levels: a prognostic marker for patients with head and neck cancer? Head Neck Oncol 2010; 2: 21.[http://dx.doi.org/10.1186/1758-3284-2-21] [PMID: 20673375]

[77]   Choudhary MM, France TJ, Teknos TN, Kumar P. Interleukin-6 role in head and neck squamous cell carcinoma progression. World J Otorhinolaryngol Head Neck Surg 2016; 2(2): 90-7.[http://dx.doi.org/10.1016/j.wjorl.2016.05.002] [PMID: 29204553]

[78]   Scheff NN, Ye Y, Bhattacharya A, et al. Tumor necrosis factor alpha secreted from oral squamous cell carcinoma contributes to cancer pain and associated inflammation. Pain 2017; 158(12): 2396-409.[http://dx.doi.org/10.1097/j.pain.0000000000001044] [PMID: 28885456]

[79]   Normando AGC, Rocha CL, de Toledo IP, et al. Biomarkers in the assessment of oral mucositis in head and neck cancer patients: a systematic review and meta-analysis. Support Care Cancer 2017; 25(9): 2969-

88.[http://dx.doi.org/10.1007/s00520-017-3783-8] [PMID: 28623401]

[80] G D, Nandan SRK, Kulkarni PG. G DSalivary Tumour Necrosis Factor-α as a Biomarker in Oral Leukoplakia and Oral Squamous Cell Carcinoma. Asian Pac J Cancer Prev 2019; 20(7): 2087-93.[http://dx.doi.org/10.31557/APJCP.2019.20.7.2087] [PMID: 31350970]

[81] Selimovic D, Wahl RU, Ruiz E, *et al.* Tumor necrosis factor-α triggers opposing signals in head and neck squamous cell carcinoma and induces apoptosis *via* mitochondrial- and non-mitochondrial-dependent pathways. Int J Oncol 2019; 55(6): 1324-38.[http://dx.doi.org/10.3892/ijo.2019.4900] [PMID: 31638203]

[82] Powrózek T, Mlak R, Brzozowska A, Mazurek M, Gołębiowski P, Małecka-Massalska T. Relationship between TNF-α -1031T/C gene polymorphism, plasma level of TNF-α, and risk of cachexia in head and neck cancer patients. J Cancer Res Clin Oncol 2018; 144(8): 1423-34.[http://dx.doi.org/10.1007/s00432-018-2679-4] [PMID: 29802455]

[83] Lin YW, Huang ST, Wu JC, *et al.* Novel HDGF/HIF-1α/VEGF axis in oral cancer impacts disease prognosis. BMC Cancer 2019; 19(1): 1083.[http://dx.doi.org/10.1186/s12885-019-6229-5] [PMID: 31711427]

[84] Schlüter A, Weller P, Kanaan O, *et al.* CD31 and VEGF are prognostic biomarkers in early-stage, but not in late-stage, laryngeal squamous cell carcinoma. BMC Cancer 2018; 18(1): 272.[http://dx.doi.org/10.1186/s12885-018-4180-5] [PMID: 29523110]

[85] Zang J, Li C, Zhao LN, *et al.* Prognostic value of vascular endothelial growth factor in patients with head and neck cancer: A meta-analysis. Head Neck 2013; 35(10): 1507-14.[http://dx.doi.org/10.1002/hed.23156] [PMID: 22987573]

[86] Zhu X, Zhang F, Zhang W, He J, Zhao Y, Chen X. Prognostic role of epidermal growth factor receptor in head and neck cancer: a meta-analysis. J Surg Oncol 2013; 108(6): 387-97.[http://dx.doi.org/10.1002/jso.23406] [PMID: 24038070]

[87] Gisterek I, Kornafel J. Naczyniowo-śródbłonkowy czynnik wzrostu w nowotworach głowy i szyi. Pol Merkuriusz Lek 2006; 20(116): 242-4.

[88] Vassilakopoulou M, Psyrri A, Argiris A. Targeting angiogenesis in head and neck cancer. Oral Oncol 2015; 51(5): 409-15.[http://dx.doi.org/10.1016/j.oraloncology.2015.01.006] [PMID: 25680863]

[89] Argiris A, Li S, Savvides P, *et al.* Phase iii randomized trial of chemotherapy with or without bevacizumab in patients with recurrent or metastatic head and neck cancer. J Clin Oncol 2019; 37(34): 3266-74.[http://dx.doi.org/10.1200/JCO.19.00555] [PMID: 31618129]

[90] Guthrie GJ. The systemic inflammation-based neutrophil-lymphocyte ratio: experience in patients with cancer 2013 Oct; 88 (1): 218-30. [http://dx.doi.org/10.1016/j.critrevonc.2013.03.010]

[91] Nakamura T, Gaston CL, Reddy K, Iwata S, Nishio J. Inflammatory biomarkers in cancer. Mediators Inflamm 2016; 2016: 7282797.[http://dx.doi.org/10.1155/2016/7282797] [PMID: 27843202]

Inflammation and Current HPV Status in Head and Neck Malignancy

Roman Carlos Zamora[1], [*], Jose Gutiérrez Jodas[2], Norhafiza Mat Lazim[3]

[1] Department of Otorhinolaryngology-Head and Neck Surgery Hospital Universitario Reina Sofia, Cordoba Spain. Direction: Avenida Menendez Pidal, s/n, Postal code 14004, Cordoba, Spain

[2] Department of Otorhinolaryngology-Head and Neck Surgery, Hospital Universitario Reina Sofia, Cordoba, Spain, Avenida Menendez Pidal, s/n, Postal code 14004Cordoba, Spain

[3] Department of Otorhinolaryngology-Head and Neck Surgery, School of Medical Sciences, Universiti Sains Malaysia, Health Campus 16150, Kubang Kerian, Kelantan, Malaysia

Abstract

Head and neck malignancy is on the rise, where the majority of the tumors are squamous cell carcinoma (HNSCC). Previously, alcohol and tobacco are reported to be the well-established risk factors for HNSCC development. Currently, the HPV driven HNSCC has shown an increase in incidence globally, with oropharyngeal and oral cavity carcinoma predominating at certain geographic locations. HPV associated oropharyngeal squamous cell carcinoma commonly occurs in Europe and certain Western countries. They have different biological profiles compared to HPV-negative HNSCC. HPV-positive HNSCC patients have different characteristics and prognosis, which remarkably affect the management of this subset of patients. HPV is a significant inflammatory agent that can promote carcinogenesis *via* multiple critical mechanisms that are discussed in the chapters. Targeting HPV for future research is a great promising avenue for the discovery of novel screening, diagnostic, and therapeutic targets.

Keywords: Alcohol and tobacco, Chronic inflammation, Head and neck cancer survival, Head and neck carcinoma, Human Papillomavirus (HPV), Prognosis, Treatment outcomes.

---

* **Corresponding author Roman Carlos Zamora:** Department of Otorhinolaryngology-Head and Neck Surgery Hospital Universitario Reina Sofia, Cordoba Spain. Direction: Avenida Menendez Pidal, s/n, Postal code 14004, Cordoba, Spain; Tel: +34634219251; E-mail: romanchos@hotmail.com

INTRODUCTION

This chapter focuses on chronic inflammation, HPV, and its relation to head and neck malignancy, as well as its various treatment and preventive options. It is well documented that chronic inflammation in the complex world of the immune system plays an important role in malignancy. Currently, the tendency of

treatment options for HNSCC patients is becoming less invasive, more conservative, and aims to have a more molecular approach. This can be ideally achieved by incorporating inflammation markers as promising therapeutic agents in the near future. Prevention plays an important role in combatting HNSCC.

As early as the 1800s, the perception of inflammation associated with cancer has been thought of but not demonstrated. In recent years, molecular studies have been able to show that inflammation contributes to the survival and proliferation of malignant cells [1]. Many of the well-established risk factors for head and neck malignancy are associated with inflammation. For instance, the environmental carcinogens such as sharp tooth and periodontitis for oral cavity carcinoma, Epstein Barr virus (EBV) for nasopharyngeal carcinoma (NPC), wood dust exposure for sinonasal malignancy and human papillomavirus (HPV) for oropharyngeal carcinoma. HPV-related HNSCC is significant as this tumor group has a different biological profile and treatment outcomes compared to HPV-negative tumors.

CHRONIC INFLAMMATION AND HEAD AND NECK ORAL CARCINOMA

Squamous cell carcinoma is the most common malignant lesion in the oral cavity. There is a significant increase in oral cancer incidence in young people, with 350,000-400,000 new cases worldwide per year. Bacteria, viruses, and fungi have been implicated and highly related to certain cancers [2]. For these reasons alone, it is important to gather more research and investigations about the risk factors of head and neck squamous cell carcinoma (HNSCC) in patients under 45 years old [3]. The oral cavity contains many bacterial species, with some of them being able to produce oral pathology. In recent years, the relationship between oral flora and head and neck cancer has been a subject of interest. Emerging evidence suggests that chronic inflammation could play an important role in the development of cancer. Importantly, studies have shown that periodontitis can promote carcinogenesis and lead to oral cavity cancers.

There is a strong association between head and neck carcinoma risk and oral leukoplakia, oral fibrosis, and repetitive dental ulcer injury [4]. There is a complex inflammatory process involved in the progression of premalignant lesions to squamous cell carcinoma. The role of T-cells (Tregs) and tumor-associated macrophages in immunohistochemical staining of cytokines showed that there was an increase in disease progression in premalignant oral lesions. In the early stages of premalignant lesions, IL-10 was seen to be increasing [5]. All of these inflammatory markers play a crucial role in the pathogenesis of head and

neck malignancy, and some have been discussed in the other chapters in this book.

Generally, during the progression of oral dysplasia, IL-4$^+$ macrophages were seen from premalignant lesions. However, TGF-β1$^+$ macrophages were seen in oral squamous cell carcinoma (OSCC) in less quantity than premalignant lesions as well as the expression of IFN-γ. These findings suggest that chronic inflammation promotes tumorigenesis in OSCC, rather than initializing it [5]. Overpopulation of pathogenic oral bacteria may be secondary to poor oral hygiene. This, in turn, can switch the chronic inflammation process and progression into OSCC. Three species of oral bacteria associated with an increased risk of oral squamous carcinoma were *Fusobacterium nucleatum*, *Prevotella tannerae*, and *Prevotella intermedia*. Additionally, it was also seen that alcohol, cigarettes, and poor oral hygiene were associated with an increase in oral pathogenic bacteria. Salivary IL1β was associated with a rise in periodontal-pathogenic bacteria and OSCC risk, which in turn can be influenced by genetic factors and lifestyle. Critically, all these results suggested that good oral hygiene may reduce OSCC risk and should be part of a prevention campaign [6].

The risk of cancer can potentially be predicted through alterations seen in the oral microbiota. Further understanding can be achieved by molecular advances in monitoring the role of oral microbiota and oral carcinogenesis [7]. For example, the formation of *8-oxo-7,8-dihydro-2'-deoxyguanosine* and *8-nitroguanine* are mutagenic DNA lesions associated with inflammation-related cancers. The formation of these mutagenic DNA has been seen in precancerous lesions due to infection and pro-inflammatory factors. Several studies have suggested that cancer development is triggered by inflammation associated-DNA damage in cancer stem-like cells. An increase in oxidative stress due to dysfunction of anti-oxidative proteins, DNA methylation, and microRNA dysregulation can lead to carcinogenesis. One example is Epstein-Barr virus-related nasopharyngeal carcinoma, in which quantitative RT-PCR analysis confirmed the downregulation of miR-497 in cancer tissues and plasma. These findings can be useful biomarkers in liquid biopsy for prevention and early detection [8] of HNSCC.

C-reactive protein (CRP) is an acute-phase protein that serves as a marker for inflammation and the progression of various cancers. A study by Metgud *et al.* compared CRP in saliva and serum in 20 normal individuals, 20 patients with OSCC, and 20 patients with oral premalignant lesions to assess as a prognostic indicator for OSCC. Mean CRP levels were more elevated in patients with premalignant lesions and OSCC compared to controls [9]. Oral cancer has become an important problem in many parts of the world, with more cases seen in developing countries. This is the reason why molecularly targeted prevention of oral cancer and the link to chronic inflammation is important. Other inflammatory mediators that play a role in oral cancer development, apart from the aforementioned, include VEGF, prostaglandin pathways, p53, inflammatory cytokines, reactive oxygen, and nitrogen species. Currently, the cytology and biopsy can make the diagnosis of HNSCC, and this can be combined with testing of inflammatory biomarkers that could be beneficial for early detection of HNSCC [10].

Alcohol and tobacco, human papillomavirus (HPV), or Epstein-Barr viruses (EBV) can start and maintain a chronic inflammation through genomic alterations or viral oncoproteins *via phosphatidylinositol 3-kinase* (PI3K) and *transcription factor nuclear factor-kappa B* (NF-κB). Various ongoing studies at molecular therapies targeting signaling in cancer cells are being developed to explore better ways of controlling cancer. One example is the immune checkpoint inhibitors in combination with inflammatory cells in the immune system [11]. It is important to understand cancer development comes from activated oncogenes or dysfunctional tumor suppressor genes. However, these factors alone are not sufficient for the development of carcinogenesis. Importantly, the infiltration of immune cells facilitates neoplasm development by enabling tumors to evade the host immune response. Structural support to developing tumors is provided by the alteration of the extracellular matrix in inflammation. Hypoxia induces DNA damage and is tumorigenic, while tissue vasculature is important for maintaining the microenvironment that supplies cell division and metastatic spread. Inflammation and its ecosystem provide support for tissue homeostasis and repair, which is important to be understood in order to produce a potential treatment target for head and neck cancers [12]. Chronic inflammatory mediators have pleiotropic effects, *i.e.*, they can favor carcinogenesis but can also limit tumor growth by stimulating immune effector mechanisms. The role of IL-1-signaling and stress protein involvement is an important mechanism in the development of anti-cancer immunity and anti-apoptotic functions. Chronic infection by various means, like reflux, viral or bacterial infection can cause up to 25% of human malignancies [13].

A study by Ambatipudi and colleagues assessed if DNA methylation derived systemic inflammation indices are associated with head and neck cancer development and survival. The multivariate logistic regression study showed that elevated Neutrophil-to-Lymphocyte ratio (NLR) is associated with increased odds of being an HNSCC case (OR = 3.25, 95% CI = 2.14-5.34, $P = 4 \times 10^{-7}$) while the contrary was observed with Lymphocyte-to-Monocyte ratio (LMR), OR = 0.88, 95% CI = 0.81-0.90, $P = 2 \times 10^{-3}$. It was seen that HPV16-E6 seropositive HNSCC cases had an elevated LMR and a lower NLR when compared to seronegative patients. Results showed that lower LMR but not lower levels of NLR were associated with an increased risk of death [14]. In another study by Wang *et al.* in inflammation-related DNA damage and cancer stem cell markers in nasopharyngeal carcinoma, several cancer stem/progenitor cell markers (CD44v6, CD24, and ALDH1A1) were studied. It was seen that CD44v6 and ALDH1A1 were significantly increased in cancer cells of primary NPC specimens in comparison to chronic nasopharyngitis. No significant difference was observed between chronic nasopharyngitis tissue and NPC in the case of CD24. The study concluded that CD44v6 and ALDH1A1 could be stem cell markers for NPC [15].

One study aimed to determine the expression of beta-defensins in nasal polyposis and chronic tonsillitis as well as to determine the relationship between the malignant process in tonsils and inflammation. In cases of chronic inflammation, the study showed large secretions of human beta defensins, while limited in malignant transformation. Endothelial nitric oxide synthase (eNOS) and nitric oxide molecule are involved in cell cycle regulation, cell proliferation and apoptosis results confirmed that eNOS is present in the upper airway in chronic inflammation and cancer [16]. It can be said that specific transcription factors enhance the expression of genes and have the ability to regulate the survival and proliferation of malignant cells. There is a link between inflammation and cancer. In the stroma of established cancers, there is a state of exaggerated inflammation and suppression of immune responses. There is no denying that precancerous lesions (oral submucous fibrosis, oral lichen planus), dento-gingival bacterial plaques, chronic periodontitis, chronic tonsillitis, *etc.*, have inflammation as a common factor [17].

Oropharyngeal Carcinoma Associated with HPV

The malignancy of the aerodigestive tract represents about 600,000 new cases per year. It is well known that alcohol, tobacco and HPV are significant etiology factors. About 40-80% of head and neck malignancies are associated with HPV [18]. The risk of developing oral and oropharyngeal carcinoma is four times higher in patients with infected HPV. The relationship between HPV and oropharyngeal carcinoma has been recognized in 2009 [19]. The incidence of oropharyngeal carcinoma (OPSCC) associated with HPV has been increased in recent years. It is estimated that approximately 70-80% of OPSCCs in North America and Europe are related to HPV infection [20]. Oral HPV 16 detection was associated with incident HNSCC with a positive association for OPSCC [21]. Of note, the OPSCCs associated with HPV have higher survival than HPV negative. At present, the therapeutic approach is based on minimizing treatment, without decreasing overall survival, and conducting prevention campaigns through health education and vaccination campaigns.

Human Papilloma Virus (HPV)

The HPV virus belongs to the papillomaviridiae family. It is a DNA virus and more than 300 subtypes have been identified. The strains with the greatest oncogenic potential are HPV 16 and 18 [22]. It is well known that HPV is transmitted to the oropharynx through oral sex and profound tongue base kissing. The risk of infection increases with the number of couples and if there is an association with HIV. Most people eliminate HPV within one to two years but in some, the infection persists and becomes a chronic infection with the risk of developing carcinoma. The HPV infection occurs in the squamous epithelium of the oropharynx, in its basal stratum. A correct union and inhibition of certain proteins take place that allows the integration of viral DNA with the cellular DNA. Subsequently, this generates cellular changes that actívate cell proliferation.

HPV has a double-stranded DNA of 8000 base pairs being divided into three regions; E, L, and log control regíón, each of which will originate a certain group of proteins [23]. The E6 and E7 region encode oncoproteins that inactivate proteins that regulate the cell cycle, p16, p53, and pRB. These oncoproteins can be categorized into high and low risk. The low-risk oncoprotein does not have activity because they are inactivated mutations, this being the cause of the different oncogenicity among the different HPV [24].

Mutation of the p16 proteins inhibits the cell cycle and phosphorylation of pRB inactivity, which leads to a phase change of the cell cycle from G1 to S. The p53 protein is responsible for cell control, DNA repair and apoptosis control. The inactivation of p53 is caused by the E6AP proteins that maintain the binding between p53-E6, inactivating p53 results in chromosomal and genomic instability. The E7 oncoprotein ensures a correct replication of the viral DNA by inactivating the 'pocket' proteins which are the pRB, p100, and p130 [24].

HPV affects the basal layer of the stratified epithelium of the oropharynx. The viral DNA, E1 and E2 proteins are integrated into the cellular DNA. With times the proliferation takes place with genome amplification and multiplication occurs. This is carried out due to the activity of E6 and E7 proteins that inactivate p53 and pRB. This mechanism that HPV has to enter into the DNA of the host cells prevents an immune reaction to be eliminated. The elimination of the virus is carried out when the cells reach the most superficial stratum which is the regression phase. The infection can be perpetuated for years if the regression phase is not completed. This is called the abortion cycle. This interruption in the cycle is due to failure of control of the E2 protein on the E6 and E7 causing the viral DNA unable to complete its cycle, thus generating genetic alteration and DNA instability with the consequent cell proliferation.

EPIDEMIOLOGY OF THE HPV RELATED HNSCC

There have been different studies that showed an increasing trend of OPSCC related HPV. The majority of this study was conducted in the US and Western Europe. In Stockholm [25] there is an increase in the prevalence of 0.7/100,000 between 1970-1979 to 1.65/100,000 between 2000-2006. In the US [26], there is an increase from 2.8/100,000 to 3.6/100,000 between the years 1988-2004. Whereas in Denmark [27] an increase in the annual incidence of 2.7% between 2000 and 2010. Although at present, it is not considered an epidemic, it is evident that there is an increase in the incidence of related HPV with OPSCC. The etiology of this increase is currently is unknown, although it could be justified by the greater number of sexual practices, the decrease in tonsillectomy in children or by a greater attempt to reach an etiological diagnosis in relation to HPV.

The association of HPV and OPSCC is considered a sexually transmitted disease, with oral sex being the main risk factor. The number of partners throughout life, early oral sex before the age of 18, deep tongue kissing, marijuana use, HPV infection of the anogenital tract and smoking are associated risk factors to the development of OPSCC and HPV [28, 29]. When comparing patients with OPSCC associated with HPV with non-associated HPV, it is observed that they are younger patients (<60 years), with lower consumption of tobacco and alcohol, higher sexual practices and higher socioeconomic status. With regard to gender, there is a greater proportion of men than women in the US and Europe. A population study of the National Cancer Database (NCDB) conducted during the period 2010 to 2014 showed a higher positive HPV in men than in women for both OPSCC (66% *vs* 50%) and OCSCC (16% *vs* 11%) [30]. HPV OPSCC positive in women appear at a later age and in an earlier stage than in men. Generally, sexual habits, lifestyle, tobacco and alcohol consumption cannot fully explain the differences of the prevalence of HPV-related HNSCC between the sexes. There should be other critical factors that are unknown. For instance, the hormonal factor, whereby the level of estrogen and progestogens fluctuation is inversely correlated with the development of OPSCC. Women who develop menopause before age 52 and those who become pregnant after age 35 have a higher risk of developing OPSCC associated HPV [30]. The race is another important factor to consider, although the most frequent HPV in all types of OPSCC is 16, African descent has been linked to HPV type 17. This difference is critical in relation to survival, since it is lower in the black race regardless of stage, applied treatment and sex. Racial disparity in the prognosis of cancer is strongly related to the genetic and epigenetic diversity, a greater metabolic propensity of obesity and the state of chronic inflammation of black people, as well as differences in innate immunity [31].

CLINICAL OVERVIEW OF HPV ASSOCIATED OROPHARYNGEAL CARCINOMA

Survival of OPSCC patients depends mainly on the stage at the time of diagnosis. In the earliest stages, symptoms are very scarce which is why this type of tumor is often diagnosed at late stages. Among the most frequent symptoms include odynophagia, dysphagia, otalgia, trismus and pharyngeal body sensation which are seen in advanced-stage diseases. The HPV positive OPSCC mainly harbor the virus within the palatine and lingual tonsils, which is a critical reservoir for HPV. As aforementioned, this group of patients has a specific profile. They are young and having multiple sexual partners, have a high socioeconomic status associated with tobacco and alcohol consumption.

It is common to find large cervical metastases and small tumors in the oropharynx which is difficult to spot in a routine examination of the oropharynx. In order to locate these small tumors, especially those smaller than 1 cm that is undetectable with white, the narrow band imaging (NBI) and autofluorescence based endoscopic imaging can be used. The NBI is currently used for the diagnosis of superficial carcinomas, assessing the hidden lesions, method of surveillance for patient post treatment and study of intraoperative resection margin [32]. In the Di Maia meta-analysis, the grouped sensitivity and specificity of NBI in patients with cervical metastases of HNSCC with unknown primary was 0.83 (99% CI, 0.54-0.95) and 0.88 (99% CI, 0.005-0.86). PET- CT is necessary for accurate staging of OPSCC. This will give information on the extent of the tumors, presence of cervical metastases, distant metastases and is highly useful for planning for radiotherapy and monitoring treatment response and evidence of recurrent diseases [33].

DIAGNOSTIC METHODS IN THE ASSESSMENT OF HPV

Of note, the diagnosis of HPV associated with oropharyngeal carcinoma is essential for its classification, treatment, and prognosis. There are currently more than 125 commercially available techniques for the detection of HPV. It is one of the most numerous diagnostic techniques available, but it is also less regulated. Generally, they can be broadly categorized into four types:

1. Determination of p16 protein.
2. DNA analysis by *in situ* hybridization
3. DNA analysis by PCR
4. Analysis of E6/E7 viral transcription RNA by reverse transcriptase PCR.

Classification HPV+ Oropharyngeal Carcinoma

The American Joint Committee on Cancer (AJCC) published the 8th edition on head and neck cancer staging in 2017 [34], introducing novel modifications with respect to the previous classification. The 7th edition classification system classified the majority of the OPSCC associated with HPV in stages III and IV. The introduction of the 8th edition has clearly differentiated between HPV positive and HPV negative.

The differentiation implies changes in stage, prognosis and treatment. The OPSCC associated or not with HPV have been classified based on overexpression of the p16 protein. The p16 is a widely available marker, inexpensive and easy to interpret. The cut-off point for overexpression of p16 is diffuse tumor expression (more than 75%) and with at least moderate staining intensity (+2/3). The new classification eliminates Tis (carcinoma *in situ*) in the OPSCC p16+, because there is no basement membrane in the epithelium of lingual and palatine tonsils. The OPSCC p16+ is the only carcinoma of the head and neck that maintain the T0 category. The other difference is in the classification of neck metastasis. For new classification, stage N1 encompasses ipsilateral neck metastasis less than 6cm, in contrast to the 7th edition classification which classifies N1 as single ipsilateral adenopathy less than 3cm. Additionally, presence of neck nodes in the OPSCC p16 positive cases larger than 6 cm are closely related to detrimental effects on survival [35]. The 8th edition classification system is more practical whereby it classifies the OPSCC HPV positive and OPSCC HPV negative based on the therapeutic and survival outcomes [34].

TREATMENT OF OROPHARYNGEAL CARCINOMA ASSOCIATED WITH HPV

In the past, the treatment of the OPSCC has been based on the use of radical radiotherapy and chemotherapy. This is because open transmandibular surgery carries high morbidities with mortality and swallowing deficit and lower survival compared to chemoradiation. Swallowing impairment secondary to treatment is one of the main sequelae that patients with OPSCC experienced. The chemoradiation, even though it has benefits, the local and systemic adverse effects are also substantial. It can also cause significant swallowing and mastication impairment due to fibrosis induced trismus. During period of radiotherapy, 62% of OPSCC patients require gastrostomy [36]. Interestingly, in order to reduce the morbidity associated with treatment without affecting survival, Trans Oral Ultrasonic (TOUSS), Transoral Laser Microsurgery (TLM) and Transoral Robotic Surgery (TORS) are being evaluated.

TOUSS was designed as a 'no robot' endoscopic transoral procedure, which is inspired by the laparoscopic approach of abdominal surgeons using a unique port, the mouth. TOUSS uses the Gyrus FK retractor, Olympus endoscope system and ultrasonic device such as the Thunderbeat (Fig. 1). This allows an endoscopic approach of the oropharynx at a much less cost than any other robotic system. This technique also gives an excellent oncological and functional result with minimal surgical complication. In a series by Fernandez *et al*. the majority of the OPSCC treated with TOUSS in stage T1 and T3 did not reveal any surgical complications. Only two patients in the series presented with post-surgical bleeding that was endoscopically controlled in the operation room. The resection margins were mostly negative for all surgical specimens [37]. TORS is another technique known for years through the robotic platform (Fig. 2). The best known is the Da Vinci Robot system. The indications of TORS for OPSCC have been extended to stage T3 and T4 without differentiating their association or not with HPV. The functional results are quite satisfactory. Choosing a candidate for transoral surgery will depend on T and N stage of the tumor that requires resection of the tongue base for more than 50% and the patient indicated for adjuvant chemoradiation [38]. In order to reduce the toxicity of chemoradiation and surgery, different therapeutic de-intensifications are being conducted. To evaluate whether lowering the dose of radiotherapy and substituting chemotherapeutic agents with lower toxicity and using minimally invasive techniques, the same oncological results are achieved as with the standard treatment. Another study evaluated the reduced dose of IMRT with or without cisplatin in the treatment of the patient with advanced oropharyngeal carcinoma [39].

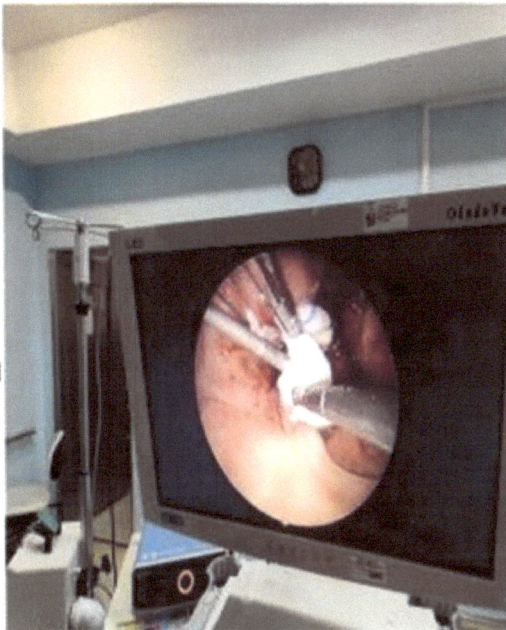

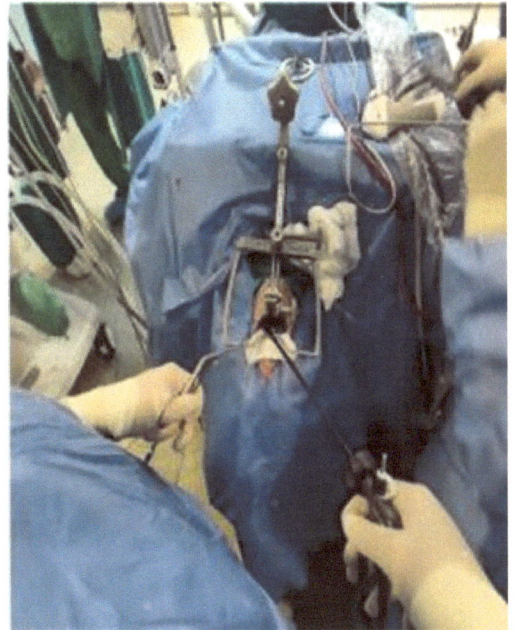

Fig. (1))
Images showing TOUSS procedure is being performed.

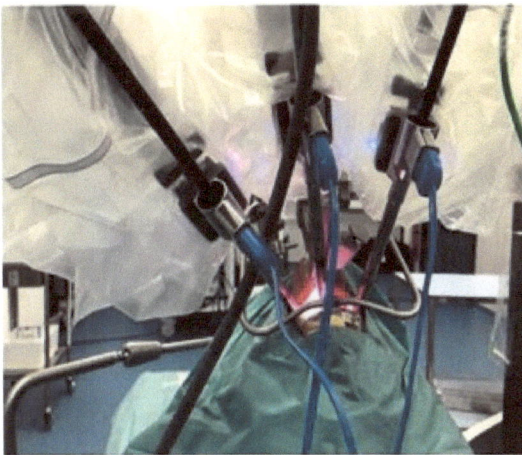

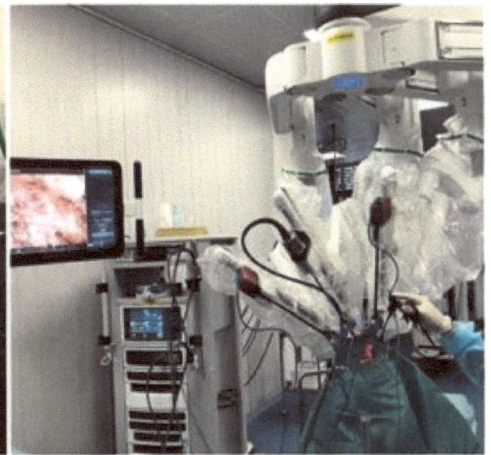

Fig.   **(2))**
Images of TORS.

Chemotherapy De-Intensification Trials

The oncology RTOG group conducted a study which comprise of 182 centers in the USA and Canada incorporating HPV positive OPSCC patients. This study aims to evaluate whether cetuximab in combination with radiation can achieve greater survival and lower toxicity in stage III and IV OPSCC patients compared to the standard cisplatin treatment [40]. The result showed that the survival was lower with cetuximab and the toxicity was similar using both cetuximab and platinum regimes. It has been shown that a lower dose of IMRT produce favorable results with less late toxicities and a statistically significant improvement in swallowing solids can be achieved. This finding supports the hypothesis that a dose of 55 Gray or less is likely to affect swallowing function [41]. Avoiding the adjuvant chemotherapy in patients with extracapsular extension is another strategy to minimize the morbidity associated with the treatment. The Washington University group reported that the presence of extracapsular extension does not affect disease free survival. In their series of 151 patients with HPV positive OPSCC treated with TORS, the 3-year survival of patients with and without extracapsular extension was 89% (95% CI 84%-95% and 94% (95% CI 83%-100%) respectively [42].

The results of the trials should provide more information and adequate risk stratification and the selection of adjuvant treatment in the future. A proper selection of adjuvant treatment de-intensification is essential to obtain excellent results. Therefore, deintensification outside a clinical trial is currently not recommended. A better understanding of the molecular alterations underlying the HPV associated disease should be elucidated to provide more opportunities for targeted therapies with less toxicity. If these approaches are adequate, the quality of life of patients should improve significantly [43].

PREVENTION OF HPV INFECTION

HPV serotypes 16 and 18 are responsible for the majority of cases of anal cancers and a significant proportion of oropharyngeal, vulvar, and vaginal cancer. There are currently three types of HPV vaccination. First is the quadrivalent HPV vaccine aka Gardasil which targets HPV types 6, 11, 16 and 18. Secondly is the 9-valent vaccine (Gardasil 9) which contains the serotypes HPV 6, 11, 16,18, 31, 33, 45, 52 and 58. Thirdly is the bivalent vaccine which is known as Cervarix that can be used for HPV types 16 and 18.

At this juncture, the vaccination indications in women are clearly documented. WHO recommends that only vaccination against HPV to girls between 9-14 years of age. This is the age before sexual activity is active. This can offer a vaccine coverage greater than 80% to reduce the HPV infection in boys [44]. In certain geographic locations, for instance, in the US, the vaccine is indicated in both girls and boys. Even though there are numerous studies that showed the vaccine may be efficacious for reducing the prevalence of HPV in the oropharynx [45-47], currently, the prevention of oropharyngeal carcinoma is not an indication of vaccination. Thus the prevention program can consists of education and awareness programs targetting the high-risk groups.

TREATMENT AND PREVENTION OF HPV ASSOCIATED HEAD AND NECK MALIGNANCIES

Current Treatment for HPV HNSCC

HPV positive head and neck malignancy represent a unique disease that has a different clinical presentation, treatment approach and prognosis compared to tobacco-associated head and neck cancers [48]. Generally, the treatment of head and neck cancer consists of surgery, endoscopic assisted procedures, chemoradiation and immune-targeted therapy. The multimodality treatment approach always gives the best treatment outcomes. The final treatment of head and neck carcinoma will depend on the site of the tumor, the tumor stage and grade, presence of lymph nodes involvement, distant metastases, patient's comorbidity and the availability of the expertise. The main aim of managing head and neck cancer patients is to eradicate the tumor as well as to improve the patient's quality of life [49].

A comprehensive assessment is necessary in order to accurately stage head and neck cancer. This is normally achieved by details clinical examination, imaging procedures and blood workup. Most of the time patients are reviewed at the outpatient clinic with all the findings and treatment plans explained to the patient and the family members. The final decision will depend on patient consent whether to proceed with surgery, chemoradiation or other choices of treatment. Conventionally, head and neck cancer is categorized into 3 main groups: early-stages tumor, late-stage tumor, recurrent disease or metastatic diseases. Stage 1 and II head and neck carcinoma are generally treated with single modality therapy *i.e.* either surgery or radiation. The cure rates for this group of patients are excellent, provided the patient fully comply with the treatment regimes. For late stage cancer, the multimodality treatment approach is required for better therapeutic outcomes. The patient will need to have surgery with adjuvant radiation or sometimes chemoradiation in combination with targeted therapy, in selected advanced disease and metastatic tumor [49].

Chemoradiation plays a critical role in the treatment of HPV positive oropharyngeal carcinoma. This is particularly true if the tumor belongs to stage III or IV disease. Currently, the de-escalation treatment has become the research focus on managing oropharyngeal carcinoma [50, 51]. This is due to the fact that these subsets of patients have a better prognosis and they are younger patient groups. Thus, the necessity to reduce the treatment-related morbidities is critical as these patients will have longer life ahead. The common chemotherapy agent that is used in head and neck malignancy includes cisplatin, bleomycin, Adriamycin, methotrexate and fluorouracil. Imperatively, most of advanced head and neck cancer is treated with the combined modality approach and involves multidisciplinary care.

Numerous studies also try to elicit which treatment strategy will have better outcomes. The surgery *versus* radiation or with concomitant chemoradiation. Different studies reported different therapeutic responses in reference to the different treatment protocols. Sinha *et al* reported that there is no difference in outcomes between the primary surgical and non-surgical therapy of oropharyngeal carcinoma [52]. Planned neck dissection has been compared with radiotherapy +/- chemotherapy has positive effects on OPSCC patients, especially stage III and IV disease with varied responses [53, 54]. Another study assessed the transoral robotic surgery in comparison with radiotherapy for early-stage OPSCC [55]. Oliver *et al.* reported that concomitant chemoradiation together with surgery has superior therapeutic outcomes in contrast to radiation plus surgery in advanced stage III and IV tumor [56, 57].

HPV positive HNSCC is a unique tumor which has different characteristic profiles compare to tobacco associate HNSCC [58]. Generally, it is associated with male patients, non-alcohol and a non-smoker, better treatment response and highly associate with p16 overexpression or the expression of E6 and E7 transcripts. Oropharyngeal cancer has been known to associate with HPV positive and the treatment can be improved with the application of chemotherapy. Selected oropharyngeal cancer did not show p16 overexpression [59]. Some other markers have been explored such as β-catenin expression [60, 61].

The enhanced treatment of cancer should also have effective assessment methods in order to get an earlier diagnosis. This is necessary so that treatment can be started early to prevent recurrent disease and metastatic spread. Nowadays, the best method of assessing the presence of p16 is by immunohistochemical staining. With the advent of technology and refinement in reagents and testing kits, the assessment of p16 also has escalated in this era of tissue engineering and biomedicine. More precise techniques have been identified and are under robust study. Now, the tissues from the fine needle aspiration cytology can be tested for the presence of p16 at ease and are highly reliable. The cost of testing also has been reduced dramatically. The p16 has been proved to be a versatile surrogate marker for HPV status, as it is can be tested even in tissue with cellular degeneration. The cost for immunostaining is also low and it has a high sensitivity that can make it an effective standalone test for HPV [62].

From our clinical practice, up to this date, there is no single therapy that is effective for treating head and neck cancer. Conventionally, the most common practice of treatment is the combination of surgery and chemoradiation. Regardless of many studies, the outcomes and complications from the treatment remain the same with the results of poor quality of life of most head and neck cancer patients. The subset of HPV positive head and neck carcinoma affects the younger patient population and has a better prognosis, which mandates treatment with less side effects and morbidity. Some of the new techniques include reduction of radiation dose, the use of targeted immunotherapy replacing the standard cisplatin chemotherapy and usage of transoral robotic surgery.

NEW POTENTIAL TREATMENT APPROACH

Historically, evidence highlight that the tonsillar crypts harbor the HPV particles and is significant during the early phase of carcinogenesis. With the availability of current biomarkers and therapeutic techniques such as nanotechnology and artificial intelligence, the disease can be detected early and targeted treatment can focus on eliminating of this initial focus of infection. In addition, with robust sequencing technology, multiple newer methods have been developed to delineate the true effects of HPV, for assessment of saliva and serum tumor DNA as a potential effective therapeutic approach [63].

Several biomarkers that can be used to predict the response to treatment in the HPV positive oropharyngeal carcinoma include tumor infiltrating lymphocytes and low MHC class I [64]. In addition to the HPV DNA oncoprotein E6 and E7 and RNA [65]. The antibodies to E6 HPV 16 have shown good prospect as biomarkers for risk stratification of OPSCC and its prognosis. The addition of immune-targeted therapy in the management armamentarium of OPSCC has been documented to show strong positive treatment outcomes. Incorporation of angiogenic inhibitor *i.e.* VEGF blockade to chemotherapy regimes was reported to improve locoregional recurrence and overall survival [66]. In recent years, many more researches have focus on the utility of the inflammatory and immune biomarkers as part of therapeutic approach in order to improve head and neck cancer prognosis and survival. In addition, the GFR status has critical sequelae on prognostication and treatment response of HPV positive OPSCC [67].

Importantly, the HPV genome has also been consistently found in the lymph nodes metastases of patient with primary head and neck malignancy. This genomic finding can be combined with the inflammatory markers and with latest technology refinement, it can be developed into an agent or system that able to give prognostication, monitor disease progression and predict treatment response of head and neck malignancy. Indeed, the HPV is critical in sustaining the malignant phenotype of the tumor. Numerous studies reported that the active HPV genome are present in every phase of clinical progression including distant metastases [62]. As we all know, the HPV positive oropharyngeal carcinoma is mostly caused by HPV type 16 and 18. It has been shown that the vaccines that prevent HPV 16 oral infection can halt the formation of oropharyngeal carcinoma and can be used in a mass screening. Numerous studies on the vaccination program against HPV 16 and 18 showed different therapeutic responses. In future, hopefully more potent vaccines and other targeted approach can be developed in order to combat HPV positive OPSCC in the early stage of its development.

The other interesting biomarkers is the expression of p16 which has been consistently applied as a surrogate marker for HPV related head and neck cancer. This is due to the fact that p16 overexpression reflects the biologically active HPV that is present in the tumor [68]. Other vital HPV biomarkers includes HPV DNA, antibodies to HPV 16 capsid protein L1, oncoproteins expression such as antibodies to E6 and E7 proteins of HPV [69]. There are different results showed by different studies on the role of E7 and E6 oncoproteins and these biomarkers. For instance, a study measures the HPV positivity by looking at HPV-16 E6 at pretreatment and post treatment level and compared with the survival rates, showed that patient with E6 positive at pre and post treatment phases carries better survival advantages [70]. These E6 and E7 biomarkers serves as a critical immune target for the development of novel vaccines that can be specifically directed against the HPV. Of note, the development of therapeutic vaccine that can be used to reduce the progressing tumors and to prevent recurrent disease with recent trials of these vaccines showed promising outcomes [70].

Recent evidences have emerged that showed that the presence of HPV is not necessarily translate to the circulating active HPV. Latest study uses the reverse transcriptase RT-PCR which is rather a complex process to assess the presence of HPV oncoproteins that can be used as a gold standard test for diagnosing HNSCC [71]. The widespread use of HPV DNA testing based on the modern automation techniques that able to increase the volume of the cases tested and enhanced reproducibility will escalate the laboratory diagnostic techniques. Other example includes the assessment method based on the viral mRNA transcription *via* RNA ISH allows detection of HPV virus particles that present even in low numbers in the HNSCC [72]. In the oropharyngeal carcinoma, the assessment of HPV DNA and overexpression of p16 was highly associated with HPV mRNA expression. Recent studies showed that the combination of these two biomarkers is a reliable surrogate marker for detecting active HPV in malignant tissues and is useful for prognostication [73]. Thus, we can conclude that with advancing laboratory diagnostic technology and enhancement in genomic profiling, a promising effective treatment protocol for head and neck malignancy is coming to reality, as we speak.

IMPLICATIONS OF NEW TREATMENT APPROACH

In clinical practice, any form of detection procedures must be highly reliable, cost effectives and technically feasible. There are many factors that can influence the success of developing a versatile kits or therapeutic agents. The related health institutions, availability of expertise and personnel, cost and financial funds, are few examples that are required to support the progression of research and enhance the treatment of head and neck cancer patients. For instance, relevant expertise and complex tissue processing that are required for mRNA E6 and E7 oncoproteins detection, which limits its routine use as the HPV diagnostic tool. Current methods of testing HPV shows some variation across the laboratory depending on the preference, cost and availability of the tools of interest. The methods of choice also depend on types of targets detection which can includes viral oncoprotein, HPV DNA or RNA, cellular protein or HPV specific serum antibodies [72].

Emerging evidences reported that patients with seropositive E6 and E7 have reduction in mortality rates regardless of DNA status, in contrast to patients with seronegative E6 and E7. The status of p16 expression is only available when E6 an E7 serologic status was known. Critically, HNSCC patients who had E6 or E7 seropositive but negative p16 overexpression do not have survival advantageous [69]. In addition, Hoffmann *et al*. stated that from their studies there was false positive and false negative result of p16 overexpression in relation to HPV positivity, hence concluded that the p16 alone cannot be used as a biomarker for HPV related HNSCC [73]. The other important biomarker that has been used in the prediction of treatment response of HNSCC is a checkpoint inhibitor namely PD-L1 expression which can be used independent from p16. As such, positivity of p16 or PD-L1 can be used to predict treatment response to the targeted therapy like nivolumab [74]. These variation warrants more research and clinical trials which translate to more expertise, personnel, and cost involved.

PREVENTION OF HEAD AND NECK MALIGNANCY

The mechanism of head and neck malignancy is complex. Multiple factors such as lifestyle habits, dietary factors, genetic alteration, carcinogenic insults, and selected environmental stimuli act in combination in promoting carcinogenesis. Previously, the importance of tobacco and alcohol consumption as significant risk factors of head and neck malignancy is well known and has gained interest from the scientific community worldwide. Now the emergence of HPV as another significant risk factor of tonsillar and base of tongue cancer has shifted the research focus to this oncogenic virus. Recent research has shown that there is a critical relationship between these risk factors, as multiple cascades of biological and molecular events are necessary for the initiation and formation of head and neck cancer. For instance, exposure to the carcinogenic materials in tobacco and alcohol causes somatic changes that interfere with the RB gene of selected HNSCC that results in p16 overexpression. This is somewhat similar to the p16 expression that was induced by HPV infection [69].

The comprehensive management of head and neck cancer should comprise an early screening and prevention program. In addition, a refined treatment protocol, frequent follow-up schemes and committed involvement of patients and family members will ensure the success of the management of HNSCC. For instance, in the case of HPV positive OPSCC, the prevention strategy and program should involve lifestyle modifications in order to reduce the risk factors of OPSCC. The younger generation should be advice on the risk of sexual behavior and having multiple partners and encourage to adopt healthy lifestyles early in the lifetime. This younger subpopulation should be educated on significance of the diagnosis of cancer that can lead to unwanted treatment-related morbidities. The necessity of undergoing surgery or chemoradiation together with frequent follow-up will alter a patient's routine and impact the quality of life. This is especially true as most head and neck cancer are diagnosed at advanced stages and require a multimodality treatment approach and carry a poor prognosis.

At this juncture, several vaccines have been identified and use in the prevention program of HPV-related HNSCC. The two vaccines that are currently available are the bivalent type (Cervarix) and the tetravalent (Gardasil) [75]. These vaccines are effective if used in young patients who have not had sexual activities. These vaccines have been reported to have high efficacy against the two significant subtypes of HPV (HPV16 and HPV 18) in clinical trials [76]. The vaccines confer protection through the generation of type-specific neutralizing antibodies against the virus particle. In addition, the vaccines also reported showing cross sensitivity to other types of HPV (HPV 31 and HPV45) [77]. A broader spectrum of vaccines type against HPV is in the investigation phase [78]. Despite the intense research that is being conducted, the currently available Cervarix and Gardasil should be made available locally at low cost, especially targeting the high-risk areas worldwide This vaccination program should become part of the screening and prevention program and has been proven effective.

Different studies claimed different responses of the vaccination scheme. Most of the studies have a focus on the prevention of cervical cancer. While these marketed vaccines prevent anogenital HPV infection, their impact on the natural history of oropharyngeal HPV is unknown [79]. Until recently, there were no studies to evaluate the effect of vaccines on HPV-associated OPSCC prevention. The observational results on the effect of the vaccine on HPV oral infections are encouraging and because most HPV-related OPSCC are caused by high-risk HPV16, it is likely that the vaccination would prevent oral HPV infections and consequently the development of OPSCCs [80]. This is in lieu of the successful development of HPV prevention vaccines, Cervarix® and Gardasil®.

FUTURE DIRECTION AND ITS IMPACTS ON SOCIOECONOMIC

Although the human papillomavirus has long been detected in squamous cell carcinomas of the head and neck (HNSCC), assessment of its site-specific prevalence has been impeded by variance in detection methodologies. At this point, the techniques to be employed for determining the HPV status of head and neck cancers is controversial, due to variations in available methods in terms of cost, sensitivity, technicality, specificity, and reliability. Three common methods of detection are currently used are Polymerase Chain Reaction (PCR), *in situ* hybridization (ISH), and p16 immunohistochemistry (IHC) [81].

At this juncture, we have seen the emergence of multiple potential biomarkers, assessment tools and gadgets, nanotechnology and so forth that can be forge into the discovery of potent screening devices, treatment agents, or markers for recurrent or progressive disease. This is vital especially in the vast difference of HPV positive OPSCC to HPV negative OPSCC. A large number of NPC gene expression profiles have emerged in public databases. It is challenging to integrate these data from several datasets to yield maximal information. Researchers have employed meta-analysis of transcriptomic data by integrating them from multiple studies to successfully identify new prognostic and diagnostic markers for cancer and other diseases [82]. The development of potential complementary genomic and inflammatory biomarkers is expected to escalate the whole management spectrum of head and neck cancer. In coming years, more enhanced diagnostic laboratory techniques are expected to make a major breakthrough with the availability of nanotechnology and artificial intelligence that has been practiced in the medical and health sciences arena.

CONCLUSION

Head and neck squamous cell carcinoma is a critical tumor that have high rates of recurrent and metastases. A subset of this tumor, the HPV-related HNSCC behaves differently and displays different treatment outcomes. Recently, numerous studies and clinical trials on oropharyngeal carcinoma HPV-positive patients have shown remarkable improvement not only in assessment but also in the therapeutic outcomes of these subsets of patients. Targeting inflammation and its markers for screening, diagnosis and treatment are a viable and practical approach in order to manage this tumor better. This can be achieved by a thorough understanding of the roles of inflammation and its association with HNSCC and HPV positive HNSCC. The committed support from the scientific community and availability of financial reserves also play dominant roles in ensuring an enhanced management of all head and neck oncology patients.

CONSENT FOR PUBLICATION

Not applicable.

CONFLICT OF INTEREST

The author declares no conflict of interest, financial or otherwise.

ACKNOWLEDGEMENTS

Declared none.

REFERENCES

[1]   Khan S, Jain M, Mathur V, Feroz SM. Chronic inflammation and cancer: paradigm on tumor progression, metastasis and therapeutic intervention. Gulf J Oncolog 2016; 1(20): 86-93.[PMID: 27050184]

[2]   Gholizadeh P, Eslami H, Yousefi M, Asgharzadeh M, Aghazadeh M, Kafil HS. Role of oral microbiome on oral cancers, a review. Biomed Pharmacother 2016; 84: 552-8.[http://dx.doi.org/10.1016/j.biopha.2016.09.082] [PMID: 27693964]

[3]   Liu X, Gao XL, Liang XH, Tang YL. The etiologic spectrum of head and neck squamous cell carcinoma in young patients. Oncotarget 2016; 7(40): 66226-38.[http://dx.doi.org/10.18632/oncotarget.11265] [PMID: 27528225]

[4]   Li S, Lee YC, Li Q, et al. Oral lesions, chronic diseases and the risk of head and neck cancer. Oral Oncol 2015; 51(12): 1082-7.[http://dx.doi.org/10.1016/j.oraloncology.2015.10.014] [PMID: 26526128]

[5]   Sun Y, Liu N, Guan X, Wu H, Sun Z, Zeng H. Immunosuppression induced by chronic inflammation and the progression to oral squamous cell carcinoma. Mediators Inflamm 2016; 2016: 5715719.[http://dx.doi.org/10.1155/2016/5715719] [PMID: 28053372]

[6]   Hsiao JR, Chang CC, Lee WT, et al. The interplay between oral microbiome, lifestyle factors and genetic polymorphisms in the risk of oral squamous cell carcinoma. Carcinogenesis 2018; 39(6): 778-87.[http://dx.doi.org/10.1093/carcin/bgy053] [PMID: 29668903]

[7]   Le Bars P, Matamoros S, Montassier E, et al. The oral cavity microbiota: between health, oral disease, and cancers of the aerodigestive tract. Can J Microbiol 2017; 63(6): 475-92.[http://dx.doi.org/10.1139/cjm-2016-0603] [PMID: 28257583]

[8]   Murata M. Inflammation and cancer. Environ Health Prev Med 2018; 23(1): 50.[http://dx.doi.org/10.1186/s12199-018-0740-1] [PMID: 30340457]

[9]   Metgud R, Bajaj S. Altered serum and salivary C-reactive protein levels in patients with oral premalignant lesions and oral squamous cell carcinoma. Biotech Histochem 2016; 91(2): 96-101.[http://dx.doi.org/10.3109/10520295.2015.1077393] [PMID: 26529498]

[10]   Patel JB, Shah FD, Joshi GM, Patel PS. Clinical significance of inflammatory mediators in the pathogenesis of oral cancer. J Cancer Res Ther 2016; 12(2): 447-57.[http://dx.doi.org/10.4103/0973-1482.147765] [PMID: 27461592]

[11]   Clavijo PE, Allen CT, Schmitt NC, Van Waes C. Inflammation and head and neck squamous cell carcinoma. In: Burtness B, Golemis EA, eds. Molecular Determinants of Head and Neck Cancer Burtness B, Golemis EA. 2018353-64.[http://dx.doi.org/10.1007/978-3-319-78762-6_13]

[12]   Bonomi M, Patsias A, Posner M, Sikora A. The Role of Inflammation in Head and Neck Cancer. In: Aggarwal BB, Sung B, Gupta SC, eds. Inflammation and Cancer Aggarwal BB, Sung B, Gupta SC. 2014107-27.[http://dx.doi.org/10.1007/978-3-0348-0837-8_5]

[13]   Multhoff G, Molls M, Radons J. Chronic inflammation in cancer development. Front Immunol 2012; 2: 98.[http://dx.doi.org/10.3389/fimmu.2011.00098] [PMID: 22566887]

[14]   Ambatipudi S, Langdon R, Richmond RC, et al. DNA methylation derived systemic inflammation indices are associated with head and neck cancer development and survival. Oral Oncol 2018; 85: 87-94.[http://dx.doi.org/10.1016/j.oraloncology.2018.08.021] [PMID: 30220325]

[15]   Wang S, Ma N, Zhao W, et al. Inflammation-related dna damage and cancer stem cell markers in nasopharyngeal carcinoma. Mediators Inflamm 2016; 2016: 9343460.[http://dx.doi.org/10.1155/2016/9343460] [PMID: 27647953]

[16]   Pacova H, Astl J, Martinek J. The pathogenesis of chronic inflammation and malignant transformation in the human upper airways: the role of beta-defensins, eNOS, cell proliferation and apoptosis. Histol Histopathol 2009; 24(7): 815-20.[PMID: 19475527]

[17]   Feller L, Altini M, Lemmer J. Inflammation in the context of oral cancer. Oral Oncol 2013; 49(9): 887-92.[http://dx.doi.org/10.1016/j.oraloncology.2013.07.003] [PMID: 23910564]

[18]   Viens LJ, Henley SJ, Watson M, et al. Human papillomavirus-associated cancers - United States, 2008-2012. MMWR Morb Mortal Wkly Rep 2016; 65(26): 661-6.[http://dx.doi.org/10.15585/mmwr.mm6526a1] [PMID: 27387669]

[19]   Grosse Y, Baan R, Straif K, et al. A review of human carcinogens--Part A: pharmaceuticals. Lancet Oncol 2009; 10(1): 13-4.[http://dx.doi.org/10.1016/S1470-2045(08)70286-9] [PMID: 19115512]

[20] O'Sullivan B, Huang SH, Su J, *et al.* Development and validation of a staging system for HPV-related oropharyngeal cancer by the International Collaboration on Oropharyngeal cancer Network for Staging (ICON-S): a multicentre cohort study. Lancet Oncol 2016; 17(4): 440-51.[http://dx.doi.org/10.1016/S1470-2045(15)00560-4] [PMID: 26936027]

[21] Agalliu I, Gapstur S, Chen Z, *et al.* Associations of oral α-, β-, and γ-human papillomavirus types with risk of incident head and neck cancer. JAMA Oncol 2016; 2(5): 599-606.[http://dx.doi.org/10.1001/jamaoncol.2015.5504] [PMID: 26794505]

[22] zur Hausen H. Papillomaviruses causing cancer: evasion from host-cell control in early events in carcinogenesis. J Natl Cancer Inst 2000; 92(9): 690-8.[http://dx.doi.org/10.1093/jnci/92.9.690] [PMID: 10793105]

[23] Sano D, Oridate N. The molecular mechanism of human papillomavirus-induced carcinogenesis in head and neck squamous cell carcinoma. Int J Clin Oncol 2016; 21(5): 819-26.[http://dx.doi.org/10.1007/s10147-016-1005-x] [PMID: 27339270]

[24] Roman A, Munger K. The papillomavirus E7 proteins. Virology 2013; 445(1-2): 138-68.[http://dx.doi.org/10.1016/j.virol.2013.04.013] [PMID: 23731972]

[25] Combes JD, Chen AA, Franceschi S. Prevalence of human papillomavirus in cancer of the oropharynx by gender. Cancer Epidemiol Biomarkers Prev 2014; 23(12): 2954-8.[http://dx.doi.org/10.1158/1055-9965.EPI-14-0580] [PMID: 25205515]

[26] Chaturvedi AK, Engels EA, Pfeiffer RM, *et al.* Human papillomavirus and rising oropharyngeal cancer incidence in the United States. J Clin Oncol 2011; 29(32): 4294-301.[http://dx.doi.org/10.1200/JCO.2011.36.4596] [PMID: 21969503]

[27] Carlander AF, Gronhoj Larsen C, Jensen DH, Garnaes E, Kiss K, Andersen L. Continuing rise in oropharyngeal cancer in a high HPV prevalence area: A Danish population-based study from 2011 to 2014. European J Cancer 2017; 70: 75-82.

[28] Chaturvedi AK, D'Souza G, Gillison ML, Katki HA. Burden of HPV-positive oropharynx cancers among ever and never smokers in the U.S. population. Oral Oncol 2016; 60: 61-7.[http://dx.doi.org/10.1016/j.oraloncology.2016.06.006] [PMID: 27531874]

[29] Taberna M, Mena M, Pavón MA, Alemany L, Gillison ML, Mesía R. Human papillomavirus-related oropharyngeal cancer. Ann Oncol 2017; 28(10): 2386-98.[http://dx.doi.org/10.1093/annonc/mdx304] [PMID: 28633362]

[30] Amin MB, Greene FL, Edge SB. The eighth edition AJCC cancer staging manual: continuing to build a bridge from a population-based to a more "personalized" approach to cancer staging. CA: A Cancer J Clinicians 2017; 67(2): 93-9.

[31] Özdemir BC, Dotto GP. Racial Differences in Cancer Susceptibility and Survival: More Than the Color of the Skin? Trends Cancer 2017; 3(3): 181-97.[http://dx.doi.org/10.1016/j.trecan.2017.02.002] [PMID: 28718431]

[32] Ni XG, Wang GQ. The role of narrow band imaging in head and neck cancers. Curr Oncol Rep 2016; 18(2): 10.[http://dx.doi.org/10.1007/s11912-015-0498-1] [PMID: 26769115]

[33] Yoo J, Henderson S, Walker-Dilks C. Evidence-based guideline recommendations on the use of positron emission tomography imaging in head and neck cancer. Clin Oncol (R Coll Radiol) 2013; 25(4): e33-66.[http://dx.doi.org/10.1016/j.clon.2012.08.007] [PMID: 23021712]

[34] Edge SB, Byrd DR, Carducci MA, Compton CC, Fritz A, Greene F. AJCC cancer staging manual. 2010.

[35] Lydiatt WM, Patel SG, O'Sullivan B. Head and neck cancers-major changes in the american joint committee on cancer eighth edition cancer staging manual. CA Cancer J Clin 2017; 67(2): 122-37.

[36] Bhayani MK, Hutcheson KA, Barringer DA, *et al.* Gastrostomy tube placement in patients with oropharyngeal carcinoma treated with radiotherapy or chemoradiotherapy: factors affecting placement and dependence. Head Neck 2013; 35(11): 1634-40.[http://dx.doi.org/10.1002/hed.23200] [PMID: 23322563]

[37] Fernandez-Fernandez MM, Montes-Jovellar L, Parente Arias PL, Ortega Del Alamo P. TransOral endoscopic UltraSonic Surgery (TOUSS): a preliminary report of a novel robotless alternative to TORS. European archives of oto-rhino-laryngology: official journal of the European Federation of Oto-Rhino-Laryngological Societies (EUFOS): affiliated with the German Society for Oto-Rhino-Laryngology -. Head Neck Surg 2015; 272(12): 3785-91.

[38] Hutcheson KA, Holsinger FC, Kupferman ME, Lewin JS. Functional outcomes after TORS for oropharyngeal cancer: a systematic review. European archives of oto-rhino-laryngology: official journal of the European Federation of Oto-Rhino-Laryngological Societies (EUFOS): affiliated with the German Society for Oto-Rhino-Laryngology -. Head Neck Surg 2015; 272(2): 463-71.

[39]   Psyrri A, Rampias T, Vermorken JB. The current and future impact of human papillomavirus on treatment of squamous cell carcinoma of the head and neck. Ann Oncol 2014; 25(11): 2101-15.[http://dx.doi.org/10.1093/annonc/mdu265] [PMID: 25057165]

[40]   Gillison ML, Trotti AM, Harris J, *et al.* Radiotherapy plus cetuximab or cisplatin in human papillomavirus-positive oropharyngeal cancer (NRG Oncology RTOG 1016): a randomised, multicentre, non-inferiority trial. Lancet 2019; 393(10166): 40-50.[http://dx.doi.org/10.1016/S0140-6736(18)32779-X] [PMID: 30449625]

[41]   Eisbruch A, Schwartz M, Rasch C, *et al.* Dysphagia and aspiration after chemoradiotherapy for head-and-neck cancer: which anatomic structures are affected and can they be spared by IMRT? Int J Radiat Oncol Biol Phys 2004; 60(5): 1425-39.[http://dx.doi.org/10.1016/j.ijrobp.2004.05.050] [PMID: 15590174]

[42]   Sinha P, Lewis JS, Jr, Piccirillo JF, Kallogjeri D, Haughey BH. Extracapsular spread and adjuvant therapy in human papillomavirus-related, p16-positive oropharyngeal carcinoma. Cancer 2012; 118(14): 3519-30.[http://dx.doi.org/10.1002/cncr.26671] [PMID: 22086669]

[43]   Chow LQM. Head and neck cancer. N Engl J Med 2020; 382(1): 60-72.

[44]   Human papillomavirus vaccines: WHO position paper, May 2017-Recommendations. Vaccine 2017; 35(43): 5753-5.[http://dx.doi.org/10.1016/j.vaccine.2017.05.069] [PMID: 28596091]

[45]   Mehanna H, Bryant TS, Babrah J, *et al.* Human papillomavirus (HPV) vaccine effectiveness and potential herd immunity for reducing oncogenic oropharyngeal HPV-16 prevalence in the United Kingdom: a cross-sectional study. Clin Infect Dis 2019; 69(8): 1296-302.[http://dx.doi.org/10.1093/cid/ciy1081] [PMID: 30590469]

[46]   Chaturvedi AK, Graubard BI, Broutian T, *et al.* Prevalence of oral hpv infection in unvaccinated men and women in the United States, 2009-2016. JAMA 2019; 322(10): 977-9.[http://dx.doi.org/10.1001/jama.2019.10508] [PMID: 31503300]

[47]   Bi D, Apter D, Eriksson T, Hokkanen M, Zima J, Damaso S. Safety of the AS04-adjuvanted human papillomavirus (HPV)-16/18 vaccine in adolescents aged 12-15 years: end-of-study results from a community-randomized study up to 6.5 years. Hum Vaccin Immunother 2019; •••: 1-12.[http://dx.doi.org/10.1080/21645515.2019.1692557] [PMID: 31829767]

[48]   Ducatman BS. The role of human papillomavirus in oropharyngeal squamous cell carcinoma. Arch Pathol Lab Med 2018; 142(6): 715-8.[http://dx.doi.org/10.5858/arpa.2018-0083-RA] [PMID: 29848036]

[49]   Whang SN, Filippova M, Duerksen-Hughes P. Recent progress in therapeutic treatments and screening strategies for the prevention and treatment of hpv-associated head and neck cancer. Viruses 2015; 7(9): 5040-65.[http://dx.doi.org/10.3390/v7092860] [PMID: 26393639]

[50]   Mirghani H, Amen F, Blanchard P, *et al.* Treatment de-escalation in HPV-positive oropharyngeal carcinoma: ongoing trials, critical issues and perspectives. Int J Cancer 2015; 136(7): 1494-503.[http://dx.doi.org/10.1002/ijc.28847] [PMID: 24622970]

[51]   Cleary RK, Cmelak AJ. Evolving treatment paradigms for oropharyngeal squamous cell carcinoma. J Glob Oncol 2018; 4: 1-9.[http://dx.doi.org/10.1200/JGO.2016.006304]

[52]   Sinha P, Karadaghy OA, Doering MM, Tuuli MG, Jackson RS, Haughey BH. Survival for HPV-positive oropharyngeal squamous cell carcinoma with surgical *versus* non-surgical treatment approach: A systematic review and meta-analysis. Oral Oncol 2018; 86: 121-31.[http://dx.doi.org/10.1016/j.oraloncology.2018.09.018] [PMID: 30409292]

[53]   Hasegawa M, Maeda H, Deng Z, *et al.* Prediction of concurrent chemoradiotherapy outcome in advanced oropharyngeal cancer. Int J Oncol 2014; 45(3): 1017-26.[http://dx.doi.org/10.3892/ijo.2014.2504] [PMID: 24969413]

[54]   Bulsara VM, Worthington HV, Glenny AM, Clarkson JE, Conway DI, Macluskey M. Interventions for the treatment of oral and oropharyngeal cancers: surgical treatment. Cochrane Database Syst Rev 2018; 12(12): CD006205.

[55]   Howard J, Masterson L, Dwivedi RC, *et al.* Minimally invasive surgery *versus* radiotherapy/chemoradiotherapy for small-volume primary oropharyngeal carcinoma. Cochrane Database Syst Rev 2016; 12(12): CD010963.[http://dx.doi.org/10.1002/14651858.CD010963.pub2] [PMID: 27943254]

[56]   Oliver RJ, Clarkson JE, Conway DI, *et al.* CSROC Expert PanelInterventions for the treatment of oral and oropharyngeal cancers: surgical treatment. Cochrane Database Syst Rev 2007; (4)CD006205.[http://dx.doi.org/10.1002/14651858.CD006205.pub2] [PMID: 17943894]

[57]   Furness S, Glenny AM, Worthington HV, *et al.* Interventions for the treatment of oral cavity and oropharyngeal cancer: chemotherapy. Cochrane Database Syst Rev 2010; (9)CD006386.[http://dx.doi.org/10.1002/14651858.CD006386.pub2] [PMID: 20824847]

[58]   Tanaka TI, Alawi F. Human Papillomavirus and Oropharyngeal Cancer. Dent Clin North Am 2018; 62(1):

111-20.[http://dx.doi.org/10.1016/j.cden.2017.08.008] [PMID: 29126488]

[59] Masand RP, El-Mofty SK, Ma XJ, Luo Y, Flanagan JJ, Lewis JS, Jr. Adenosquamous carcinoma of the head and neck: relationship to human papillomavirus and review of the literature. Head Neck Pathol 2011; 5(2): 108-16.[http://dx.doi.org/10.1007/s12105-011-0245-3] [PMID: 21305368]

[60] Qian G, Hu Z, Xu H, *et al.* A novel prediction model for human papillomavirus-associated oropharyngeal squamous cell carcinoma using p16 and subcellular β-catenin expression. J Oral Pathol Med 2016; 45(6): 399-408.[http://dx.doi.org/10.1111/jop.12378] [PMID: 26493274]

[61] Nwanze J, Cohen C, Schmitt AC, Siddiqui MT. β-catenin expression in oropharyngeal squamous cell carcinomas: comparison and correlation with p16 and human papillomavirus *in situ* hybridization. Acta Cytol 2015; 59(6): 479-84.[http://dx.doi.org/10.1159/000443602] [PMID: 26849661]

[62] Holmes BJ, Maleki Z, Westra WH. The fidelity of p16 staining as a surrogate marker of human papillomavirus status in fine-needle aspirates and core biopsies of neck node metastases: implications for hpv testing protocols. Acta Cytol 2015; 59(1): 97-103.[http://dx.doi.org/10.1159/000375148] [PMID: 25765380]

[63] Timbang MR, Sim MW, Bewley AF, Farwell DG, Mantravadi A, Moore MG. HPV-related oropharyngeal cancer: a review on burden of the disease and opportunities for prevention and early detection. Hum Vaccin Immunother 2019; 15(7-8): 1920-8.[http://dx.doi.org/10.1080/21645515.2019.1600985] [PMID: 31050595]

[64] Dalianis T. Human papillomavirus and oropharyngeal cancer, the epidemics, and significance of additional clinical biomarkers for prediction of response to therapy (Review). Int J Oncol 2014; 44(6): 1799-805.[http://dx.doi.org/10.3892/ijo.2014.2355] [PMID: 24676623]

[65] D'Souza G, Clemens G, Troy T, *et al.* Evaluating the utility and prevalence of hpv biomarkers in oral rinses and serology for HPV-related oropharyngeal cancer. Cancer Prev Res (Phila) 2019; 12(10): 689-700.[http://dx.doi.org/10.1158/1940-6207.CAPR-19-0185] [PMID: 31420362]

[66] Chan KK, Glenny AM, Weldon JC, Furness S, Worthington HV, Wakeford H. Interventions for the treatment of oral and oropharyngeal cancers: targeted therapy and immunotherapy. Cochrane Database Syst Rev 2015; (12)CD010341.[http://dx.doi.org/10.1002/14651858.CD010341.pub2] [PMID: 26625332]

[67] Nakano T, Yamamoto H, Nakashima T, *et al.* Molecular subclassification determined by human papillomavirus and epidermal growth factor receptor status is associated with the prognosis of oropharyngeal squamous cell carcinoma. Hum Pathol 2016; 50: 51-61.[http://dx.doi.org/10.1016/j.humpath.2015.11.001] [PMID: 26997438]

[68] Deng Z, Hasegawa M, Aoki K, *et al.* A comprehensive evaluation of human papillomavirus positive status and p16INK4a overexpression as a prognostic biomarker in head and neck squamous cell carcinoma. Int J Oncol 2014; 45(1): 67-76.[http://dx.doi.org/10.3892/ijo.2014.2440] [PMID: 24820457]

[69] Liang C, Marsit CJ, McClean MD, *et al.* Biomarkers of HPV in head and neck squamous cell carcinoma. Cancer Res 2012; 72(19): 5004-13.[http://dx.doi.org/10.1158/0008-5472.CAN-11-3277] [PMID: 22991304]

[70] Smith EM, Rubenstein LM, Ritchie JM, *et al.* Does pretreatment seropositivity to human papillomavirus have prognostic significance for head and neck cancers? Cancer Epidemiol Biomarkers Prev 2008; 17(8): 2087-96.[http://dx.doi.org/10.1158/1055-9965.EPI-08-0054] [PMID: 18708401]

[71] Masand RP, El-Mofty SK, Ma XJ, Luo Y, Flanagan JJ, Lewis JS, Jr. Adenosquamous carcinoma of the head and neck: relationship to human papillomavirus and review of the literature. Head Neck Pathol 2011; 5(2): 108-16.[http://dx.doi.org/10.1007/s12105-011-0245-3] [PMID: 21305368]

[72] Bishop JA, Ma XJ, Wang H, *et al.* Detection of transcriptionally active high-risk HPV in patients with head and neck squamous cell carcinoma as visualized by a novel E6/E7 mRNA *in situ* hybridization method. Am J Surg Pathol 2012; 36(12): 1874-82.[http://dx.doi.org/10.1097/PAS.0b013e318265fb2b] [PMID: 23060353]

[73] Deng Z, Hasegawa M, Aoki K, *et al.* A comprehensive evaluation of human papillomavirus positive status and p16INK4a overexpression as a prognostic biomarker in head and neck squamous cell carcinoma. Int J Oncol 2014; 45(1): 67-76.[http://dx.doi.org/10.3892/ijo.2014.2440] [PMID: 24820457]

[74] Wang J, Sun H, Zeng Q, *et al.* HPV-positive status associated with inflamed immune microenvironment and improved response to anti-PD-1 therapy in head and neck squamous cell carcinoma. Sci Rep 2019; 9(1): 13404.[http://dx.doi.org/10.1038/s41598-019-49771-0] [PMID: 31527697]

[75] Testi D, Nardone M, Melone P, Cardelli P, Ottria L, Arcuri C. HPV and oral lesions: preventive possibilities, vaccines and early diagnosis of malignant lesions. Oral Implantol (Rome) 2016; 8(2-3): 45-51.[http://dx.doi.org/10.11138/orl/2015.8.2.045] [PMID: 27555904]

[76] Draper E, Bissett SL, Howell-Jones R, *et al.* A randomized, observer-blinded immunogenicity trial of Cervarix(®) and Gardasil(®) Human Papillomavirus vaccines in 12-15 year old girls. PLoS One 2013; 8(5): e61825.[http://dx.doi.org/10.1371/journal.pone.0061825] [PMID: 23650505]

[77] Godi A, Bissett SL, Miller E, Beddows S. Relationship between humoral immune responses against HPV16, HPV18, HPV31 and HPV45 in 12-15 year old girls receiving cervarix$^{®}$ or gardasil$^{®}$ vaccine. PLoS One 2015; 10(10): e0140926.[http://dx.doi.org/10.1371/journal.pone.0140926] [PMID: 26495976]

[78] Schellenbacher C, Roden RBS, Kirnbauer R. Developments in L2-based human papillomavirus (HPV) vaccines. Virus Res 2017; 231: 166-75.[http://dx.doi.org/10.1016/j.virusres.2016.11.020] [PMID: 27889616]

[79] Gildener-Leapman N, Ferris RL, Bauman JE. Promising systemic immunotherapies in head and neck squamous cell carcinoma. Oral Oncol 2013; 49(12): 1089-96.[http://dx.doi.org/10.1016/j.oraloncology.2013.09.009] [PMID: 24126223]

[80] Aldalwg MAH, Brestovac B. Human papillomavirus associated cancers of the head and neck: an Australian perspective. Head Neck Pathol 2017; 11(3): 377-84.[http://dx.doi.org/10.1007/s12105-017-0780-7] [PMID: 28176136]

[81] Whang SN, Filippova M, Duerksen-Hughes P. Recent progress in therapeutic treatments and screening strategies for the prevention and treatment of hpv-associated head and neck cancer. Viruses 2015; 7(9): 5040-65.[http://dx.doi.org/10.3390/v7092860] [PMID: 26393639]

[82] Janvilisri T. Omics-based identification of biomarkers for nasopharyngeal carcinoma. Dis Markers 2015; 2015: 762128.[http://dx.doi.org/10.1155/2015/762128] [PMID: 25999660]

Treatment of Head and Neck Cancer and Relation to Inflammation

Rohaizam Japar Jaafar[1,*], Zulkifli Yusof[1], Zakinah Yahaya[2]

[1] Hospital Sultanah Bahiyah, Alor Setar, Kedah, Malaysia
[2] Hospital Kuala Lumpur, Kuala Lumpur, Malaysia

Abstract

Over the past decades, the survival rate of head and neck cancers has not significantly changed. Recently, the importance of the inflammatory responses in head and neck cancer has been a hot topic and of increasing interest. There has been suspicion about the relationship between inflammation and carcinogenesis, and thus, many works had proven these relations. Manipulation of the inflammatory mediators has been experimented with, to reduce the tumor burden, treat as well as prevent the cancer occurrence or second primary. This chapter summarizes the relationship between inflammation and cancer, emphasizing epidemiological and clinical evidence and proposing the current potential targets of anti-inflammatory agents for the therapeutic approach of head and neck cancer (HNC). We hope this knowledge will help us combat carcinogenesis and reduce the morbidity of the current conventional treatment for a better quality of life.

Keywords: Head and neck cancer, Inflammation, Treatment.

* **Corresponding author Rohaizam Japar Jaafar:** Hospital Sultanah Bahiyah, Alor Setar, Kedah, Malaysia; Tel: +60126306022; E-mail: rohaizamjaafar@me.com

INTRODUCTION

The investigation toward inflammatory-associated carcinogenesis and approaches to reach the inflammatory targets is a relatively new area in cancer research [1]. When Rudolf Virchow introduced the term inflammation-related carcinogenesis in 1863, many epidemiological studies and research support the theory only years later [1, 2]. To date, inflammation is widely recognized as a hallmark for carcinogenesis. The idea for inflammation-related malignancies allows us to target the inflammatory response as therapeutic management of cancer at the molecular level.

The role of medical treatment in head and neck cancer has evolved over the years with a better understanding of tumor genetics and biology. Although it is a clear

connection that an inflammation leading to cancer; for example, hepatitis due to hepatitis B virus or C or toxic compounds as the initiation in the development of hepatocellular carcinoma, association between chronic esophagitis and Barrett's metaplasia with esophageal cancer, chronic pancreatitis and pancreatic cancer, inflammatory breast cancer as a result of unresolved breast inflammation and Helicobacter pylori infection with gastric adenocarcinoma [2], but the inflammation-related head and neck cancer is still new. Understanding inflammatory pathway blockage, overexpression of inflammatory mediators and targeting the cancer microenvironment can be the promising approach for head and neck cancer treatment.

In 2008, about 16.1% of newly diagnosed cancers were related to infections [3], while epidemiologic studies indicate that at least 20% of all cancers begin as a direct consequence of chronic inflammatory processes [2]. Undoubtedly, inflammation-related oncogenesis is complex; it involves numerous cells and mediators through multiple mechanisms. There is a crosstalk between two pathways, the extrinsic pathway, driven by non-cancerous cells and the environment, and the intrinsic pathway, which is driven by oncogenes expression. The extrinsic insult such as infection, obesity, smoking, alcohol, microparticles, for example, silica and asbestos, and chronic inflammatory diseases is an established risk factor related to chronic inflammation [2, 3]. For example, cigarette smoking is proven to modulate an immune response. The effects are complex; both pro-inflammatory and suppressive effects may be initiated. Nevertheless, it contains toxins and bacterial lipopolysaccharide responsible for mucosal damage, and molecular derangements leading to oncogenesis by increasing cytogenic abnormalities, inactivation of tumor suppressor genes, and changes in the intracellular signaling pathway. As a direct consequence, smoking impairs immunity in the oral cavity, promotes gingival and periodontal disease and oral cancer. Smoking is also a risk factor in developing premalignant lesions, including leukoplakia and erythroplakia, which can progress to invasive carcinomas [4].

On the other hand, the intrinsic factor can be triggered by mutations, recruitment, and activation of inflammatory cells [4, 5]. It directly affects the initiation, angiogenesis, cell migration, progression, and aggressiveness of the tumor. At a molecular level, this process activates the apoptotic pathway either by down-regulate pro-apoptotic or up-regulate anti-apoptotic molecules. Inflammatory cytokines are major inducers that play a vital role in oncogenesis, and even there is emerging evidence that tumor cells and tumor-associated leucocytes can produce inflammatory cytokines and chemokines by themselves [5]. The inflammatory cytokines are tumor necrosis factor-α (TNF-α), interleukin- 1β (IL-1β) and interleukin-6 (IL-6), and chemokines are prostaglandins, oncogenes, cyclooxygenase-2, inducible nitric oxide synthase, 5-lipoxygenase, matrix metalloproteinases, vascular endothelial growth factor, hypoxia-inducible factor-1α, nuclear factor-κβ (NF-κβ), nuclear factor of activated T-cells, signal transducers and activators of transcription 3-STAT3, activator protein-1 (AP-1), cAMP, and enhancer-binding protein. Additionally, activation of various kinases, including Iκβ kinase (IKK), protein kinase-C, mitogen-activated protein kinase, and phosphoinositide-3 kinase/protein kinase B (PI3K)/AKT, participates in inflammation-related oncogenesis [6⁻10]. Anti-inflammatory agents are believed to alter the tumor microenvironment, reduce cell migration, increase apoptosis, and increasing sensitivity to other therapy [3, 6].

There are several genetic alterations associated with chronic inflammation in head and neck cancer (HNC). An example of the interplay between inflammation and genetic alteration is HPV-related oropharyngeal squamous cell carcinoma. They present at a younger age, who is non-smoker and do not consume alcohol. HPV-16 DNA has been found in up to 72%, and inactivation of p16 is a frequent event witnessed in >80% of oropharyngeal tumour specimens [11⁻13]. The HPV integrates into host DNA expresses oncoproteins E6 to target the tumor suppressor genes p53 and E7, which act on the pRb for ubiquitin-mediated intracellular degradation, inactivate the normal cell cycle resulting in oncogenic transformation [11]. HPV-16 and HPV-18 are the most common oncogenic variant [14, 15]. Notably, it has been found that 50% of all oropharyngeal tumor specimens contain p53 mutations [16].

Another example is the Epstein-Barr virus. It is known to have a causal relationship in lymphoma, nasopharyngeal carcinoma, and gastric carcinoma, in which it mainly infects human lymphocytes and oropharyngeal epithelial cells. Multiple and diverse pathways are involved in EBV-related oncogenesis. The interaction of virus and host genes during its latency period leads to G1/S phase transition and inhibition of cell apoptosis. The latent proteins and miRNAs encoded by EBV activates the oncogenes such as Bcl-2 and MYC, activate signaling pathways such as NF-κB, JAK/STAT, and PI3K/Akt, and inhibit tumor suppressor genes such as p53, PTEN, and p16^{INK4A}. EBV is known to facilitate the oncogenic courses with specific oncogene activation [17].

In this chapter, we would like to list several strategies, possibly to reduce the tumor burden, treat and prevent cancer. There is an increasing number of FDA-approved anti-inflammatory agents concerning cancer. Since monotherapy or conventional modality insufficiently to eradicate cancer, a combination supposedly to be introduced [6]. The majority of agents target rapidly proliferating cells, resulting in cell death. Others can alter the tumour or the therapeutic agents' pharmacokinetics and pharmacodynamics on the molecular level to increase apoptosis's efficacy. For example, steroid administration can change the pharmacokinetics of chemotherapeutic drugs to decrease their toxicity and increase their activity in the tumour leading to differences in the concentration, half-life, and clearance of the active metabolite. The anti-inflammatory agents may also have synergistic effects to sensitize cancer cells to conventional cancer treatment. While these compounds may eventually prove their utility, more emphasis should be placed on the agents for clinical use to bring about the best benefit for the patients [6].

STRATEGIES AND THERAPEUTIC TARGETS

Non-selective Agent to Arrest Inflammation

Aspirin and NSAIDs

In 1897, Hoffmann discovered acetylsalicylic acid in a pure and stable form and was registered under the name "Aspirin" two years later. It came from 'a'cetyl, and 'spir' came from the plant in which salicylic acid had initially been isolated, *spirea ulmania*. Only a decades later, in 1971, Sir John Vane discovered aspirin as a prostaglandin synthetase inhibitor. Eventually, there is emerging evidence showing the benefits of aspirin in cancer and led to the discovery of NSAIDs as chemoprevention agents [18‑20]. Although the use of NSAIDs such as aspirin, ibuprofen, indomethacin, and celecoxib in the long term has been associated with the reduced risk of developing colorectal, esophageal, lung, gastric, breast, prostate and ovarian cancer and cancer-related mortality by 20% to 25%, its role in preventing head and neck cancer remains investigational [2, 6, 20‑23]. Experimental studies show that NSAIDs can arrest tumor growth in HNSCC, showing the potential to reduce the risk of second primary and as a chemopreventive agent [4].

NSAIDs non-selectively inhibit COX of the arachidonic acid metabolism pathway and inflammatory mediators such as prostaglandins and leukotrienes [24]. Prostaglandin E2 is produced by PGE synthase causes increased cell proliferation, inhibition of apoptosis, and stimulation of angiogenesis. It is synthesized in multiple-steps. Arachidonic acid is first released from membrane-bound phospholipids by phospholipase A2, then converted to prostaglandin H2 mediated by COX and finally PGE2. This step recognition is essential to target the synthesis of PGE2 [20]. A two-step model has been implicated by Haddad *et al.* suggesting the inactivation of PGE2 located in the developing tumor microenvironment is first mediated by the PGT, which engages carrier-mediated membrane transport of prostaglandins (PGE2, PGF2a, and PGD2) from the extracellular to the cytoplasm and the second step involves catabolization of 15-hydroxyprostaglandin dehydrogenase (15-PGDH) in the cytoplasm and inactivates PGE2 [25].

The binding of prostaglandin to their receptors results in the activation of adenylyl cyclase resulting cyclic AMP (cAMP). PGE2 and elevated COX-2 contributes to carcinogenesis and cancer progression [26-29]. There are two isoforms of COX, which one of those have differences in the therapeutic and side effects. Prostaglandins produced by COX-1 play a role in platelet function, renal tubules, and gastrointestinal epithelium, whereas COX- 2 is involved in pain and inflammation [30]. It has been shown that COX-2 has an essential role in the biology of HNSCC [31]. COX-2 is the most common anti-cancer inflammatory target, although numerous other targets such as NF- κB, cytokines/cytokines receptors, chemokines/receptors, FGF/R, and VEGF have also been examined. Several studies have suggested that the anti-tumor activity of COX-2 inhibitors is at least partly unrelated to their inhibition of cyclooxygenase [6]. The correlation between COX-2 expression and head and neck tumor indicates size and prognosis [31].

The mechanism by which NSAIDs inhibit tumor development is thought through the inhibition of COX-2 and, consequently the synthesis of PGs [31]. The elevated COX-2 has been postulated through induced EGFR- mediated activation of the cell survival cascade (AKT/c- FLIP/COX-2) and regulates the tumor microenvironment through IL-17 results in anti-apoptotic activity and promote macrophage differentiation, respectively [32, 33]. Inhibition of several transduction pathways, including Wnt–β catenin, PIK3CA/ AKT/PTEN, and NF-κB, has been postulated because patients with PIK3 mutations and those with mutations within the NF-κB pathway could have reduced cancer risk after use of NSAIDs [34-36]. On the other hand, high-dose aspirin is also thought to induce apoptosis through COX-independent mechanisms such as activation of caspases, p38 MAP kinase, and ceramide pathway, releasing mitochondrial cytochrome C and regulating several different targets, for example, ALOX15, PAWR (pro-apoptotic gene), and BCL2L1 (anti-apoptotic gene) [37].

As high as 40% improvement and reduced recurrence seen with colorectal carcinoma using COX-2 inhibitors (rofecoxib and celecoxib) and current phase 3 clinical study recommended it as adjuvant therapy, but there is a mixed result of NSAIDs usage in preventing head and neck cancer [34, 38]. In 2006, Jayaprakash *et al.* and Caponigro *et al.* reported a risk reduction across all the primary tumors with higher risk reduction for oral cavity and oropharyngeal cancers. Moderate smokers or moderate drinkers have the most significant risk reduction, and the protective effect was higher in women [39]. As opposed to that, Bonomi *et al.* showed a significant reduction in HNSCC risk with aspirin use for laryngeal cancers [4]. Although *in-vitro* studies suggest an anti-tumor effect of COX inhibitors in head and neck cancer, Gillespie in 2007 found no difference in head and neck cancer recurrence or overall survival in COX inhibitor users compared to non-users [40]. A few years later, Ahmadi *et al.* stated that NSAIDs use was associated with a 75% reduction in risk of developing HNSCC, while Becker *et al.*, with large scale epidemiology study came out indicating that aspirin and NSAID use do not affect overall HNSCC risk. However, he suggests that regular ibuprofen use may be beneficial in HNSCC prevention [21, 23]. Kim *et al.* concluded that celecoxib's cytotoxicity effects are unpredictable and may vary in a clinical setting. This warrants further investigations as a combined alternative [41].

Bin Yang *et al.* showed that COX-2 expression could be a prognostic factor correlated with a high risk of lymph node metastasis. An advanced TNM stage in HNSCC indicates poor overall survival, recurrence-free survival and disease- free survival in patients with HNSCC [42] but a year later, Kim *et al.* indicating that aspirin and NSAIDs do not affect survival, recurrence, or second cancer occurrence in patients with HNSCC. The cumulative aspirin dose before HNSCC diagnosis did not affect survival outcomes [43]. Recently, Hedberg *et al.* concluded that regular NSAIDs usage, irrespective of HPV status, likely confers a statistically and clinically significant advantage in DSS as well as OS in patients with PIK3CA-altered HNSCC, through the PI3K and COX pathways [44].

A few authors have proposed a combination of treatment. COX-2 inhibitors have demonstrated synergy when combined with EGFR inhibitors in preclinical models [45, 46]. Based on a recent *in-vivo* study using combined EGFR and COX-2 in very high-risk dysplastic oral leukoplakia patients, a preliminary data of a Phase I study of daily celecoxib, combined with weekly docetaxel, cisplatin and concurrent radiotherapy in patients with locally advanced HNSCC have shown significant combined regimes to target both pathways [47]. Crosstalk between COX-2 and EGFR signaling pathways in HNSCC suggests that a combined approach is justified and more effective inhibiting growth and angiogenesis rather than monotherapy [41, 48, 49].

Celecoxib, with erlotinib and reirradiation, was shown to be a feasible and clinically active regimen in a population of patients with recurrent HNSCC who had a poor prognosis [48]. A combination of apricoxib with erlotinib in non- small-cell lung cancer showed a 60% disease control rate [50]. Apricoxib, compared to celecoxib in HNSCC setting, showed better up-regulation of E-cadherin expression and down-regulation of vimentin, which was implicated as a sensitivity marker to EGFR TKI [51]. Targeted therapy combination Huang *et al.* investigated a combined treatment of nimotuzumab and celecoxib in poorly differentiated NPC with promising results [52].

Not surprisingly, in oral premalignant lesions (OPL), the COX-2 is overexpressed too. However, clinical trials using non-steroidal anti-inflammatory drugs (NSAIDs) to inhibit COX-2 have not been very successful in the chemoprevention of OPL. Ketorolac, as an oral rinse, a non-selective COX inhibitor, failed to show any significant reduction in oral leukoplakia. As a specific inhibitor of COX-2, Celecoxib failed to control oral premalignant lesions too [53]. Celecoxib was ineffective in controlling oral premalignant lesions in a recent randomized controlled trial [54].

Nevertheless, due to their non-selective isozymes, long-term NSAID can result in unwanted and paradoxical effects, including renal failure and gastrointestinal bleeding, peptic ulcers, and intestinal inflammation that may increase cancer risk. Furthermore, NSAIDs also can cause potentially life-threatening thromboembolic complications, for example, pulmonary embolism, myocardial infarction, and stroke. Few selective COX-2 inhibitors have been withdrawn from the market (rofecoxib in 2004 and valdecoxib in 2005) except celecoxib that is still available in the United States and Europe [20, 55⁻60].

Steroids

Although there are no formal studies investigating steroid as monotherapy in head and neck cancer, but rather as a co-administration to reduces edema and pain. Steroids are believed to interact with DNA-regulators genes, which results in apoptosis *via* TP53-independent signal transduction pathways. It modulates, enhances, or activates up or down-regulation of proliferation, enhances cellular glutathione and ABCB1 expression, induces of metallothionein synthesis, and stimulate O6-methylguanine-DNA methyl-transferase activity which responsible for DNA repair [60].

The intermediate and long-acting corticosteroids have been investigated for its potential therapeutic and chemoprotective effects. Dexamethasone, hydrocortisone, and prednisolone have been tested for its anti-inflammatory function by inhibition of various cytokines production [61]. Several *in-vivo* studies demonstrated that dexamethasone treatment could decrease tumor growth in renal, breast, lung, and hematological malignancies [61⁻63]. It is reported that dietary dexamethasone administration to exposed mice to tobacco smoke leads to a decrease in lung tumor incidence for more than 60% [2, 61].

Again, pretreatment with dexamethasone can enhance the effects of conventional therapies in animal studies. A co-administration of dexamethasone in an animal model with glioma, breast, lung, and colon cancers led to a 2-4- fold increment in the efficacy of carboplatin and/or gemcitabine [36, 64, 65]. In a recent clinical trial, patients with relapsed multiple myeloma, dexamethasone combined with carfilzomib, and lenalidomide showed significantly improved progression-free survival of the patients [62]. In clinical settings, high-dose dexamethasone (up to 16 mg twice a day) before chemotherapy improved the efficacy of chemotherapy drugs [36].

Statins

Statins are common and usually prescribed for dyslipidemia. Its role repeatedly demonstrated an onco-protective, radiosensitizing, and pro-differentiating effects in head and neck cancer *in vitro*. A phase I clinical trial has demonstrated stable disease in HNC with very high-dose lovastatin. In a retrospective large cohort study suggesting significant overall survival and disease-free survival in patients with the larynx, hypopharynx, and nasopharynx SCC concomitantly taking statins the time of cancer diagnosis [66].

Statins have usually been used as an adjunct treatment combined with 5-fluorouracil, cisplatin, and doxorubicin, although monotherapy as a chemopreventive approach has been reported [67, 68]. Statins have the pro-apoptotic effect by inhibiting HMG-CoA reductase, thus arrest the synthesis of isoprenoids that is essential for membrane localization and activation of signaling proteins such as ras, rho, and rac [69]. Besides, a downregulation of the RAF/MEK/ ERK pathway, inhibition of degradation of cell-cycle regulators p21 and p27, c-Myc activation, and proinflammatory pathways (NF-kB and COX2) further increased its apoptotic effects [70].

A real benefit of statin usage as head and neck anticancer still questionable and not as a standard treatment yet as it requires a high dose to achieve the effects. Some experimental studies showed a protective effect for colorectal, lung, liver, breast, and renal cell carcinoma while others do not [71⁻82]. In 2014, Diakos *et al.* reported a 90% risk reduction of inflammatory bowel disease-related colorectal cancer if co-treatment with statin [83, 84]. Of note, some authors still believe the promising effects of statins as adjunct treatments at a safer dose.

Targeted Strategies in the Tumor Microenvironment *Via* Cytokines, Chemokines and Specific Enzymes Manipulation

Several cytokines and growth factors also activate signal pathways that promote the malignant phenotype. TNF-α, IL-1, HGF, and their receptors promote activation of the mitogen-activated protein kinase-activator protein-1 (MAPK- AP-1), nuclear factor-kappa B (NF-κB), and phosphati-dylinositol-3 kinase (PI3K)/Akt pathways [85]. The knowledge of immunomodulatory directed towards specific cytokines and chemokines has been an increased role in cancer therapy. As initial works are targeted for a non-cancer inflammatory disease with anti-TNF α and anti-interleukin-6 therapies, there has been a little experience in patients with cancer [86]. A recent discovery of the signaling pathways, especially transforming growth factor-β (TGF-β) and PTEN/PI3K/Akt/mTOR pathways, allows us to understand head and neck oncogenesis [87].

Cytokines include interleukins (ILs), interferons (IFNs), tumor necrosis factors (TNFs), and growth factors. Cytokine plays an essential role in the initiation, regulation, and maintenance of inflammatory and immune responses. They are divided into pro-inflammatory (*e.g.*, IL-1, IL-6, IL-8, TNF-α, and IFN-γ) and anti-inflammatory *e.g.*, IL-4, IL-10, TGF-β, and vascular endothelial growth factor (VEGF). It is understood that high levels of pro-inflammatory cytokines play a role in the development of HNSCC [88]. High levels of IL-1a, IL-6, IL-8, granulocyte-macrophage colony-stimulating factor (GM-CSF), growth-regulated oncogene-(a) GRO1, VEGF, and hepatocyte growth factor (HGF) have been involved in the development of HNSCC [89].

Pro-inflammatory cytokines are produced by macrophages, B and T lymphocytes, endothelial cells, and fibroblasts involved in the promotion of cell proliferation, induction of angiogenesis, autophagy, and inhibition of apoptosis. TNF-α and interferon-γ induce autophagy, a cellular degradation process involving the amino acid recycling for cellular survival and proliferation [90⁻92]. Anti-inflammatory cytokines such as IL-10 are produced by CD8+T cells inhibits NF-κB signaling through IκB kinases and unbinding NF-κB DNA [93⁻95]. In clinical practice, it shows that low levels of cytokines and growth factors are associated with response to therapy and high levels are associated with poor outcomes in patients with HNSCC receiving chemotherapy and radiation [96].

CXCR4 is the most studied chemokine receptor. The antagonists, plerixafor is now in clinical use in non-Hodgkin lymphoma and multiple myeloma undergoing autologous stem cell transplantation. Trabectedin, a new cytotoxic drug, has shown selective cytotoxicity to tumor-associated macrophages and circulating monocytes *via* caspase-8-dependent apoptosis and inhibits inflammatory mediators such as CCL2, interleukin-6, and CXCL8 in soft-tissue sarcoma and ovarian cancer [97⁻100].

IL-1β: IL-1β is one of an essential inflammatory regulator that promotes tumor progression through an accumulation of MDSCs which inhibit anti-cancer activity [101⁻103]. This is showed with an experimental study using IL-1R–deficient mice with breast carcinoma that have a delayed accumulation of MDSC and reduced primary and metastatic tumor progression [104]. Although the IL-1 antagonist has been used in the clinic to treat rheumatoid arthritis and autoinflammatory syndromes [101], its usage for anti-cancer still on trial. Anankira, a recombinant IL-1R antagonist, is used in phase 2 clinical trial for multiple myeloma, showed improved disease stability. Currently, Anakinra is being tested for advanced pancreatic, breast and colon cancer [102, 103].

_IL-6_: IL-6 promotes oral oncogenesis by enhanced secretion of matrix metalloproteinases 1 and 9 and activate STAT-1 and STAT-3 phosphorylation *via* IL-6 receptors and Janus family kinases (JAk). Moreover, IL-1β also stimulates Snail-1 and inhibits Cdh1 expression in HNSCC and further enhanced IL-8 and VEGF expression, which all of this causes neo-angiogenesis, tumor infiltration, and metastasis [105⁻116]. Chen and Bigbee reported an elevation of IL-6 levels in serum and saliva of patients with head and neck cancers to have a significant relation with staging and response to therapy [117, 118]. Recently, IL-6 becomes a potential target for cancer prevention. Toclizumab, an FDA-approved anti-IL-6 receptor monoclonal antibody, is being tested in combination with albumin-bound paclitaxel plus gemcitabine for pancreatic cancer [3] while Siltuximab has been tested in ovarian, prostate and renal cancer, with some promising result [107, 108].

TNF-α: Although TNF-α is a critical pro-inflammatory cytokine, its role in carcinogenesis is controversial. TNF-α acts *via* two receptors TNFR1 and TNFR2. TNF-R1 (p60) is the initiator, expressed in all cell types and contains the death domain (DD) that is important in apoptosis whereas TNF-R2 (p80) is expressed mainly in immune cells and does not contain the death domain (DD) [119⁻122]. It is postulated that the tumor-promoting mechanism is based on ROS and RNS, which can induce DNA damage and facilitate oncogenesis in a complex cascade [123⁻125]. Infliximab, a recombinant IgG1 monoclonal antibody specific for TNF-α was initially developed for rheumatoid arthritis, but is now undergoing phase 2 studies in breast and renal cell cancer [100, 126]. Therapeutic use TNF-α cascade manipulation such as Etanercept, Adalimumab, Golimumab, and Certolizumab has shown limited clinical response in TNFα- regulated cytokines in ovarian, breast, pancreatic, and renal cancers [3, 127].

Controversy remains regarding the use of anti-TNF-α drugs given emerging toxicities and possible association with the development of new malignancies [100]. Significant side effects of this anti-TNF-α agents are an infection such as tuberculosis, varicella, and other opportunistic infections, and more importantly, a malignancy itself. The risk of non-Hodgkin's lymphoma and skin cancer has been reported with TNF-α blocker. Therefore, its use needs to be carefully assessed because of the divergent outcomes [128⁻130].

***NF-κB, STAT-3, HIF-1*:** NF-κB and its pro-inflammatory cytokines (tumor necrosis factor (TNF)-α, IL-1β, IL-6, and IL-8) are activated in HNSCC tumor specimens [1, 131]. NF-κB promotes leukocyte chemoattractant proteins ligand (CXCL-12, CCL-2, and CCL-3), COX-2, and endothelial adhesion molecules such as E-selectin, vascular cell adhesion molecule 1 and intercellular adhesion molecule 1, that leads to inflammatory reactions [132, 133]. Nevertheless, NF-κB has a dual effect on inflammation. One, the activation of NF-κB, activates cytotoxic response against cancer cells NF-κB, and second, the activation increases the expression of ROS or inducible NO synthase resulting in cell proliferation, anti-apoptosis and genetic instability which promotes oncogenesis [1, 134⁻136]. Therefore, blocking NF-κB function in HNSCC will arrest tumor growth and reduce the expression of other chemokines-associated-pro- inflammatory molecules such as IL-6 and IL-8 [1, 131]. Inhibition of NF-κB is also known to sensitize cancer cells to TNF-α treatment [137⁻139].

NF-κB signaling is interconnected with STAT3 and HIF-1 pathways, co-regulating with numerous oncogenic and inflammatory genes [140⁻143]. STAT- 3 is stimulated and activated by IL-6, IL-11, IL-12 IL23, and various growth factors, mediates a protumorigenic response in the tumor microenvironment. Therefore, inhibition STAT-3 indirectly mediate tumor regression and provides a rational strategy to block carcinogenesis at an early stage [144⁻146].

HIF-1α is mediated by the recruitment of the NF-κB complex to the HIF-1α promoter. HIF-1α promotes chemoresistance, angiogenesis, invasiveness, metastasis, resistance to cell death, altered metabolism, and genomic instability [147, 148].

Immunotherapy in Head and Neck Cancer: An Immunotherapeutic Approach and Current Trials

In contrast to the inflammatory modulators, as we have discussed earlier, the critical strategy of an immunotherapeutic agent is to augment the immune response against tumor cells, facilitate the various immune cells and target directly towards the malignant cells. Current trials of immune therapeutic-based approaches predominantly comprise immune checkpoint inhibitors, adoptive cell transfer, and vaccines [149]. Most of these agents are still under trials [149, 150] and might not be included in our discussion.

Checkpoint Inhibitors

Checkpoint inhibitors are antibodies that bind to the checkpoint receptor on the T-cell and prevent it from binding to the inhibitory ligand on the tumor cell, which triggers the immune response. The immune checkpoint receptors cytotoxic T-lymphocyte-associated protein 4 (CTLA-4) and PD ligand are the most common targets in the clinical trials [149, 151]. A favorable outcome has been observed using these agents, and these are some of the examples used in head and neck cancers.

Ipilimumab blocks the CTLA-4 receptor, which prevents T-cell inhibition and enables an effective response against the tumor. A combined treatment of Ipilimumab and nivolumab for malignant melanoma [152] and non-small-cell lung carcinoma [153] showed a tolerable safety profile and encouraging response rate than Ipilimumab as a single agent [154]. A randomized, double-blind, phase II study of Nivolumab combined with Ipilimumab *versus* placebo in recurrent/metastatic squamous cell carcinoma of the head and neck (SCCHN) is currently ongoing [155].

Pembrolizumab binds to the PD-1 receptor on the T cell and blocks the binding of the PD-1 ligand on the tumor cell, thus prevents immune suppression of the PD-1 ligand. Based on encouraging results in KEYNOTE-012 [156, 157] and KEYNOTE-055 trials [158]. Pembrolizumab was the first FDA-approved drug for patients with progressive recurrent or metastatic SCC of the head and neck on or after treatment with platinum-containing chemotherapy. An undergoing phase III trial measures progression-free survival and overall survival of pembrolizumab in first-line treatment of recurrent/metastatic HNSCC compare pembrolizumab as monotherapy *versus* combination with chemotherapy [159]. The safety and efficacy of pembrolizumab given with chemoradiation (CRT) are yet to be determined in KEYNOTE-412 [160].

Nivolumab has a similar mechanism of action as pembrolizumab. It blocks the interaction of the PD-1 receptor ligand with the tumor and T cells to prevent suppression of the immune response. CheckMate 141 evaluated the efficacy, safety, and quality of life of nivolumab monotherapy *versus* standard single agent of the investigator's choice (IC) in patients with recurrent/metastatic HNSCC. Nivolumab demonstrates significant overall survival and a favorable safety profile after long term follow-up [161]. Nivolumab was approved by the FDA and the National Institute of Health and Care Excellence (NICE) and Scottish Medicines Consortium (SMC) in the UK to treat progressive recurrent or metastatic SCC of the head and neck, or after platinum-based therapy.

Durvalumab works through the PD-1 receptor/ligand pathway. It inhibits the binding of PD-L1. A randomized, multicenter, global, phase 2 trial (CONDOR) of durvalumab monotherapy *versus* durvalumab in combination with tremelimumab (anti-CTLA-4), in patients with recurrent or metastatic SCC of the head and neck and low PD-L1 expression showed similar efficacy and durvalumab as a monotherapy showed an acceptable toxicity profile [162].

Adoptive Cell Transfer

Adoptive cell therapy (ACT) is a complex process that involves harvesting autogenous tumor-infiltrating lymphocytes, grow it *in-vitro*, and tested against the tumor to establish their tumor-killing properties. The expanded immune cells with direct anticancer activity are then implanted back into the patient. A promising outcome has been observed with melanoma, cervical cancer, hematological malignancies, bile duct cancer, and neuroblastoma but yet to be used in cancer of the head and neck [163]. A phase I/II Trial of T-cell receptor gene therapy targeting HPV-16 E7 +/- PD-1 Blockade for HPV-associated-cancers to determine a safe and efficacy of E7 TCR cells for metastatic HPV-16+ cancers is still recruiting [164].

Vaccination

Traditionally, vaccination works by exposing the immune system to a weakened virus, which allows for the production of antibodies without exposure to actual virulent pathogens. Then, memory B cells are activated if there is the presence of a future infection. In a cancer setting, a vaccine given once the cancers have already developed is called therapeutic vaccines. The activation of cytotoxic T cells or induce the antibody production towards the cancer cells might delay or stop the cancer growth, tumor shrinkage, or prevent a recurrence.

While vaccination in HPV-related HNSCC is mainly speculative, a randomized, double-blind trial (FUTURE II) of HPV-6/11/16/18 vaccine *versus* placebo shows a significant reduction of high-grade cervical intraepithelial neoplasia related to HPV-16 or HPV-18 in the vaccination group [165]. Also, HPV-related vulvar intraepithelial neoplasia showed that almost 50% of patients responded well to the therapeutic vaccination at one year [166].

A phase I/II vaccine (HARE-40) to indicate a recommended safe and tolerable dose of HPV vaccine in patients with previously treated HPV16+ HNC and advanced HPV16+ cancer (head and neck, anogenital, penile or cervical) is still recruiting [167].

CONCLUSION

In conclusion, inflammation is a complex process involving many mediators that facilitates tumor progression through multiple mechanisms. The treatment of HNSCC is new and involves the manipulation of different pathways, cytokines, and chemokines. The selected targets, as mentioned, are promising and demonstrated the potential to arrest oncogenesis. However, the complete picture of the dynamic crosstalk among tumor cells, immune cells, and inflammation still has room for further investigations.

Nevertheless, the effects of anti-inflammatory agents on normal and malignant tissues are unpredictable and complicated. We believe several new clinical and pre-clinical trials are underway at this time of writing, investigating a more appropriate and competent agent to use as monotherapy or combinations.

Head and neck cancer (HNC) is a complex disease with challenging outcomes despite advances in surgery, radiotherapy, and chemotherapy. Molecular targeted therapies seem appealing; however, but most cancers involve multiple abnormal pathways that we think a combination of agents may appropriate. Rapidly emerging immunotherapy helps us shift towards non-surgical treatments, which may result in less morbidity and better outcomes. Currently, trials with immune-modulating agents have been conducted with promising results in the radical setting. Finally, a multidisciplinary team is crucial, and the success of these approaches depends on close collaboration between clinicians.

CONSENT FOR PUBLICATION

Not applicable.

CONFLICT OF INTEREST

The authors confirm that the content of this chapter have no conflict of interest.

ACKNOWLEDGEMENTS

Declared none.

REFERENCES

[1]   Samadi AK, Bilsland A, Georgakilas AG, *et al.* A multi-targeted approach to suppress tumor-promoting inflammation. Semin Cancer Biol 2015; 35 (Suppl.): S151-84.[http://dx.doi.org/10.1016/j.semcancer.2015.03.006] [PMID: 25951989]

[2]   Todoric J, Antonucci L, Karin M. Targeting inflammation in cancer prevention and therapy. Cancer Prev Res (Phila) 2016; 9(12): 895-905.[http://dx.doi.org/10.1158/1940-6207.CAPR-16-0209] [PMID: 27913448]

[3]   Nakamura K, Smyth MJ. Targeting cancer-related inflammation in the era of immunotherapy. Immunol Cell Biol 2017; 95(4): 325-32.[http://dx.doi.org/10.1038/icb.2016.126] [PMID: 27999432]

[4]   Bonomi M, Patsias A, Posner M, Sikora A. The role of inflammation in head and neck cancer. Adv Exp Med Biol 2014; 816: 107-27.[http://dx.doi.org/10.1007/978-3-0348-0837-8_5] [PMID: 24818721]

[5]   Balkwill F, Mantovani A. Inflammation and cancer: back to Virchow? Lancet 2001; 357(9255): 539-45.[http://dx.doi.org/10.1016/S0140-6736(00)04046-0] [PMID: 11229684]

[6]   Rayburn ER, Ezell SJ, Zhang R. Anti-inflammatory agents for cancer therapy. Mol Cell Pharmacol 2009; 1(1): 29-43.[http://dx.doi.org/10.4255/mcpharmacol.09.05] [PMID: 20333321]

[7]   Aggarwal BB, Gehlot P. Inflammation and cancer: how friendly is the relationship for cancer patients? Curr Opin Pharmacol 2009; 9(4): 351-69.[http://dx.doi.org/10.1016/j.coph.2009.06.020] [PMID: 19665429]

[8]   Balkwill F, Mantovani A. Cancer and inflammation: implications for pharmacology and therapeutics. Clin Pharmacol Ther 2010; 87(4): 401-6.[http://dx.doi.org/10.1038/clpt.2009.312] [PMID: 20200512]

[9]   Kundu JK, Surh YJ. Nrf2-Keap1 signaling as a potential target for chemoprevention of inflammation-associated carcinogenesis. Pharm Res 2010; 27(6): 999-1013.[http://dx.doi.org/10.1007/s11095-010-0096-8] [PMID: 20354764]

[10]   Bishayee A. The role of inflammation and liver cancer. Adv Exp Med Biol 2014; 816: 401-35.[http://dx.doi.org/10.1007/978-3-0348-0837-8_16] [PMID: 24818732]

[11]   Chung CH, Gillison ML. Human papillomavirus in head and neck cancer: its role in pathogenesis and clinical implications. Clin Cancer Res 2009; 15(22): 6758-62.[http://dx.doi.org/10.1158/1078-0432.CCR-09-0784] [PMID: 19861444]

[12]   Ang KK, Harris J, Wheeler R, *et al.* Human papillomavirus and survival of patients with oropharyngeal cancer. N Engl J Med 2010; 363(1): 24-35.[http://dx.doi.org/10.1056/NEJMoa0912217] [PMID: 20530316]

[13]   Reed AL, Califano J, Cairns P, *et al.* High frequency of p16 (CDKN2/MTS-1/INK4A) inactivation in head and neck squamous cell carcinoma. Cancer Res 1996; 56(16): 3630-3.[PMID: 8705996]

[14]   Tumban E. A current update on human papillomavirus-associated head and neck cancers. Viruses 2019; 11(10): E922.[http://dx.doi.org/10.3390/v11100922] [PMID: 31600915]

[15]   Perez-Ordoñez B, Beauchemin M, Jordan RC. Molecular biology of squamous cell carcinoma of the head and neck. J Clin Pathol 2006; 59(5): 445-53.[http://dx.doi.org/10.1136/jcp.2003.007641] [PMID: 16644882]

[16]   Poeta ML, Manola J, Goldwasser MA, *et al.* TP53 mutations and survival in squamous-cell carcinoma of the head and neck. N Engl J Med 2007; 357(25): 2552-61.[http://dx.doi.org/10.1056/NEJMoa073770] [PMID: 18094376]

[17]   Yin H, Qu J, Peng Q, Gan R. Molecular mechanisms of EBV-driven cell cycle progression and oncogenesis. Med Microbiol Immunol (Berl) 2019; 208(5): 573-83.[http://dx.doi.org/10.1007/s00430-018-0570-1] [PMID: 30386928]

[18]   Jack DB. One hundred years of aspirin. Lancet 1997; 350(9075): 437-9.[http://dx.doi.org/10.1016/S0140-6736(97)07087-6] [PMID: 9259670]

[19]   Usman MW, Luo F, Cheng H, Zhao JJ, Liu P. Chemopreventive effects of aspirin at a glance. Biochim Biophys Acta 2015; 1855(2): 254-63.[PMID: 25842298]

[20]   Kanda Y, Osaki M, Okada F. Chemopreventive strategies for inflammation-related carcinogenesis: current status and future direction. Int J Mol Sci 2017; 18(4): E867.[http://dx.doi.org/10.3390/ijms18040867] [PMID: 28422073]

[21]   Ahmadi N, Goldman R, Seillier-Moiseiwitsch F, Noone AM, Kosti O, Davidson BJ. Decreased risk of squamous cell carcinoma of the head and neck in users of nonsteroidal anti-inflammatory drugs. Int J Otolaryngol 2010; 2010: 424161.[http://dx.doi.org/10.1155/2010/424161] [PMID: 20628564]

[22]   Reddanna P. Anti-inflammatory drugs for cancer prevention and treatment: emerging options. J Cancer Sci Ther 2012; 4: xxvii-i.

[23]   Becker C, Wilson JC, Jick SS, Meier CR. Non-steroidal anti-inflammatory drugs and the risk of head and neck cancer: A case-control analysis. Int J Cancer 2015; 137(10): 2424-31.[http://dx.doi.org/10.1002/ijc.29601] [PMID: 25974157]

[24]   Roxburgh CS, McMillan DC. Cancer and systemic inflammation: treat the tumour and treat the host. Br J

Cancer 2014; 110(6): 1409-12.[http://dx.doi.org/10.1038/bjc.2014,90] [PMID: 24548867]

[25] Haddad Y, Choi W, McConkey DJ. Delta-crystallin enhancer binding factor 1 controls the epithelial to mesenchymal transition phenotype and resistance to the epidermal growth factor receptor inhibitor erlotinib in human head and neck squamous cell carcinoma lines. Clin Cancer Res 2009; 15(2): 532-42.[http://dx.doi.org/10.1158/1078-0432.CCR-08-1733] [PMID: 19147758]

[26] Chen EP, Smyth EM. COX-2 and PGE2-dependent immunomodulation in breast cancer. Prostaglandins Other Lipid Mediat 2011; 96(1-4): 14-20.[http://dx.doi.org/10.1016/j.prostaglandins.2011.08.005] [PMID: 21907301]

[27] Buchanan FG, Wang D, Bargiacchi F, DuBois RN. Prostaglandin E2 regulates cell migration via the intracellular activation of the epidermal growth factor receptor. J Biol Chem 2003; 278(37): 35451-7.[http://dx.doi.org/10.1074/jbc.M302474200] [PMID: 12824187]

[28] Dannenberg AJ, Subbaramaiah K. Targeting cyclooxygenase-2 in human neoplasia: rationale and promise. Cancer Cell 2003; 4(6): 431-6.[http://dx.doi.org/10.1016/S1535-6108(03)00310-6] [PMID: 14706335]

[29] Cooper JS, Pajak TF, Forastiere AA, et al. Radiation Therapy Oncology Group 9501/IntergroupPostoperative concurrent radiotherapy and chemotherapy for high-risk squamous-cell carcinoma of the head and neck. N Engl J Med 2004; 350(19): 1937-44.[http://dx.doi.org/10.1056/NEJMoa032646] [PMID: 15128893]

[30] Wong RSY. Role of Nonsteroidal Anti-Inflammatory Drugs (NSAIDs) in Cancer Prevention and Cancer Promotion. Adv Pharmacol Sci 2019; 2019: 3418975.[http://dx.doi.org/10.1155/2019/3418975] [PMID: 30838040]

[31] Wilson JC, Anderson LA, Murray LJ, Hughes CM. Non-steroidal anti-inflammatory drug and aspirin use and the risk of head and neck cancer: a systematic review. Cancer Causes Control 2011; 22(5): 803-10.[http://dx.doi.org/10.1007/s10552-011-9751-6] [PMID: 21409528]

[32] Xu X, Wells A, Padilla MT, Kato K, Kim KC, Lin Y. A signaling pathway consisting of miR-551b, catalase and MUC1 contributes to acquired apoptosis resistance and chemoresistance. Carcinogenesis 2014; 35(11): 2457-66.[http://dx.doi.org/10.1093/carcin/bgu159] [PMID: 25085901]

[33] Li W, Zhang B, Li H, et al. TGF β1 mediates epithelial mesenchymal transition via β6 integrin signaling pathway in breast cancer. Cancer Invest 2014; 32(8): 409-15.[http://dx.doi.org/10.3109/07357907.2014.933235] [PMID: 25019211]

[34] Diakos CI, Charles KA, McMillan DC, Clarke SJ. Cancer-related inflammation and treatment effectiveness. Lancet Oncol 2014; 15(11): e493-503.[http://dx.doi.org/10.1016/S1470-2045(14)70263-3] [PMID: 25281468]

[35] Wang H, Li M, Rinehart JJ, Zhang R. Dexamethasone as a chemoprotectant in cancer chemotherapy: hematoprotective effects and altered pharmacokinetics and tissue distribution of carboplatin and gemcitabine. Cancer Chemother Pharmacol 2004; 53(6): 459-67.[http://dx.doi.org/10.1007/s00280-003-0759-9] [PMID: 14752578]

[36] Leggas M, Kuo KL, Robert F, et al. Intensive anti-inflammatory therapy with dexamethasone in patients with non-small cell lung cancer: effect on chemotherapy toxicity and efficacy. Cancer Chemother Pharmacol 2009; 63(4): 731-43.[http://dx.doi.org/10.1007/s00280-008-0767-x] [PMID: 18500521]

[37] Elwood PC, Gallagher AM, Duthie GG, Mur LA, Morgan G. Aspirin, salicylates, and cancer. Lancet 2009; 373(9671): 1301-9.[http://dx.doi.org/10.1016/S0140-6736(09)60243-9] [PMID: 19328542]

[38] Steinbach G, Lynch PM, Phillips RK, et al. The effect of celecoxib, a cyclooxygenase-2 inhibitor, in familial adenomatous polyposis. N Engl J Med 2000; 342(26): 1946-52.[http://dx.doi.org/10.1056/NEJM200006293422603] [PMID: 10874062]

[39] Jayaprakash V, Rigual NR, Moysich KB, et al. Chemoprevention of head and neck cancer with aspirin: a case-control study. Arch Otolaryngol Head Neck Surg 2006; 132(11): 1231-6.[http://dx.doi.org/10.1001/archotol.132.11.1231] [PMID: 17116820]

[40] Gillespie MB, Moody MW, Lee FS, et al. Head and neck cancer recurrence and mortality in nonselective cyclooxygenase inhibitor users. Arch Otolaryngol Head Neck Surg 2007; 133(1): 28-31.[http://dx.doi.org/10.1001/archotol.133.1.28] [PMID: 17224518]

[41] Kim YY, Lee EJ, Kim YK, et al. Anti-cancer effects of celecoxib in head and neck carcinoma. Mol Cells 2010; 29(2): 185-94.[http://dx.doi.org/10.1007/s10059-010-0026-y] [PMID: 20082220]

[42] Yang B, Jia L, Guo Q, Ren H, Hu Y, Xie T. Clinicopathological and prognostic significance of cyclooxygenase-2 expression in head and neck cancer: A meta-analysis. Oncotarget 2016; 7(30): 47265-77.[http://dx.doi.org/10.18632/oncotarget.10059] [PMID: 27323811]

[43] Kim SA, Roh JL, Kim SB, Choi SH, Nam SY, Kim SY. Aspirin use and head and neck cancer survival: an observational study of 11,623 person-years follow-up. Int J Clin Oncol 2018; 23(1): 52-

8.[http://dx.doi.org/10.1007/s10147-017-1165-3] [PMID: 28725937]

[44] Hedberg ML, Peyser ND, Bauman JE, *et al.* Use of nonsteroidal anti-inflammatory drugs predicts improved patient survival for *PIK3CA*-altered head and neck cancer. J Exp Med 2019; 216(2): 419-27.[http://dx.doi.org/10.1084/jem.20181936] [PMID: 30683736]

[45] Chen Z, Zhang X, Li M, *et al.* Simultaneously targeting epidermal growth factor receptor tyrosine kinase and cyclooxygenase-2, an efficient approach to inhibition of squamous cell carcinoma of the head and neck. Clin Cancer Res 2004; 10(17): 5930-9.[http://dx.doi.org/10.1158/1078-0432.CCR-03-0677] [PMID: 15355926]

[46] Chung JH, Rho JK, Xu X, *et al.* Clinical and molecular evidences of epithelial to mesenchymal transition in acquired resistance to EGFR-TKIs. Lung Cancer 2011; 73(2): 176-82.[http://dx.doi.org/10.1016/j.lungcan.2010.11.011] [PMID: 21168239]

[47] Caponigro F, Milano A, Basile M, Ionna F, Iaffaioli RV. Recent advances in head and neck cancer therapy: the role of new cytotoxic and molecular-targeted agents. Curr Opin Oncol 2006; 18(3): 247-52.[http://dx.doi.org/10.1097/01.cco.0000219253.53091.fb] [PMID: 16552236]

[48] Kao J, Genden EM, Chen CT, *et al.* Phase 1 trial of concurrent erlotinib, celecoxib, and reirradiation for recurrent head and neck cancer. Cancer 2011; 117(14): 3173-81.[http://dx.doi.org/10.1002/cncr.25786] [PMID: 21246519]

[49] Gross ND, Bauman JE, Gooding WE, *et al.* Erlotinib, erlotinib-sulindac *versus* placebo: a randomized, double-blind, placebo-controlled window trial in operable head and neck cancer. Clin Cancer Res 2014; 20(12): 3289-98.[http://dx.doi.org/10.1158/1078-0432.CCR-13-3360] [PMID: 24727329]

[50] Reckamp K, Gitlitz B, Chen LC, *et al.* Biomarker-based phase I dose-escalation, pharmacokinetic, and pharmacodynamic study of oral apricoxib in combination with erlotinib in advanced nonsmall cell lung cancer. Cancer 2011; 117(4): 809-18.[http://dx.doi.org/10.1002/cncr.25473] [PMID: 20922800]

[51] St John MA, Wang G, Luo J, *et al.* Apricoxib upregulates 15-PGDH and PGT in tobacco-related epithelial malignancies. Br J Cancer 2012; 107(4): 707-12.[http://dx.doi.org/10.1038/bjc.2012.203] [PMID: 22828609]

[52] Huang J, Yuan X, Pang Q, *et al.* Radiosensitivity enhancement by combined treatment of nimotuzumab and celecoxib on nasopharyngeal carcinoma cells. Drug Des Devel Ther 2018; 12: 2223-31.[http://dx.doi.org/10.2147/DDDT.S163595] [PMID: 30038488]

[53] Mulshine JL, Atkinson JC, Greer RO, *et al.* Randomized, double-blind, placebo-controlled phase IIb trial of the cyclooxygenase inhibitor ketorolac as an oral rinse in oropharyngeal leukoplakia. Clin Cancer Res 2004; 10(5): 1565-73.[http://dx.doi.org/10.1158/1078-0432.CCR-1020-3] [PMID: 15014005]

[54] Papadimitrakopoulou VA, William WN, Jr, Dannenberg AJ, *et al.* Pilot randomized phase II study of celecoxib in oral premalignant lesions. Clin Cancer Res 2008; 14(7): 2095-101.[http://dx.doi.org/10.1158/1078-0432.CCR-07-4024] [PMID: 18381950]

[55] McGettigan P, Henry D. Cardiovascular risk with non-steroidal anti-inflammatory drugs: systematic review of population-based controlled observational studies. PLoS Med 2011; 8(9): e1001098.[http://dx.doi.org/10.1371/journal.pmed.1001098] [PMID: 21980265]

[56] Shishodia S. Molecular mechanisms of curcumin action: gene expression. Biofactors 2013; 39(1): 37-55.[http://dx.doi.org/10.1002/biof.1041] [PMID: 22996381]

[57] Wang R, Guo L, Wang P, *et al.* Chemoprevention of cancers in gastrointestinal tract with cyclooxygenase 2 inhibitors. Curr Pharm Des 2013; 19(1): 115-25.[PMID: 22950494]

[58] Wilken R, Veena MS, Wang MB, Srivatsan ES. Curcumin: A review of anti-cancer properties and therapeutic activity in head and neck squamous cell carcinoma. Mol Cancer 2011; 10: 12.[http://dx.doi.org/10.1186/1476-4598-10-12] [PMID: 21299897]

[59] Cerella C, Sobolewski C, Dicato M, Diederich M. Targeting COX-2 expression by natural compounds: a promising alternative strategy to synthetic COX-2 inhibitors for cancer chemoprevention and therapy. Biochem Pharmacol 2010; 80(12): 1801-15.[http://dx.doi.org/10.1016/j.bcp.2010.06.050] [PMID: 20615394]

[60] Rutz HP. Effects of corticosteroid use on treatment of solid tumours. Lancet 2002; 360(9349): 1969-70.[http://dx.doi.org/10.1016/S0140-6736(02)11922-2] [PMID: 12493280]

[61] Witschi H, Espiritu I, Ly M, Uyeminami D. The chemopreventive effects of orally administered dexamethasone in Strain A/J mice following cessation of smoke exposure. Inhal Toxicol 2005; 17(2): 119-22.[http://dx.doi.org/10.1080/08958370590899712] [PMID: 15764489]

[62] Arai Y, Nonomura N, Nakai Y, *et al.* The growth-inhibitory effects of dexamethasone on renal cell carcinoma *in vivo* and *in vitro*. Cancer Invest 2008; 26(1): 35-40.[http://dx.doi.org/10.1080/07357900701638418] [PMID: 18181043]

[63] Gong H, Jarzynka MJ, Cole TJ, *et al.* Glucocorticoids antagonize estrogens by glucocorticoid receptor-mediated activation of estrogen sulfotransferase. Cancer Res 2008; 68(18): 7386-

17

93.[http://dx.doi.org/10.1158/0008-5472.CAN-08-1545] [PMID: 18794126]

[64] Wang H, Li M, Rinehart JJ, Zhang R. Pretreatment with dexamethasone increases antitumor activity of carboplatin and gemcitabine in mice bearing human cancer xenografts: *in vivo* activity, pharmacokinetics, and clinical implications for cancer chemotherapy. Clin Cancer Res 2004; 10(5): 1633-44.[http://dx.doi.org/10.1158/1078-0432.CCR-0829-3] [PMID: 15014014]

[65] Wang H, Wang Y, Rayburn ER, Hill DL, Rinehart JJ, Zhang R. Dexamethasone as a chemosensitizer for breast cancer chemotherapy: potentiation of the antitumor activity of adriamycin, modulation of cytokine expression, and pharmacokinetics. Int J Oncol 2007; 30(4): 947-53.[http://dx.doi.org/10.3892/ijo.30.4.947] [PMID: 17332934]

[66] Lebo NL, Griffiths R, Hall S, Dimitroulakos J, Johnson-Obaseki S. Effect of statin use on oncologic outcomes in head and neck squamous cell carcinoma. Head Neck 2018; 40(8): 1697-706.[http://dx.doi.org/10.1002/hed.25152] [PMID: 29934959]

[67] Sassano A, Platanias LC. Statins in tumor suppression. Cancer Lett 2008; 260(1-2): 11-9.[http://dx.doi.org/10.1016/j.canlet.2007.11.036] [PMID: 18180097]

[68] Xiao H, Yang CS. Combination regimen with statins and NSAIDs: a promising strategy for cancer chemoprevention. Int J Cancer 2008; 123(5): 983-90.[http://dx.doi.org/10.1002/ijc.23718] [PMID: 18548583]

[69] Gehrke T, Scherzad A, Hackenberg S, *et al.* Additive antitumor effects of celecoxib and simvastatin on head and neck squamous cell carcinoma *in vitro*. Int J Oncol 2017; 51(3): 931-8.[http://dx.doi.org/10.3892/ijo.2017.4071] [PMID: 28713941]

[70] Bonovas S, Filioussi K, Tsavaris N, Sitaras NM. Use of statins and breast cancer: a meta-analysis of seven randomized clinical trials and nine observational studies. J Clin Oncol 2005; 23(34): 8606-12.[http://dx.doi.org/10.1200/JCO.2005.02.7045] [PMID: 16260694]

[71] Blais L, Desgagné A, LeLorier J. 3-Hydroxy-3-methylglutaryl coenzyme A reductase inhibitors and the risk of cancer: a nested case-control study. Arch Intern Med 2000; 160(15): 2363-8.[http://dx.doi.org/10.1001/archinte.160.15.2363] [PMID: 10927735]

[72] Graaf MR, Beiderbeck AB, Egberts AC, Richel DJ, Guchelaar HJ. The risk of cancer in users of statins. J Clin Oncol 2004; 22(12): 2388-94.[http://dx.doi.org/10.1200/JCO.2004.02.027] [PMID: 15197200]

[73] Friis S, Poulsen AH, Johnsen SP, *et al.* Cancer risk among statin users: a population-based cohort study. Int J Cancer 2005; 114(4): 643-7.[http://dx.doi.org/10.1002/ijc.20758] [PMID: 15578694]

[74] Olsen JH, Johansen C, Sørensen HT, *et al.* Lipid-lowering medication and risk of cancer. J Clin Epidemiol 1999; 52(2): 167-9.[http://dx.doi.org/10.1016/S0895-4356(98)00147-4] [PMID: 10201659]

[75] Kaye JA, Jick H. Statin use and cancer risk in the General Practice Research Database. Br J Cancer 2004; 90(3): 635-7.[http://dx.doi.org/10.1038/sj.bjc.6601566] [PMID: 14760377]

[76] Poynter JN, Gruber SB, Higgins PD, *et al.* Statins and the risk of colorectal cancer. N Engl J Med 2005; 352(21): 2184-92.[http://dx.doi.org/10.1056/NEJMoa043792] [PMID: 15917383]

[77] Khurana V, Bejjanki HR, Caldito G, Owens MW. Statins reduce the risk of lung cancer in humans: a large case-control study of US veterans. Chest 2007; 131(5): 1282-8.[http://dx.doi.org/10.1378/chest.06-0931] [PMID: 17494779]

[78] Farwell WR, Scranton RE, Lawler EV, *et al.* The association between statins and cancer incidence in a veterans population. J Natl Cancer Inst 2008; 100(2): 134-9.[http://dx.doi.org/10.1093/jnci/djm286] [PMID: 18182618]

[79] Khurana V, Caldito G, Ankem M. Statins might reduce risk of renal cell carcinoma in humans: case-control study of 500,000 veterans. Urology 2008; 71(1): 118-22.[http://dx.doi.org/10.1016/j.urology.2007.08.039] [PMID: 18242378]

[80] Schönbeck U, Libby P. Inflammation, immunity, and HMG-CoA reductase inhibitors: statins as antiinflammatory agents? Circulation 2004; 109(21) (Suppl. 1): II18-26.[http://dx.doi.org/10.1161/01.CIR.0000129505.34151.23] [PMID: 15173059]

[81] Tsan YT, Lee CH, Ho WC, Lin MH, Wang JD, Chen PC. Statins and the risk of hepatocellular carcinoma in patients with hepatitis C virus infection. J Clin Oncol 2013; 31(12): 1514-21.[http://dx.doi.org/10.1200/JCO.2012.44.6831] [PMID: 23509319]

[82] Lochhead P, Chan AT. Statins and colorectal cancer. Clin Gastroenterol Hepatol 2013; 11(2): 109-18.[http://dx.doi.org/10.1016/j.cgh.2012.08.037] [PMID: 22982096]

[83] Bonovas S, Filioussi K, Flordellis CS, Sitaras NM. Statins and the risk of colorectal cancer: a meta-analysis of 18 studies involving more than 1.5 million patients. J Clin Oncol 2007; 25(23): 3462-8.[http://dx.doi.org/10.1200/JCO.2007.10.8936] [PMID: 17687150]

18

[84] Samadder NJ, Mukherjee B, Huang SC, *et al.* Risk of colorectal cancer in self-reported inflammatory bowel disease and modification of risk by statin and NSAID use. Cancer 2011; 117(8): 1640-8.[http://dx.doi.org/10.1002/cncr.25731] [PMID: 21472711]

[85] Van Waes C. Nuclear factor-kappaB in development, prevention, and therapy of cancer. Clin Cancer Res 2007; 13(4): 1076-82.[http://dx.doi.org/10.1158/1078-0432.CCR-06-2221] [PMID: 17317814]

[86] Germano G, Allavena P, Mantovani A. Cytokines as a key component of cancer-related inflammation. Cytokine 2008; 43(3): 374-9.[http://dx.doi.org/10.1016/j.cyto.2008.07.014] [PMID: 18701317]

[87] Molinolo AA, Amornphimoltham P, Squarize CH, Castilho RM, Patel V, Gutkind JS. Dysregulated molecular networks in head and neck carcinogenesis. Oral Oncol 2009; 45(4-5): 324-34.[http://dx.doi.org/10.1016/j.oraloncology.2008.07.011] [PMID: 18805044]

[88] Wang F, Arun P, Friedman J, Chen Z, Van Waes C. Current and potential inflammation targeted therapies in head and neck cancer. Curr Opin Pharmacol 2009; 9(4): 389-95.[http://dx.doi.org/10.1016/j.coph.2009.06.005] [PMID: 19570715]

[89] Lee TL, Yang XP, Yan B, *et al.* A novel nuclear factor-kappaB gene signature is differentially expressed in head and neck squamous cell carcinomas in association with TP53 status. Clin Cancer Res 2007; 13(19): 5680-91.[http://dx.doi.org/10.1158/1078-0432.CCR-07-0670] [PMID: 17908957]

[90] Thompson PA, Khatami M, Baglole CJ, *et al.* Environmental immune disruptors, inflammation and cancer risk. Carcinogenesis 2015; 36 (Suppl. 1): S232-53.[http://dx.doi.org/10.1093/carcin/bgv038] [PMID: 26106141]

[91] Trivedi PP, Jena GB, Tikoo KB, Kumar V. Melatonin modulated autophagy and Nrf2 signaling pathways in mice with colitis-associated colon carcinogenesis. Mol Carcinog 2016; 55(3): 255-67.[http://dx.doi.org/10.1002/mc.22274] [PMID: 25598500]

[92] Yoshida GJ. Therapeutic strategies of drug repositioning targeting autophagy to induce cancer cell death: from pathophysiology to treatment. J Hematol Oncol 2017; 10(1): 67.[http://dx.doi.org/10.1186/s13045-017-0436-9] [PMID: 28279189]

[93] Sun J, Madan R, Karp CL, Braciale TJ. Effector T cells control lung inflammation during acute influenza virus infection by producing IL-10. Nat Med 2009; 15(3): 277-84.[http://dx.doi.org/10.1038/nm.1929] [PMID: 19234462]

[94] Schottelius AJ, Mayo MW, Sartor RB, Baldwin AS, Jr. Interleukin-10 signaling blocks inhibitor of kappaB kinase activity and nuclear factor kappaB DNA binding. J Biol Chem 1999; 274(45): 31868-74.[http://dx.doi.org/10.1074/jbc.274.45.31868] [PMID: 10542212]

[95] Schetter AJ, Heegaard NH, Harris CC. Inflammation and cancer: interweaving microRNA, free radical, cytokine and p53 pathways. Carcinogenesis 2010; 31(1): 37-49.[http://dx.doi.org/10.1093/carcin/bgp272] [PMID: 19955394]

[96] Allen C, Duffy S, Teknos T, *et al.* Nuclear factor-kappaB-related serum factors as longitudinal biomarkers of response and survival in advanced oropharyngeal carcinoma. Clin Cancer Res 2007; 13(11): 3182-90.[http://dx.doi.org/10.1158/1078-0432.CCR-06-3047] [PMID: 17545521]

[97] Germano G, Mantovani A, Allavena P. Targeting of the innate immunity/inflammation as complementary anti-tumor therapies. Ann Med 2011; 43(8): 581-93.[http://dx.doi.org/10.3109/07853890.2011.595732] [PMID: 21756064]

[98] Onuffer JJ, Horuk R. Chemokines, chemokine receptors and small-molecule antagonists: recent developments. Trends Pharmacol Sci 2002; 23(10): 459-67.[http://dx.doi.org/10.1016/S0165-6147(02)02064-3] [PMID: 12368070]

[99] Ryan CW, Desai J. The past, present, and future of cytotoxic chemotherapy and pathway-directed targeted agents for soft tissue sarcoma. Am Soc Clin Oncol Educ Book 2013386-93.[http://dx.doi.org/10.14694/EdBook_AM.2013.33.e386] [PMID: 23714556]

[100] Germano G, Frapolli R, Belgiovine C, *et al.* Role of macrophage targeting in the antitumor activity of trabectedin. Cancer Cell 2013; 23(2): 249-62.[http://dx.doi.org/10.1016/j.ccr.2013.01.008] [PMID: 23410977]

[101] Bunt SK, Sinha P, Clements VK. Inflammation induces myeloid-derived suppressor cells that facilitate tumor progression. J Immunol (Baltimore, Md 1950) 2006; 176(1): 284-90.

[102] Kroemer G, Galluzzi L, Kepp O, Zitvogel L. Immunogenic cell death in cancer therapy. Annu Rev Immunol 2013; 31: 51-72.[http://dx.doi.org/10.1146/annurev-immunol-032712-100008] [PMID: 23157435]

[103] Lust JA, Lacy MQ, Zeldenrust SR, *et al.* Induction of a chronic disease state in patients with smoldering or indolent multiple myeloma by targeting interleukin 1beta-induced interleukin 6 production and the myeloma proliferative component. Mayo Clin Proc 2009; 84(2): 114-22.[http://dx.doi.org/10.4065/84.2.114] [PMID:

19

19181644]

[104] Bunt SK, Yang L, Sinha P, Clements VK, Leips J, Ostrand-Rosenberg S. Reduced inflammation in the tumor microenvironment delays the accumulation of myeloid-derived suppressor cells and limits tumor progression. Cancer Res 2007; 67(20): 10019-26.[http://dx.doi.org/10.1158/0008-5472.CAN-07-2354] [PMID: 17942936]

[105] Worden B, Yang XP, Lee TL, *et al.* Hepatocyte growth factor/scatter factor differentially regulates expression of proangiogenic factors through Egr-1 in head and neck squamous cell carcinoma. Cancer Res 2005; 65(16): 7071-80.[http://dx.doi.org/10.1158/0008-5472.CAN-04-0989] [PMID: 16103054]

[106] Lee TL, Yeh J, Friedman J, *et al.* A signal network involving coactivated NF-kappaB and STAT3 and altered p53 modulates BAX/BCL-XL expression and promotes cell survival of head and neck squamous cell carcinomas. Int J Cancer 2008; 122(9): 1987-98.[http://dx.doi.org/10.1002/ijc.23324] [PMID: 18172861]

[107] Aghajan M, Li N, Karin M. Obesity, autophagy and the pathogenesis of liver and pancreatic cancers. J Gastroenterol Hepatol 2012; 27 (Suppl. 2): 10-4.[http://dx.doi.org/10.1111/j.1440-1746.2011.07008.x] [PMID: 22320909]

[108] Heinrich PC, Behrmann I, Haan S, Hermanns HM, Müller-Newen G, Schaper F. Principles of interleukin (IL)-6-type cytokine signalling and its regulation. Biochem J 2003; 374(Pt 1): 1-20.[http://dx.doi.org/10.1042/bj20030407] [PMID: 12773095]

[109] St John MA, Dohadwala M, Luo J, *et al.* Proinflammatory mediators upregulate snail in head and neck squamous cell carcinoma. Clin Cancer Res 2009; 15(19): 6018-27.[http://dx.doi.org/10.1158/1078-0432.CCR-09-0011] [PMID: 19789323]

[110] Nibali L, Fedele S, D'Aiuto F, Donos N. Interleukin-6 in oral diseases: a review. Oral Dis 2012; 18(3): 236-43.[http://dx.doi.org/10.1111/j.1601-0825.2011.01867.x] [PMID: 22050374]

[111] Hirano T, Ishihara K, Hibi M. Roles of STAT3 in mediating the cell growth, differentiation and survival signals relayed through the IL-6 family of cytokine receptors. Oncogene 2000; 19(21): 2548-56.[http://dx.doi.org/10.1038/sj.onc.1203551] [PMID: 10851053]

[112] Sundelin K, Roberg K, Grénman R, Håkansson L. Effects of cytokines on matrix metalloproteinase expression in oral squamous cell carcinoma in vitro. Acta Otolaryngol 2005; 125(7): 765-73.[http://dx.doi.org/10.1080/00016480510027484] [PMID: 16012040]

[113] Berishaj M, Gao SP, Ahmed S. Stat3 is tyrosine- phosphorylated through the interleukin- 6/glycoprotein 130/Janus kinase pathway in breast cancer. Breast Cancer Res 2007; 9(3): R32.

[114] Bollrath J, Phesse TJ, von Burstin VA, *et al.* gp130-mediated Stat3 activation in enterocytes regulates cell survival and cell-cycle progression during colitis-associated tumorigenesis. Cancer Cell 2009; 15(2): 91-102.[http://dx.doi.org/10.1016/j.ccr.2009.01.002] [PMID: 19185844]

[115] Liu Y, Liu A, Li H, Li C, Lin J. Celecoxib inhibits interleukin-6/interleukin-6 receptor-induced JAK2/STAT3 phosphorylation in human hepatocellular carcinoma cells. Cancer Prev Res (Phila) 2011; 4(8): 1296-305.[http://dx.doi.org/10.1158/1940-6207.CAPR-10-0317] [PMID: 21490132]

[116] Bianchi M, Broggini M, Balzarini P, Franchi S, Sacerdote P. Effects of nimesulide on pain and on synovial fluid concentrations of substance P, interleukin-6 and interleukin-8 in patients with knee osteoarthritis: comparison with celecoxib. Int J Clin Pract 2007; 61(8): 1270-7.[http://dx.doi.org/10.1111/j.1742-1241.2007.01453.x] [PMID: 17590218]

[117] Chen Z, Malhotra PS, Thomas GR, *et al.* Expression of proinflammatory and proangiogenic cytokines in patients with head and neck cancer. Clin Cancer Res 1999; 5(6): 1369-79.[PMID: 10389921]

[118] Bigbee WL, Grandis JR, Siegfried JM. Multiple cytokine and growth factor serum biomarkers predict therapeutic response and survival in advanced-stage head and neck cancer patients. Clin Cancer Res 2007; 13(11): 3107-8.[http://dx.doi.org/10.1158/1078-0432.CCR-07-0746] [PMID: 17545511]

[119] Locksley RM, Killeen N, Lenardo MJ. The TNF and TNF receptor superfamilies: integrating mammalian biology. Cell 2001; 104(4): 487-501.[http://dx.doi.org/10.1016/S0092-8674(01)00237-9] [PMID: 11239407]

[120] Tartaglia LA, Goeddel DV. Two TNF receptors. Immunol Today 1992; 13(5): 151-3.[http://dx.doi.org/10.1016/0167-5699(92)90116-O] [PMID: 1322675]

[121] Aggarwal BB. Signalling pathways of the TNF superfamily: a double-edged sword. Nat Rev Immunol 2003; 3(9): 745-56.[http://dx.doi.org/10.1038/nri1184] [PMID: 12949498]

[122] Ashkenazi A, Dixit VM. Death receptors: signaling and modulation. Science 1998; 281(5381): 1305-8.[http://dx.doi.org/10.1126/science.281.5381.1305] [PMID: 9721089]

[123] Woo CH, Eom YW, Yoo MH, *et al.* Tumor necrosis factor-alpha generates reactive oxygen species *via* a cytosolic phospholipase A2-linked cascade. J Biol Chem 2000; 275(41): 32357-62.[http://dx.doi.org/10.1074/jbc.M005638200] [PMID: 10934206]

[124] Hussain SP, Hofseth LJ, Harris CC. Radical causes of cancer. Nat Rev Cancer 2003; 3(4): 276-85.[http://dx.doi.org/10.1038/nrc1046] [PMID: 12671666]

[125] Xia L, Mo P, Huang W, *et al.* The TNF-α/ROS/HIF-1-induced upregulation of FoxMI expression promotes HCC proliferation and resistance to apoptosis. Carcinogenesis 2012; 33(11): 2250-9.[http://dx.doi.org/10.1093/carcin/bgs249] [PMID: 22831955]

[126] Feldmann M, Elliott MJ, Woody JN, Maini RN. Anti-tumor necrosis factor-alpha therapy of rheumatoid arthritis. Adv Immunol 1997; 64: 283-350.[http://dx.doi.org/10.1016/S0065-2776(08)60891-3] [PMID: 9100984]

[127] Brown ER, Charles KA, Hoare SA, *et al.* A clinical study assessing the tolerability and biological effects of infliximab, a TNF-alpha inhibitor, in patients with advanced cancer. Ann Oncol 2008; 19(7): 1340-6.[http://dx.doi.org/10.1093/annonc/mdn054] [PMID: 18325912]

[128] Moreland LW, Baumgartner SW, Schiff MH, *et al.* Treatment of rheumatoid arthritis with a recombinant human tumor necrosis factor receptor (p75)-Fc fusion protein. N Engl J Med 1997; 337(3): 141-7.[http://dx.doi.org/10.1056/NEJM199707173370301] [PMID: 9219699]

[129] Wiens A, Correr CJ, Venson R, Otuki MF, Pontarolo R. A systematic review and meta-analysis of the efficacy and safety of adalimumab for treating rheumatoid arthritis. Rheumatol Int 2010; 30(8): 1063-70.[http://dx.doi.org/10.1007/s00296-009-1111-4] [PMID: 19707765]

[130] Keystone EC, Genovese MC, Klareskog L, *et al.* GO-FORWARD StudyGolimumab, a human antibody to tumour necrosis factor alpha given by monthly subcutaneous injections, in active rheumatoid arthritis despite methotrexate therapy: the GO-FORWARD Study. Ann Rheum Dis 2009; 68(6): 789-96.[http://dx.doi.org/10.1136/ard.2008.099010] [PMID: 19066176]

[131] Kross KW, Heimdal JH, Aarstad HJ. Mononuclear phagocytes in head and neck squamous cell carcinoma. Eur Arch Otorhinolaryngol 2010; 267(3): 335-44.[http://dx.doi.org/10.1007/s00405-009-1153-y] [PMID: 19967383]

[132] Hill MM, Hemmings BA. Inhibition of protein kinase B/Akt. implications for cancer therapy. Pharmacol Ther 2002; 93(2-3): 243-51.[http://dx.doi.org/10.1016/S0163-7258(02)00193-6] [PMID: 12191616]

[133] Abraham AG, O'Neill E. PI3K/Akt-mediated regulation of p53 in cancer. Biochem Soc Trans 2014; 42(4): 798-803.[http://dx.doi.org/10.1042/BST20140070] [PMID: 25109960]

[134] Giliano NY, Konevega LV, Noskin LA. Dynamics of intracellular superoxide and NO content in human endotheliocytes and carcinoma cells after treatment with NO synthase inhibitors. Bull Exp Biol Med 2010; 149(1): 78-81.[http://dx.doi.org/10.1007/s10517-010-0880-9] [PMID: 21113464]

[135] Liu PP, Liao J, Tang ZJ, *et al.* Metabolic regulation of cancer cell side population by glucose through activation of the Akt pathway. Cell Death Differ 2014; 21(1): 124-35.[http://dx.doi.org/10.1038/cdd.2013.131] [PMID: 24096870]

[136] Stambolic V, Woodgett JR. Functional distinctions of protein kinase B/Akt isoforms defined by their influence on cell migration. Trends Cell Biol 2006; 16(9): 461-6.[http://dx.doi.org/10.1016/j.tcb.2006.07.001] [PMID: 16870447]

[137] Orlowski RZ, Baldwin AS, Jr. NF-kappaB as a therapeutic target in cancer. Trends Mol Med 2002; 8(8): 385-9.[http://dx.doi.org/10.1016/S1471-4914(02)02375-4] [PMID: 12127724]

[138] Lee KY, Chang W, Qiu D, Kao PN, Rosen GD. PG490 (triptolide) cooperates with tumor necrosis factor-alpha to induce apoptosis in tumor cells. J Biol Chem 1999; 274(19): 13451-5.[http://dx.doi.org/10.1074/jbc.274.19.13451] [PMID: 10224110]

[139] Ganster RW, Taylor BS, Shao L, Geller DA. Complex regulation of human inducible nitric oxide synthase gene transcription by Stat 1 and NF-kappa B. Proc Natl Acad Sci USA 2001; 98(15): 8638-43.[http://dx.doi.org/10.1073/pnas.151239498] [PMID: 11438703]

[140] Grivennikov S, Karin E, Terzic J, *et al.* IL-6 and Stat3 are required for survival of intestinal epithelial cells and development of colitis-associated cancer. Cancer Cell 2009; 15(2): 103-13.[http://dx.doi.org/10.1016/j.ccr.2009.01.001] [PMID: 19185845]

[141] Grivennikov SI, Greten FR, Karin M. Immunity, inflammation, and cancer. Cell 2010; 140(6): 883-99.[http://dx.doi.org/10.1016/j.cell.2010.01.025] [PMID: 20303878]

[142] Nagai T, Tanaka M, Tsuneyoshi Y, *et al.* Targeting tumor-associated macrophages in an experimental glioma model with a recombinant immunotoxin to folate receptor beta. Cancer Immunol Immunother 2009; 58(10): 1577-86.[http://dx.doi.org/10.1007/s00262-009-0667-x] [PMID: 19238383]

[143] Aggarwal BB, Sethi G, Ahn KS, *et al.* Targeting signal-transducer-and-activator-of-transcription-3 for prevention and therapy of cancer: modern target but ancient solution. Ann N Y Acad Sci 2006; 1091: 151-69.[http://dx.doi.org/10.1196/annals.1378.063] [PMID: 17341611]

[144] Mankan AK, Greten FR. Inhibiting signal transducer and activator of transcription 3: rationality and rationale design of inhibitors. Expert Opin Investig Drugs 2011; 20(9): 1263-75.[http://dx.doi.org/10.1517/13543784.2011.601739] [PMID: 21751940]

[145] Pilati C, Amessou M, Bihl MP, et al. Somatic mutations activating STAT3 in human inflammatory hepatocellular adenomas. J Exp Med 2011; 208(7): 1359-66.[http://dx.doi.org/10.1084/jem.20110283] [PMID: 21690253]

[146] Kortylewski M, Xin H, Kujawski M, et al. Regulation of the IL-23 and IL-12 balance by Stat3 signaling in the tumor microenvironment. Cancer Cell 2009; 15(2): 114-23.[http://dx.doi.org/10.1016/j.ccr.2008.12.018] [PMID: 19185846]

[147] Kumar S, Mehta K. Tissue transglutaminase constitutively activates HIF-1α promoter and nuclear factor-κB via a non-canonical pathway. PLoS One 2012; 7(11): e49321.[http://dx.doi.org/10.1371/journal.pone.0049321] [PMID: 23185316]

[148] DeClerck K, Elble RC. The role of hypoxia and acidosis in promoting metastasis and resistance to chemotherapy. Front Biosci 2010; 15: 213-25.[http://dx.doi.org/10.2741/3616] [PMID: 20036816]

[149] Subramaniam SS, Paterson C, McCaul JA. Immunotherapy in the management of squamous cell carcinoma of the head and neck. Br J Oral Maxillofac Surg 2019; 57(10): 957-66.[http://dx.doi.org/10.1016/j.bjoms.2019.08.002] [PMID: 31653434]

[150] Dogan V, Rieckmann T, Münscher A, Busch CJ. Current studies of immunotherapy in head and neck cancer. Clin Otolaryngol 2018; 43(1): 13-21.[http://dx.doi.org/10.1111/coa.12895] [PMID: 28464441]

[151] Pardoll DM. The blockade of immune checkpoints in cancer immunotherapy. Nat Rev Cancer 2012; 12(4): 252-64.[http://dx.doi.org/10.1038/nrc3239] [PMID: 22437870]

[152] Larkin J, Chiarion-Sileni V, Gonzalez R, et al. Combined nivolumab and ipilimumab or monotherapy in untreated melanoma. N Engl J Med 2015; 373(1): 23-34.[http://dx.doi.org/10.1056/NEJMoa1504030] [PMID: 26027431]

[153] A multi-arm phase I safety study of nivolumab in combination with gemcitabine/cisplatin, pemetrexed/cisplatin, carboplatin/paclitaxel, bevacizumab maintenance, erlotinib, ipilimumab or as monotherapy in subjects with stage IIIB/IV non-small cell lung cancer (NSCLC)(checkmate 012) Available from: https://clinicaltrials. Gov/ct2/show/NCT01454102

[154] Hellmann MD, Rizvi NA, Goldman JW, et al. Nivolumab plus ipilimumab as first-line treatment for advanced non-small-cell lung cancer (CheckMate 012): results of an open-label, phase 1, multicohort study. Lancet Oncol 2017; 18(1): 31-41.[http://dx.doi.org/10.1016/S1470-2045(16)30624-6] [PMID: 27932067]

[155] A double-blind, randomized, two arm phase 2 study of nivolumab in combination with ipilimumab versus nivolumab in combination with ipilimumab placebo in recurrent or metastatic squamous cell carcinoma of the head and neck (SCCHN) (checkmate 714) Available from: https:// clinicaltrials.gov/ct2/show/NCT02823574

[156] Saba NF, Mody MD, Tan ES. Toxicities of systemic agents in squamous cell carcinoma of the head and neck (SCCHN): a new perspective in the era of immunotherapy. Crit Rev Oncol Hematol 2017; 115: 50-8.A.

[157] Phase IB multi-cohort study of pembrolizumab (MK-3475) in subjects with advanced solid tumors (mk-3475-012/keynote-012 Available from: https:// clinicaltrials.gov/ct2/show/

[158] A phase II clinical trial of single agent pembrolizumab (mk-3475) in subjects with recurrent or metastatic head and neck squamous cell carcinoma (hnscc) who have failed platinum and cetuximab (mk-3475-055/keynote-055) Available from: https:// clinicaltrials.gov/ct2/show/NCT02255097

[159] A phase 3 clinical trial of pembrolizumab (mk-3475) in first line treatment of recurrent/metastatic head and neck squamous cell carcinoma (mk-3475-048/keynote-048) Available from: https:// clinicaltrials.gov/ct2/show/

[160] A randomized phase iii study of pembrolizumab (mk-3475) given concomitantly with chemoradiation and as maintenance therapy versus chemoradiation alone in subjects with locally advanced head and neck squamous cell carcinoma (keynote-412) (mk-3475- 412/keynote-412) Available from: https:// clinicaltrials.gov/ct2/show/

[161] Ferris RL, Blumenschein G, Jr, Fayette J, et al. Nivolumab vs investigator's choice in recurrent or metastatic squamous cell carcinoma of the head and neck: 2-year long-term survival update of CheckMate 141 with analyses by tumor PD-L1 expression. Oral Oncol 2018; 81: 45-51.[http://dx.doi.org/10.1016/j.oraloncology.2018.04.008] [PMID: 29884413]

[162] Siu LL, Even C, Mesía R, et al. Safety and efficacy of durvalumab with or without tremelimumab in patients with pd-l1-low/negative recurrent or metastatic hnscc: the phase 2 condor randomized clinical trial. JAMA Oncol 2019; 5(2): 195-203.[http://dx.doi.org/10.1001/jamaoncol.2018.4628] [PMID: 30383184]

[163] Rosenberg SA, Restifo NP. Adoptive cell transfer as personalized immunotherapy for human cancer. Science

]   2015; 348(6230): 62-8.[http://dx.doi.org/10.1126/science.aaa4967] [PMID: 25838374]

[164   A phase i/ii trial of t cell receptor gene therapy targeting hpv-16 e7 with or without pd- 1 blockade for hpv-
]   associated cancers Available from: https:// clinicaltrials.gov/ct2/show/

[165   Future II Study GroupN Engl J Med 2007; 356: 1915-27.[http://dx.doi.org/10.1056/NEJMoa061741] [PMID:
]   17494925]

[166   Kenter GG, Welters MJ, Valentijn AR, *et al.* Vaccination against HPV-16 oncoproteins for vulvar
]   intraepithelial neoplasia. N Engl J Med 2009; 361(19): 1838-47.[http://dx.doi.org/10.1056/NEJMoa0810097]
        [PMID: 19890126]

[167   Therapeutic HPV vaccine trial +/- anti-cd40 in hpv-driven squamous cell carcinoma (HARE-40) Available
]   from: https:// clinicaltrials.gov/ct2/show/

Behind the Screen: The Emergence of New Evidence

Belayat H. Siddiquee

, , Norhafiza Mat Lazim

1 Department of Otolaryngology-Head and Neck Surgery, Bangabandhu Sheikh Mujib Medical University (BSMMU), Dhaka-1000, Bangladesh

2 Department of Otorhinolaryngology-Head and Neck Surgery, School of Medical Sciences, Universiti Sains Malaysia, Health Campus 16150, Kubang Kerian, Kelantan, Malaysia

Abstract

Head & Neck Squamous Cell Carcinoma (HNSCC) is a heterogeneous group of malignancies that collectively constitute a significant group of cancer worldwide. It affects not only the elderly patients but more so the middle age and the pediatric patient population. Around 90% of these tumors develop from the mucosal lining of the head and neck region *i.e.* Head & Neck Squamous Cell Carcinoma (HNSCC). These mainly include oral cavity carcinoma, oropharyngeal carcinoma, hypopharyngeal carcinoma, laryngeal carcinoma, sinonasal carcinoma, nasopharyngeal carcinoma, and salivary glands carcinomas. Different types of these carcinomas are prevalent at some geographic locations due to various environmental, dietary, social, and genetic factors. Head and neck cancers are critical as these affect many vital functions of the human being, such as breathing, eating, smell, hearing, and vision. Clinical and epidemiologic studies show aetio-

28

pathological relation between chronic inflammation and cancer in several organs, including the Head and Neck region. A huge number of inflammatory mediators and markers have been identified and investigated in the current genomic era. Significant inflammatory biomarkers have a potential role not only in screening and prevention but also in treatment and assessing the prognosis of HNSCC. This chapter will highlight the recent facts, the discovery of evidence of the inflammation, and biomarkers for HNSCC.

Keywords: Alcohol and smoking, Biomarkers, Head and neck malignancy, HNSCC, Human papilloma virus, Immunoscore, Inflammation and cancer, Nasopharyngeal carcinoma, Oncogenic virus.

* **Corresponding author Belayat H. Siddiquee:** Department of Otolaryngology-Head and Neck Surgery, Bangabandhu Sheikh Mujib Medical University (BSMMU), Dhaka-1000, Bangladesh; Tel: 01917374020; E-mail: drbelayat@gmail.com

INTRODUCTION

Head and neck malignancies are increasing throughout the planet. It affects not only the elderly patients but more so the middle age and the pediatric population.

In the UK, HNSCC incidence has been rising by almost a quarter in the last decade, with an estimated annual burden of 11,400 new cases. Since the early 1990s, Oropharyngeal cancers (OPCs) have seen the biggest rise among head and neck squamous cell carcinoma (HNSCC), with incidence rates is doubling yearly. In contrast, there is a 20% decrease in the incidence of laryngeal cancer in the same period, though the rate has become steady more recently []. Lifestyle factors play an important role in the etiology of these cancers. Around 75% of HNSCC have been attributed to the individual or combined effects of tobacco and alcohol consumption. Tobacco use is an established primary risk factor for HNSCC, which causes adverse outcomes, including increased overall and cancer-specific mortality and risk for developing a second primary cancer. Continued smoking is also strongly associated with treatment toxicity []. Human papillomavirus (HPV), predominantly HPV-16 infection, is also recognized as a primary risk factor for oropharyngeal cancers (OPCs), especially in younger age groups. Despite an overall decline in mortality rates of HNSCC, survival remains poor. The overall 5- year survival rate is around 50% but ranges from 33% for hypopharyngeal cancers to 60% for laryngeal cancers. People with HPV positive oropharyngeal tumors have consistently demonstrated improved survival compared to their HPV negative counterparts, although they are frequently diagnosed at a later stage [].

There is a marked difference in HNSCC incidence by gender, race, and geographical distribution. The development of HNSCC is the result of interaction among environmental factors and genetic inheritance and is, therefore, multifactorial. HNSCCs are molecularly and genetically heterogeneous diseases, encompassing a wide array of carcinogenicity involving tissue and organs of the head and neck. Over the last few decades better understanding of the etiological factors, that cause HNSCC contributes to the management of these serious diseases dramatically. Besides smoking and alcohol, other factors like viruses, chronic inflammation in the territory, nutritional elements deficiency, chronic irritations even the genetic pre-disposition drawing the attention of the researchers. Despite this lot of things are yet to be explored. Because this is often observed that having a risk factor or even several risk factors does not mean that one will get cancer, many people having an HNSCC may not have had any known risk factor exposure.

Biomarkers are biological molecules identified in the cancer tissue or blood. Research surrounding biomarkers help in opening a new horizon in the diagnosis and treatment of HNSCC. They used to correlate with the presence or absence of a disease, are prognostically related to the disease course, and sometimes predictive of a tumor's response to a specific therapy. Biomarkers should be objective, independent, and require validation by clinical testing and patient outcome. Ideally, biomarkers should be easy to analyze, quantitative, affordable, and must be subjected to quality control and assurance [].

Risk Factor Analysis

Tobacco is associated with HNSCC []. More than 70 known carcinogens were found in cigarette smoke []. Among the toxic and carcinogenic substances absorbing in the body from tobacco, exposure are tobacco-specific nitrosamines (TSNA) and polycyclic aromatic hydrocarbons (PAH), which are mostly studied with regard to carcinogenicity. TSNA found in tobacco and tobacco smoke, essentially formed during the curing and processing of tobacco. They are found both incombustible and smokeless forms of tobacco. TSNA can be formed through various chemical reactions []. Seven TSNA have been identified in tobacco products and N'- nitrosonornicotine (NNN), 4(methylnitrosamino)-1- (3-pyridyl)-1-butanol (NNAL) are two of them []. Two prospective cohorts, the Shanghai Cohort Study and the Singapore Chinese Health Study help us to gain valuable epidemiologic data regarding the use of NNN and NNAL to give information about cancer risk []. Recently, a control study was performed to see tobacco-related carcinogens in HNSCC. Urinary levels of 1-HOP, NNN, and NNAL were measured in smokers with newly diagnosed cases of HNSCC and compared to smokers without cancer. Levels of 1-HOP and NNN were raised in the smokers with the HNSCC group compared to the control group who are matched on several other variables, including age, gender, number of cigarette sticks consumed per day [].

Alcohol plays a role as a solvent to increase mucosal exposure to carcinogens and enhance cellular uptake of these. Acetaldehyde, a metabolite of alcohol can form DNA adducts that interfere with DNA synthesis and repair []. The synergistic effect of tobacco and alcohol is supported by an analysis of combined data from 17 European and American studies. The population attributable to risk was 72%, which included 4% for alcohol alone, 33% for tobacco alone and 35% attributable to both alcohol and tobacco. This effect was more than multiplicative. Similar steep rises in the risk of HNSCC among alcohol and tobacco users, especially those using high amounts of each product, have been demonstrated by Dal Maso *et al.* []. Consumption of tobacco along with alcohol increase the HNSCC risk. All smokers and alcohol users may not develop cancer, suggesting that individual variation in genetic susceptibility plays a critical role []. In general, there is a strong association between alcohol and tobacco use and the combined use of these further increases the risk [].

Although tobacco smoking and alcohol drinking are responsible for most new HNSCC cases, the prognostic role of smoking status and alcohol intake during cancer presentation is unclear, especially in HPV associated OPCs. Smoking and alcohol use both increase the mortality risk, but the magnitude of the effect is usually inconsistent. Moreover, it is not yet established whether smoking and alcohol use furnish any additional prognostic information other than the tumor, node, metastasis (TNM) staging system, which currently forms the basis for clinical decision making in HNSCC. Although there is a slight decline in HNSCC related mortality [], the survival rate is still poor. The overall 5-year survival rate is around 50%, but ranges from 33% for hypopharyngeal cancers to 60% for laryngeal cancers []. People with HPV-positive oropharyngeal tumors have consistently demonstrated better survival compared to their HPV-negative counterparts, despite the fact that they are frequently diagnosed at an advanced stage []. This is because of improved therapeutic efficacy. People with HPV-positive oropharyngeal cancers have also distinct risk factor profiles, including higher socioeconomic status and lower comorbidity which may increase survival [].

Many cancers, including the HNSCC are caused by oncogenic strains of viruses like Human papillomavirus (HPV) and Epstein - Barr virus (EBV). The HPV has two oncogenes, E6 and E7, the expression of which inactivates p53 and retinoblastoma (RB), respectively, causing perturbation of cell cycle regulation in the infected cells and is considered to be the onset of HPV-related carcinogenesis []. The detection of viral E6 and E7 transcripts is an acceptable assay for the detection of an oncogenic HPV infection in HNSCC. EB virus is a γ (gamma)-Herpes virus and a member of the Herpesviridae family. Herpes viruses consist of large, complex DNA viruses, able to encode about 100 different proteins, and are one of the largest virus groups []. This virus affects more than 90% of the adult population worldwide in some form or other. EB virus is also associated with a variety of malignant disorders. In the head and neck region, the establishment of latent transforming EB virus infection and the potential viral genetic alteration that occurs in epithelial cells may contribute to the cancer development, its growth and invasive capabilities, especially in the subclass of nasopharyngeal carcinoma []. Plasma EBV DNA analysis has proven useful in diagnosing early nasopharyngeal carcinoma in the absence of any clinical clue [].

Chronic mechanical irritation (CMI) is an important risk factor for oral cancer and is considered a potentially malignant disorder [,]. CMI of the oral mucosa is due to repeated injury by the intraoral injuring agent. Defective teeth (sharp or rough surfaces because of decay or fractures), ill-fitting dentures (sharp or rough surfaces, overextended flanges or lack of retention) and/or habitual acts (*e.g.* oral mucosa biting or sucking, tongue interposition or thrusting), acting individually or together, may all be responsible. CMI could initiate changes in the healthy mucosa or intensify existing oral diseases and also produces several alterations related to its duration and intensity. Effects usually range from a hyperproliferative epithelial response if the stimulus is mild (frictional keratosis), to several levels of tissue injury (atrophy, erosion, ulcer) if it is intense or is of longer duration (chronic traumatic ulcer), often with fibrous connective tissue growth (reactive hyperplasia, *e.g.* Denture-induced fibrous hyperplasia). Some authors have suggested that the relationship between oral cancer and CMI could be the result of the tumor's growth; the larger the tumor, the more probability of being injured. Many cases of oral cancer have been described on the site of CMI because of a broken tooth or a defective denture. Oral cancer occurs mainly in locations that could be exposed to prosthetic or dental CMI, particularly in non-smokers without other risk factors [,].

Clinical and epidemiologic studies support an association between chronic inflammation and cancer in several organs ['']. Chronic cervicitis and cervical cancer, ulcerative colitis and colorectal cancer, reflux esophagitis and esophageal cancer, and hepatitis and liver cancer are few examples. In the oral cavity, periodontitis is a chronic inflammatory disease of the structures around teeth []. The ensuing chronic inflammation induces local pathologic and anatomic changes, namely, periodontal pocket formation, clinical attachment loss, and alveolar bone loss []. If not treated, periodontitis ultimately leads to tooth loss. The pocket epithelium is characterized by continuous proliferation, the formation of rete- ridges, and ulcerations. In the connective tissue, there is more angiogenesis, chronic inflammatory infiltrate, fibrosis, and loss of tissue. The average prevalence of periodontitis among the general population is around 30% []. Periodontitis causes the continuous release of inflammatory cytokines, enzymes, and toxins into saliva. The levels of these inflammatory markers in the saliva are directly related to the extent and severity of periodontitis [,]. Periodontal pathogens and inflammatory cytokines can travel with saliva and the blood, causing inflammation and tissue injury at distant sites also [`].

Evidence strongly suggests that diet can influence the risk for HNSCC, and data shows a probable causal relationship for decreased HNSCC risk with non-starchy vegetables, fruits, and food containing carotenoids. A relation between poor oral hygiene and HNSCC has been suggested [`], but the underlying mechanism was not clear. Chronic periodontitis, an outcome of poor oral hygiene, is associated with oral premalignant lesions [] and HNSCC [,]. The potential association between chronic inflammation and HNSCC is further supported by two case-control studies suggesting a beneficial effect of nonsteroidal anti inflammatory drugs (NSAID) against HNSCC [,]. Aspirin administration in a hospital-based case-control study between patients with HNSCC and control subjects similar by age, sex, and smoking status, revealed a 25% decrease in the risk of HNSCC. Risk reduction was observed in all primary subsites, with cancers of the oral cavity and oropharynx []. The mechanism of the biological relation between chronic inflammation and cancer, although described extensively but it is evolving continuously since both are complex processes under the control of several driving factors. Bacteria and their products, including endotoxins, enzymes, and metabolic by-products, may directly induce genetic and epigenetic changes in surrounding epithelial cells [`]. They also increase the production of carcinogenic acetaldehydes [`] and nitrosamines [,]. However, the available evidence supports an indirect association through stimulation of inflammation. Host cells, including neutrophils, macrophages, lymphocytes, monocytes, fibroblasts, and epithelial cells, respond to bacteria by generating cytokines, chemokines, prostaglandins, growth factors, and other signals that provide an environment for cell survival, proliferation, migration, angiogenesis, and inhibition of apoptosis []. This environment facilitates epithelial cells for mutations and drives these mutant epithelial cells to proliferate and migrate and gives them a growth advantage. Numerous studies have confirmed the associations of several genes and proteins involved in different stages of inflammation with carcinogenesis [`]. Chronic inflammation may also act synergistically with other carcinogens to increase the risk of HNSCC. For example, breaks in the mucosal barrier due to chronic inflammation may favor enhanced penetration of other carcinogens *e.g.* tobacco, alcohol, and dietary metabolites []. High consumption of fruit and vegetable and low intake of red meat was associated with reduced risk for HNSCC [].

Exposure to the carcinogen, oral hygiene, chronic irritation to the oral mucosa, dental plaque formation, positive family history, and exposure to ultraviolet rays all play a role individually or in combination in the HNSCC development because they can modulate toxin and carcinogenic metabolism [˙]. The contribution of family factors in HNSCC development maybe because of familial aggregations of inheritable genetic factors. Several genetic polymorphisms in genes involved in the carcinogen metabolism, DNA repair, and several other processes may also have contributed to this.

Inflammation, A Hallmark of HNSCC

Inflammation in and around cancer is considered as a "hallmark of cancer". Many studies demonstrate that tumors may develop and progress within inflammatory diseases. The main steps in the development of cancer are genetic changes that make these cancer cells potential with many of the hallmarks of cancer, such as self-sufficient growth and resistance to anti-growth and pro-death signals. While the genetic changes that occur within cancer cells themselves, such as activated oncogenes or dysfunctional tumor suppressors, are responsible for many aspects of cancer development. Tumor promotion and progression are dependent on ancillary processes involving cells of the tumor environment that are not necessarily cancerous themselves. Infiltration of immune cells helps tumor development by the production of factors that facilitate carcinogenesis by enabling tumors to evade the host immune response. Small molecules including cytokines, chemokines, and growth factors play main roles in both inflammation and cancer by promoting proliferation, angiogenesis, and carcinogenesis and by recruiting immune cells. The extracellular matrix is changed in inflammation and provides structural support to developing tumors. Hypoxia is a common condition in cancers and inflamed tissues that causes DNA damage and induces tumorigenic factors. Finally, tissue vasculature is a vital part of its microenvironment, supplying oxygen, nutrients, and growth factors to rapidly dividing cells and providing a mechanism for metastatic spread [,]. Inflammation often exists in the tumor microenvironment and is induced by inflammatory mediators (cytokines, chemokines, and growth factors) produced by the tumor, stroma, and infiltrating cells. These factors modulate tissue remodeling and angiogenesis and actively help tumor cell survival and chemoresistance through autocrine and paracrine mechanisms. HNSCC has got high inflammatory and aggressive character, and they express a number of cytokines and growth factors involved in inflammation. These cytokines and growth factors activate signal transduction pathways, which regulate the expression of genes controlling growth, survival, and chemosensitivity. This is an important update on recent advances in the understanding of the mechanisms driving cancer-related inflammation in HNSCC and on targeted molecular therapies under preclinical and clinical investigations [].

There are many different pathways through which a proinflammatory diet can influence the risk of HNSCC. Diet directly contributes to the excessive production of proinflammatory biomarkers such as CRP, IL-6, white blood cell count, and homocysteine [ˉ]. The inflammation contributes to the "hallmarks of cancer" by supplying bioactive molecules to the tumor microenvironment []. Additionally, inflammatory transcription factors can be activated by inflammatory cytokines and other inflammatory biomarkers, which play a key role in both cancer initiation and promotion. Inflammatory cytokines can change the oral microbiota, which in turn can cause an increased risk of periodontitis and cancer [,].

Bacteria and their products, including endotoxins, enzymes, and metabolic by-products, may directly induce genetic and epigenetic changes in surrounding epithelial cells [ˉ]. They also intensify the production of carcinogenic acetaldehydes [ˉ] and nitrosamines [,]. However, the available evidence supports an indirect association through stimulation of inflammation. Host cells, including neutrophils, macrophages, monocytes, lymphocytes, fibroblasts, and epithelial cells, respond to bacteria by producing cytokines, chemokines, prostaglandins, growth factors, and other signals that provide an environment for cell survival, proliferation, migration, angiogenesis, and inhibition of apoptosis []. This environment favors epithelial cells to accumulate mutations and drives these mutant epithelial cells to proliferate and migrate and gives them a growth advantage. Numerous *in vivo* and *in vitro* studies have confirmed the associations of several genes and proteins responsible for different stages of inflammation with carcinogenesis [ˉ]. In addition to its independent association with HNSCC, chronic inflammation may also act synergistically with other carcinogens to increase the risk of HNSCC. For example, breaks in the mucosal barrier due to chronic inflammation may enhance the penetration of other carcinogens such as tobacco, alcohol, and dietary metabolites [,].

Pathogenesis of HNSCC Development

HNSCC represents around 90% of all head and neck cancers and arises from the mucosa of the upper aerodigestive tract, including the nose, nasopharyngeal, paranasal sinuses, oral cavity, oropharynx, hypopharynx, larynx, and also the cervical esophagus. Proper understanding of the evolving molecular pathophysiology of head & neck tumorigenesis is essential for the development of feasible as well as effective diagnostic, therapeutic, and preventative strategies. It is established that HNSCC develops by a multistage pathogenesis process as reported in the genetic progression model for colon cancer []. Molecular alterations in epithelial cells generally precede phenotypic histologic changes and accumulate along the malignant transformation process from the benign to premalignant and also invasive states. Increased understanding of the cellular and molecular features of solid tumors has further improved the pathologist's capability for diagnosis and prognosis assessment of HNSCC. Identification of known and potential tumor markers including chromosomal changes, oncogenes, and tumor suppressor genes has far-reaching implications for predicting the biological behavior of a tumor and its response to a particular therapy.

Features in Premalignant Oral Lesions

Multistage pathogenesis of cancer formation was first suggested by Vogelstein *et al.* specifically for the colon. This genetic model for tumor formation included the activation of oncogenes and inactivation of tumor suppressor genes. He coined that a minimum of four mutations was necessary for malignant transformation. Steps have been described during advancement including initiation, promotion, and progression. This pattern has been observed in many cancers including those of the brain, bladder, and also in the head and neck. Califano *et al.* reported a "Vogelgram" for HNSCC, which linked histologic features in the progression of HNSCC to specific molecular changes []. Further investigation concentrating on the transcriptional changes that occur during the progression from normal-appearing mucosa to dysplastic tissue and then invasive HNSCC [].

Cytogenic Features

Genomic alterations happening in precancerous and cancerous lesions can express themselves on different levels (chromosomal, DNA, RNA, and protein), in many ways such as point mutations, amplifications, deletions, and chromosomal alterations. Common methods to detect the presence of these changes include conventional cytogenetics, comparative genomic hybridization (CGH), spectral karyotyping, and cDNA microarrays. CGH is a technical cytogenetic process for assessing the gains or losses in DNA content (*e.g.*, chromosomal imbalances) within a tumor's entire genome. CGH does not show morphological changes between chromosomes [].

Weber *et al.* used this technique to see the average number of chromosomal imbalances in 12 oral premalignant lesions (including dysplasia and carcinomas-*in situ*) and invasive oral HNSCCs []. An average of 3.2 ± 1.2 imbalances was seen in premalignant lesions while invasive HNSCCs had a significantly higher average of 11.9 ± 1.9 (p = 0.003) imbalances. In the premalignant lesions, gains were identified on 8q and 16p, while losses were found on 3p, 5q, 13q, and 4q, 8p, and 9p. In individual biopsies from the same subject that contained both premalignancy and invasive carcinoma, most of the genomic alterations discovered in premalignancy were also found in HNSCC. Brieger *et al.* used CGH to analyze chromosomal alterations in OPCs and their surrounding benign mucosa. In the morphologically healthy mucosa collected 2 cm from the primary tumor margin, no chromosomal changes could be identified. In normal-looking mucosa located 1 cm from the tumor, the most common amplifications were in 15q and 21q. Almost all of these alterations were found in the primary tumor also [].

These cytogenetic changes are consistent with previous reports implicating molecular features appear early in head and neck tumorigenesis before histologic and phenotypic changes and also accumulate through successive stages. CGH is a very important tool, but the other aforesaid techniques are also frequently used.

Molecular Features

Microsatellite Instability

Microsatellites are repeats of non-coding DNA sequences that normally occur within the human genome. Defects in the DNA healing process may lead to microsatellites that are abnormally short or long; this process has been termed microsatellite instability (MI). MI is indirect evidence of a mismatch repaired (MMR) protein's function. A suggested mechanism relevant in HNSCC tumorigenesis is through promoter hypermethylation. When MMR promoters are hypermethylated, it provides indirect evidence of the increased possibility that promoters of tumor suppressor genes are also hypermethylated, and therefore not functional []. But when a microsatellite repeats replication error, if it goes uncorrected, a germline hereditary mutation could result in inactivation of tumor suppressor genes and uncontrolled cell and tumor growth. This idea of a mutator phenotype provides an alternate option to a multistage accumulation of genetic alterations to explain head & neck tumorigenesis.

Loss of Heterozygosity (LOH)

Mutation can inactivate an allele of a gene, *e.g.* tumor suppressor gene. When this occurs in a parent's germline cell, the inactivated allele is passed onto the offspring resulting in heterozygosity. If genomic loss takes place in the somatic cell of the offspring affecting the remaining allele, LOH occurs and tumor-suppressive function in that cell is lost. LOH assays commonly employ microsatellite analysis to assess polymorphic chromosomal regions that map in or around tumor suppressor genes.

In premalignant oral lesions, LOH at 9p21 and/or 3p14 increases the probability of malignant transformation []. Other chromosomal losses have been associated with increased risk: 4q, 8p, 11q, 13q, and 17p. Hyperplastic or dysplastic lesions with LOH at 3p and/or 9p plus one of the other above losses were found to have a 33-fold increase in cancer risk []. Lesions that are lack significant dysplasia to necessitate estimation of cancer risks, molecular markers may yet to be proved useful. Zhang *et al.* proposed a staging system incorporating assessments from both histology and LOH criteria [].

p53

A well-characterized tumor suppressor gene p53 is located on chromosome 17p. Its role is to control cell growth arrest and apoptosis. The p53 protein has a too short half-life, and thus, is difficult to detect in benign tissues. Overexpression of p53 can happen from mutation, a defect in its degradation, or from binding to other proteins. On the whole, mutations of the p53 tumor suppressor gene have been found in half of HNSCC tumors and are the most common genetic alterations found in the malignancy of human beings. The types of mutations vary from mutations, transversions, transitions, and deletions. Various proteins usually bind with p53, such as SV40 large T, which blocks its DNA binding capability. Binding with adenovirus E1B blocks p53's transcriptional activity. Finally, binding with HPV E6 targets p53 for accelerated degradation [].

Increasing frequencies of p53 alterations and genomic instability have been identified during progressive steps in HNSCC carcinogenesis. Shin *et al.* analyzed p53 expression and chromosomal polysomy *via* immunohistochemistry and chromosome *in situ* hybridization, in epithelial specimens. 19% of adjacent normal-appearing mucosa, 29% of hyper-plastic lesions, 46% of dysplastic lesions, and 58% of HNSCC tumors expressed p53. Normal-appearing mucosa lacked detectable p53 levels as expected []. These findings suggest that premalignancy is usually associated with altered p53 expression and increased genomic instability, which are possibly early markers of carcinogenesis.

Retinoic Acid Receptor-β

Retinoids (natural and synthetic derivatives of vitamin A) regulate cell growth and differentiation and have growth-suppressive effects in epithelial cells.

Retinoic acid receptorβ (RARβ), a steroid hormone receptor whose expression is suppressed in premalignant tissues and established HNSCC through an unknown mechanism.

p16/ Rb

In addition to p53, Rb is the other major tumor suppression pathway in human carcinogenesis. Rb normally suppresses cell growth by binding to E2F1 transcription factors and preventing cells from advancing from G1 into the S phase of the cell cycle (G1 arrest). Altered expression of Rb and p16 has been reported in oral carcinomas []. In fact, alterations in p16 are considered the most common genetic alteration in HNSCC []. The HPV oncoprotein E7 is known to cause inactivation of Rb.

Mitochondrial DNA

Opposing to changes in human genomic DNA, the alteration can occur in mitochondrial DNA instead. The usual site for polymorphisms and mutations is the poly-cytosine tract (C-tract) of the displacement loop of the mitochondrial genome. Ha *et al.*, tested 137 premalignant lesions for C-tract DNA changes using PCR and polyacrylamide gel electrophoresis [].

EGFR/STAT3

Overexpression of epidermal growth factor receptor (EGFR) is present in malignant, premalignant, and normal-appearing tissues from HNSCC patients, which is correlated with poor prognosis [,]. EGFR staining increased linearly in the stratum spinosum in oral leukoplakia with increasing degrees of dysplasia [].

Features in Squamous Cell Carcinoma (HNSCC)

Cytogenetic Features

A good number of molecular features found in HNSCC are due to cytogenetic changes. The conventional cytogenic study includes the preparation of metaphase spreads of cultured tumor biopsies. The frequent cytogenetic alterations in HNSCC include chromosomal gains on 3q, 8q, 9q, 20q, 7p, 11q13, and 5p. Genomic losses are more frequent than gains and being identified on 3p, 9p, 21q, 5q, 13q, 18q, and 8p []. Investigation of these alterations in untreated HNSCC specimens enables the identification of genes responsible for disease phenotypes and also improves the idea about the pathophysiology behind the disease. Both classical and molecular cytogenetic

39

mechanisms are shown in HNSCC to have a complex karyotype, with the most common change being tetraploidization. Moreover, an average number of 15 aberrations are found across the genome []. These changes usually include deletions, translocations, and isochromo-somes.

Molecular alterations are also seen in non-squamous cancers of the head and neck region. The most specific mucoepidermoid carcinoma-associated genetic alteration is the t (11;19) (q21; p13) translocation initially detected by traditional karyotyping []. This translocation generates a mucoepidermoid carcinoma translocated 1 (MECT1)–mastermind-like 2 (MAML2) gene fusion product consisting of exon 1 of MECT1 fused to exons 2–5 of MAML2 []. Patients with fusion-positive tumors are generally younger, have a lower grade tumor, with a significantly lower risk of local recurrence, metastasis, or tumor-related death. Only a few translocation-positive aggressive high-grade mucoepidermoid carcinomas have been described [].

Molecular Features

p53

Early studies have failed to identify a correlation between p53 expression and survival of HNSCC patients. When patients with laryngeal primaries were studied, positive p53 expression was significantly associated with the patient's poor outcome [,]. In studies focusing on certain types of mutations (*e.g.*, missense, nonsense), correlations were observed with prognosis [,]. Other studies to see the relation between p53 mutations and prognosis have yielded conflicting data [,]. The prevalence of p53 changes in HNSCC underscores its importance in tumorigenesis. Inactivation of this tumor suppressor gene is found to be correlated with resistance to chemotherapy []. Restoration of function *via* intratumoral injection of adenoviral p53 gene therapy (Ad-p53 or INGN-201) has demonstrated favorable results in phase I and phase II trials in patients with advanced and recurrent HNSCC [].

Telomerase Activation

Lee *et al.* measured telomerase activity *via* TRAP in the peripheral blood mononuclear cells of 120 patients (100 with HNSCC and 20 controls) []. Telomerase positivity is highly significant and correlate with higher T stage (p = 0.005); higher N stage (p = 0.002); and higher AJCC stage (p < 0.001). Multivariate analysis reveals telomerase expression is an independent predictor of survival. (p = 0.017) This is very important that the expression of a protein in the peripheral blood cells from HNSCC patients demonstrated prognostic potential. Thurnher *et al.* used a modified semiquantitative TRAP assay to assess HNSCC tumors. When stratified by the presence or absence of cervical metastases, a statistically significant difference in telomerase activity was found between the two groups []. This study shows primary feasibility in using biomarkers, such as telomerase to identify patients at high risk of cervical metastasis.

HPV

There is increasing evidence that suggests the association of high-risk HPV strains with a subset of HNSCC as an aetiological factor. Viral DNA is found in Carcinoma *in situ* (CIS), primary HNSCC, and metastatic lesions by a number of molecular techniques. DNA has been found in around 50% of oropharyngeal cancers, particularly in nonsmokers. Viral oncoproteins E6 and E7 of high-risk HPV strains 16 and 18 disrupt the p53 and Rb tumor suppressor pathways, respectively, thereby providing potential mechanisms for transformation. HPV-positive tumors usually show the following features: usually originate in the oropharynx (tonsil or tongue base), basaloid histology, positive history of tobacco and/or alcohol may or may not be present, and improved survival compared to HPV-negative counterpart []. Additionally, there is a rise in Oropharyngeal cancer incidence over the last three decades, detected in younger adults. HPV involvement has implications for the potential transmission of some HNSCC malignancies *via* Oro-genital contact and the potential application of HPV vaccines targeted at people at risk.

EGFR/STAT3

Epidermal growth factor receptor (EGFR) represents an important therapeutic target in HNSCC. Cetuximab is a chimeric monoclonal antibody that binds to the extracellular domain of EGFR. Several trials reported on the efficacy of cetuximab and platinum-based chemotherapy in recurrent and refractory HNSCC cases [,]. Response rates are approximately 10% in patients with progressive disease with combination therapy. The severity of one of the side effects, acneiform rash, is directly related to outcome and survival. The phase III trial conducted by Burtness *et al.* found increased response rates for recurrent and/or metastatic HNSCC patients treated with cisplatin and cetuximab (26%) *vs.* cisplatin and placebo (10%) (p = 0.03) []. Another class of EGFR-targeted therapy includes the tyrosine kinase inhibitors (TKIs). Gefitinib and erlotonib oral preparations TKIs, have shown clinical activity in a variety of HNSCC treatment settings [,]. Caponigro *et al.* summarize recent clinical trials for this group of targeted therapies [].

COX-2

Keratinocyte inflammation has been identified as crucial for chemical carcinogenesis in oral HNSCC. Inflammatory mediators such as prostaglandins, interleukin-1, interleukin-6, and tumor necrosis factor α are central to this process. The release of prostaglandins can cause vasodilation, alters vascular permeability, and inflammatory cell infiltration –all potential tumor-promoting effects. COX-2 is overexpressed in much oral dysplasia and HNSCC. Prostaglandin E2 (PGE2) is related to malignant transformation in HNSCC []. COX-2 inhibitors exert an anti-proliferative effect and induce apoptosis in oral cancer cell lines. Studies have revealed a decrease in PGE2 levels and dose-dependent reduction of tumor growth [].

NF-Kb

NF-kB (nuclear factor of kappa light polypeptide in B-cells), upon activation, translocate from the cytosol to the nucleus to induce transcription, leading to cell proliferation and reduced apoptosis. A clinical trial evaluating the proteasome inhibitor bortezomib in combination with cisplatin and radiotherapy for locoregionally advanced HNSCC is ongoing for which standard chemo-radiation regimens are yet to be established [].

VEGF

The contribution of angiogenesis in the progression of solid tumors is crucial. Without adequate blood supply for a relentlessly growing cancer, newly dividing tumor cells are unlikely to survive due to lacking necessary nutrients and oxygen. Vascular endothelial growth factor (VEGF) is a proangiogenic mediator, binds to corresponding receptors on endothelial cells. This results in endothelial migration, proliferation, and increased vascular permeability. High VEGF and VEGF receptor expression in HNSCC patients are associated with increased tumor proliferation rates and worse survival []. In HNSCC, angiogenesis represents a potential technique of resistance against anti-EGFR agents. Vokes *et al*. conducted a phase I-II trial of erlotinib with bevacizumab in patients with metastatic and/or recurrent incurable HNSCC [,]. Favorable results were watched with no dose-limiting toxicities.

TGF-β/Ras

Transforming growth factorβ (TGFβ) has played a crucial role in cell differentiation, tissue regeneration, and regulation of the immune system. Ras activation has been associated with malignant transformation. Ras mutations are rare in HNSCC in the western part of the world (< 5%), while Ras overexpression is much more common [].

Molecular Features in Metastatic Lesions of HNSCC

Lymph node metastasis in the neck is the single most significant prognostic predictor of HNSCC. This reduces survival by 50% on average. Immunohistochemical profiling of primary and metastatic lesions has revealed various genes implicated in metastasis. Similar gene expression profiles are found in primary tumors and their metastases, which indicates that molecular alterations occur early in the metastatic lesion. E-cadherin is a cell adhesion molecule that regulates adhesion between adjacent epithelial cells. Down-regulation of E-cadherin has been found in HNSCC patients with metastatic tumors []. Dissociation of tumor cells is suggested as a probable mechanism. Integrins are transmembrane proteins that take part in cell adhesion in addition to signal transduction. Increased cell motility and growth have been reported in HNSCC *via* upregulation of integrin α v β 6 []. Overexpression of matrix metalloproteinase-2 (MMP2) and MMP9 are associated with invasion, metastasis, and poor prognosis []. Likewise, upregulation of EGFR, proangiogenic genes such as VEGF and IL-8, and chemokine receptor-7 (CCR7) have all been implicated in HNSCC metastasis []. Detection of tumors, which are at high risk for locoregional and distal metastasis by molecular testing would have a profound impact on patients' prognosis.

Alcohol-Induced Molecular Changes

A molecular understanding of the pathogenesis of an alcohol-related HNSCC remains elusive and poorly understood. Since ethanol alone is not considered a carcinogen, most studies involving alcohol and cancer focus on its ability to increase penetration of carcinogens, interfere with DNA repair mechanisms, or cause DNA damage through acetaldehyde, the first metabolite of ethanol, which is a known carcinogen. Evidence of an association between pre-treatment alcohol use and HNSCC mortality risk is conflicting. Some studies report an inverse association between alcohol intake and survival whilst others have found little or no evidence of an effect. Consequently, it is unclear whether any association of alcohol consumption with HNSCC cancer mortality is genuine or the result of residual confounding by smoking (or other factors). Recently, it was suggested that the effects of alcohol intake on HNSCC survival may differ by treatment method and primary site but this study only included 427 individuals from a single cancer center in Japan, emphasizing the need for further research in this area [].

Applications of Altered Molecular Features Of HNSCC

Early Detection of HNSCC

Diagnosing HNSCC at an early stage is a very critical clinical step to improve outcomes. A recently developed oral rinse utilizes ELISA to detect soluble CD44 (an overexpressed protein marker) in HNSCC []. This biochemical test revealed elevated CD44 levels in 62% of the 102 HNSCC patients in the study group. This assay also picked up a few false-positives cases. Sensitivity ranged from 62% to 70% while the specificity spectrum is from 75% to 88%.

Biomarkers in Risk Assessment and Molecular Staging

Surgical Margin Assessment for Risk of Local Recurrence

Adequacy of surgical resection of HNSCC is evaluated by frozen sections from margins around the lesion. Local recurrence may occur in up to 50% of cases with histologically negative margins []. Detection of pre-malignant molecular changes in histologically cancer-free tissue will further ensure margin safety and also can guide which patient will require postoperative adjuvant therapy. Gene promoter hypermethylation is one of the common mechanisms for loss of tumor suppressor gene function. Rosas *et al*. showed that at least 56% of HNSCC are characterized by abnormal methylation of p16, MGMT, or death-associated protein kinase []. The feasibility of per-operative rapid DNA tissue extraction, rapid bisulfite treatment, and quantitative methylation-specific PCR (QMSP) for p 16 and MGMT was studied by Goldenberg *et al* []. While conventional QMSP requires about 24 hours, the rapid QMSP assay takes 5 hours and requires the simultaneous work of two persons. This approach is useful for cases requiring extensive resection and reconstruction.

Molecular Predictors of Survival

cDNA microarray technology is being utilized for outcome prediction in HNSCC patients. Belbin analyzed gene expression from 17 patients using gene chips containing 9,216 clones []. 375 differentially expressed genes, so far identified by this method enabling the investigators to classify patients into two groups. The better prognosis group had a 2-year disease-specific survival of 100%, while the inferior group had a 56% survival. This molecular assay was found to be more efficient in anticipating outcomes than standard clinical and pathological criteria. Genes identified in the unfavorable prognostic group included catalase, cytokine family members, xanthine oxidase, and phosphodiesterase genes.

MicroRNA

These are endogenous 21–22 nucleotide long non-protein-coding RNA sequences regulating target mRNA expression by complementary interaction with the 3′ untranslated region of mRNA. The extent of complementarity between microRNA and its target determines the mechanism of translational inhibition: partial complementarity will induce mRNA repression, and perfect complement-arity will cause translational inhibition. MicroRNA biogenesis and its role in carcinogenesis are studied by Gomes *et al.* [].

Histopathological Changes and their Clinical Implications

Premalignant Lesions of the Head and Neck

A precancerous epithelial lesion shows histological changes and also has an increased potential of progressing to an invasive squamous cell carcinoma. These altered situations include hyperplasia, and more ominously, mild to severe dysplasia. Clinically signs of premalignancy include leukoplakia and erythroplakia, which are not the synonyms of histologic diagnoses.

Leukoplakia

Leukoplakia is a clinical condition where a white patch or plaque cannot be rubbed off and cannot be labeled with a more specific diagnosis. The prevalence of oral leukoplakia in the US is around 2.9%, usually affecting in their fifth to seventh decades irrespective of sexes []. Seventy to ninety percent of cases are tobacco consumers, the most consistent causal factor []. The majority of white patches are due to chronic irritation (*i.e.*, tobacco or dental trauma) and, histologically, represent an irregularly thickened keratin layer ranging from simple hyper parakeratosis to an early invasive carcinoma. Therefore, leukoplakia does not correlate with the histologic diagnosis of dysplasia.

The malignant transformation potential in oral leukoplakia is well known. Studies performed in the US show an average transformation rate of 15.6% (range 13.6– 17.5%) with varying periods of follow up [,]. Malignancy is considered irreversible, but premalignancy is reversible after withdrawal or removal of the offending agent. A prospective cohort of Indian smokers, who quit smoking showed a marked decrease in the incidence of oral leukoplakia during follow-up). But no decrease could be seen among patients of oral lichen planus []. DNA content in the leukoplakia lesions has been found to be a significant predictor of local failure following surgical resection. Lesions harboring aneuploid or tetraploid DNA reflect a higher chance of recurrence compared to their normal diploid counterparts [].

Erythroplakia

Erythroplakia is characterized by a velvety appearance with distinct borders and known as the red analog of Leukoplakia. The incidence of erythroplakia is much lower than leukoplakia but is associated more frequently with malignancy. Often this is a clinical presentation of an early HNSCC. Broadly 50% of erythroplakia lesions may harbor invasive HNSCC. Leukoplakia usually shows a significant rate of spontaneous regression, erythroplakia lesions generally never.

Squamous Dysplasia

Squamous dysplasia implies to morphologic changes have taken place in the epithelial cells. Dysplasia requires a combination of architectural change with cytologic atypia. The microscopic evidence of dysplasia includes keratin pearls, "drop-shaped" rete ridges, irregular epithelial stratification, abnormally superficial mitoses, and loss of cell polarity []. The cytologic criteria used for the diagnosis and grading of dysplasia are hyperchromasia, a variation of nuclear size, shape, atypical mitotic figures, increased nuclear-cytoplasmic ratio, location of mitotic figures, and dyskeratosis.

Biologically, squamous dysplasia represents a wide spectrum and there are no specified criteria to precisely divide this range of changes into mild, moderate, or severe categories. Usually, pathologists recognize the variations in degrees of dysplasia. Nonetheless, a high degree of inter-and intra-observer variations in determining the presence and grading of squamous dysplasia existing ["]. Clinical information about the lesion does not increase agreement rates [] and associated inflammation further increases the disagreement rates. Ulceration, irradiation, and a few nutritional deficiencies (iron, folate, B12) can simulate dysplastic changes.

A classification of squamous dysplasia has been described. "Questionable or mild" dysplasia into a low-risk group and "moderate to severe" dysplasia into a high-risk group []. In mild and moderate dysplasia, the epithelial changes are limited to the lower and middle third of the surface epithelium, respectively. In severe dysplasia and Carcinoma *In- Situ* (CIS), the altered feature involves the full thickness. Severe dysplasia and CIS occasionally may not be distinguishable and should be treated in the same way.

Lichen Planus

The premalignant potential of lichen planus (LP) of the Oral cavity is uncertain because of the available conflicting data. One prospective study of Lichen Planus with a mean follow-up of 5.6 years found malignant transformation in 1.2% []. Another prospective study including patients with oral lichenoid lesions (125 subjects) and LP (67 subjects) after a mean follow-up of 4.5 years, reveals four patients with oral lichenoid lesions developed HNSCC while none with LP did. After comparing the expected against actual figures for a number of patients developing cancer, no change in LP patients was observed, while a 142-fold increase was seen in patients with oral lichenoid lesions (p = 0.04) [].

Carcinoma *In-situ* (CIS) and Early Invasive Squamous Cell Carcinoma

The concept of CIS is that malignant transformation has already taken place, but an invasion is absent. The lesion is not merely a dysplasia. The histologic hallmark of malignancy is an invasion. Invasion is easily detected when cytologically abnormal squamous epithelial cells extend into subepithelial tissues or show perineural or vascular invasion. Detection of the early invasion into the lamina propria is a common diagnostic dilemma. The loss of basement membrane material is not a very reliable feature, because an overtly invasive carcinoma can synthesize basement membrane-like material at its leading invasive edge. The histologic features of invasive HNSCC include: varying degrees of keratinization, atypical squamous cells showing nuclear atypia, increased nuclear-to-cytoplasmic ratio, increased atypical mitotic figures; hyperchromasia, basement membrane invasion, and associated inflammatory response. In the future, the molecular features will assist in the evaluation of squamous dysplasia.

Others

Submucous fibrosis is considered as an idiopathic, precancerous condition. The oral cavity is most commonly affected. Histologic picture includes epithelial atrophy, juxtaepithelial inflammation, and fibroelastic changes in the lamina propria. Malignant transformation may occur in 8%–33%. Steroid and hyaluronidase injections, or iron supplementation derive no benefit in this condition.

Sideropenic dysphagia occurs in patients with Plummer-Vinson syndrome (a triad of iron deficiency anemia, post cricoid dysphagia and upper esophageal webs,) and is characterized by significant epithelial atrophy with increased turnover rates. The clinical condition is strongly related to esophageal cancer [].

Biomarkers and Future Screening for HNSCC

Biomarkers represent important tools that contribute to the diagnosis, assess the likely course of the lesion, and predict response to treatment. They are categorized as diagnostic prognostic or predictive, respectively. Regarding HNSCC, although many biomarkers have been suggested to significantly impact diagnosis and prognosis, few of them are validated for use in clinical practice. A significant proportion of biomarkers are not introduced into clinical practice because they lack important features, such as high specificity and sensitivity, high positive predictive value, clinical relevance, and short turnaround time [].

TNM is a good prognostic system for predicting patient prognosis, but actual outcomes of patients might be frequently different than expected as per TNM stages. Some patients with small tumors may recur quickly, whereas others with metastatic disease show an unexpectedly favorable prognosis. Recently it is well-established that the immune system plays a pivotal role in the control of tumor growth [] and it has been suggested that potentially invading cancer cells are held in an equilibrium state by the mechanism of the immune system []. Subsequently, certain tumors escape and become clinically apparent. Research evidence has emphasized the need for the development of immunological biomarkers that can offer prognostic information and facilitate clinical decision-making. Lesions infiltrating immune cells, including T and B lymphocytes, macrophages, or neutrophils may exert both ways effect on tumor expansion either negatively or positively.

Knowledge about the dynamics and functional roles of different subsets of tumor infiltrating cells in the tumor-suppressive microenvironment could improve our idea of immunology and define subgroups of patients, likely to respond to immunotherapy. Cytotoxic CD8+ tumor infiltrating lymphocytes (TILs) are thought to be the major effector immune cells directed against tumor cells and have been shown to possess prognostic significance in many solid tumors [,]. On the contrary, regulatory T cells (Tregs) inhibit immune response and counteract cytotoxic T cells. Inconsistent results have been reported regarding prognostic significance of Tregs. Some studies have reported an association with poor prognosis in a variety of malignancies including breast, lung, and cervical cancers, while others are demonstrating favorable prognostic significance, *e.g.*, in colorectal cancer []. HNSCC is a disease characterized by profound immunosuppression. Several studies have reported a significantly increased density of TILS in HPV-positive as compared to in HPV-negative oropharyngeal cancers (OPCs), which implies a more potent anti-tumoral immune response in HPV- OPCs [⁻]. This is the suggested mechanism for improved outcomes in HPV- OPCs across studies.

High levels of TILs have been associated with improved survival in HPV-OPCs [,].

Patients with HPV-positive disease with low TIL levels do not show any survival advantage over the HPV-negative subjects []. On the contrary, HPV-positive patients with high TILs have superior survival [], suggesting the use of TILs as a future biomarker for HPV- positive patients. High TILs are also associated with a better prognosis in tobacco related HNSCC [,]. Moreover, levels of both CD8+ and CD3+ T cells are associated with increased overall survival after definitive chemoradiation, both in HPV-positive and HPV-negative HNSCC [,]. In another study, only stroma TILs infiltration has been associated with increased survival [].

HPV-OPCs have been shown in several studies to possess a high degree of Treg infiltration [,]. Tregs have been shown to correlate with locoregional control and favorable survival [], possibly reflecting the downregulation of inflammation which triggers carcinogenesis.

Potential Treatment Approach and Biomarkers

Despite modernized treatment strategies involving surgery, radiotherapy (RT), and/or chemotherapy (CT), the overall prognosis in advanced stages (III/IV) HNSCC patients remains unsatisfactory owing to loco-regional recurrence. Randomized trials using CT (cisplatin/carboplatin alone, or in combination with 5-Fluorouracil, methotrexate, or paclitaxel) and/or RT show increased locoregional control or survival and prevented subsequent distant metastasis by eradicating occult metastasis. Even then, increased risk of cardiac failure or the dose-limiting toxicities in cancer patients limits their clinical utilization. So major interest is being placed on the development of molecular targeted therapies for HNSCCs []. The search for new biological agents should focus on inhibitors that are likely to act on multiple targets. Otherwise, combination of different agents that target distinct specific pathways to hinder the escape of tumor cells by alternate mechanisms, resulting in more effective disease control [].

There are many markers (*e.g.* HPV16 DNA detection in tumors, serologic response to the L1, E6, and E7 proteins, and p16 immunohistochemical staining) used to detect HPV infection, but there is lackings of data comparing them in any given population. There is also no data available for disease outcome. So which marker or combination of HPV markers is preferred for predicting overall survival among HNSCC patients remains a clinical problem. Liang C, *et al.* (2012) have assessed different measurements of HPV exposure and infection, evaluating different markers (serologic response (L1, E6, E7), presence of HPV DNA in tumor detected using PCR, and p16 immunostaining [].

A higher prevalence of HPV DNA positivity has been recorded in patients with advanced-stage disease or poorly differentiated tumors compared with those who have an early stage or well/moderately differentiated HNSCC at diagnosis. Despite the higher percentage of HPV-infected HNSCC cases with advanced stage characteristics, studies have revealed that patients with HPV DNA-detected tumors have a more favorable prognosis and less disease recurrence compared to HPV-negative HNSCC, even after adjusting all other prognostic factors [].

Serological test for HPV detection has many advantages over a test that requires DNA isolation from a biopsy: It can be performed before treatment, is less invasive, faster, less expensive, and may serve as a method to monitor treatment response over the disease course. In addition, as has been recommended for ideal prognostic markers, all tumor tissue will remain available for these patients with adequate quantity for HPV testing using well-established, reliable methods [].

Immunostaining for p16 protein has recently been regarded as a practical alternative for HPV testing based on a high correlation between HPV detection and p16 overexpression. For non-oropharyngeal cancers, and even for a subset of OPCs, the possibility of encountering elevated p16 expression by non-viral related mechanisms must be considered. A false-positive rate for HPV detection based solely on p16 overexpression may be acceptable when it comes to prognostication. p16 overexpression has been associated with improved outcomes for patients with OPCs is quite independent of HPV status [].

HNSCC patients subjected to chemoradiation therapy (CT/RT) seem to cause a significant growth of Interleukin 1β and 6 (IL-1β, IL-6) and tumor necrosis factor-α (TNF-α), all positively associated with the severity of mucosal toxicity []. A surprising observation is the post-treatment increase in cytokines. This

may be related to response to treatment. Other factors to consider are post-radiation mucositis which correlates with increases in cytokines [].

Specific Markers and Its Application on HNSCC

HPV detection in HNSCC is now regarded as a powerful biomarker indicating a more favorable clinical outcome. Routine HPV assessment is becoming part of the standard pathologic evaluation of all OPCs. Both the College of American Pathologists and the American Joint Committee on Cancer have recommended routine HPV testing as part of the pathologic evaluation of resected oropharyngeal squamous cell carcinoma (OPCs) specimens for molecular tumor staging. As more is understood about the unique natural history of HPV-positive HNSCC - from viral infection to viral persistence to viral-induced malignant transformation, the practice of HPV testing will probably continue to increase. Detection of HPV is emerging as a valid biomarker for discerning the presence and progress of disease encompassing all aspects of patient care from early cancer detection to more accurate staging to selection of patients most likely to be benefitted from specific treatments, up to post-treatment tumor surveillance [].

Different biomarkers for the detection of biologically active HPV infections in HNSCC have been evaluated and compared. Among these, the most popular is overexpression of p16INK4A protein, assessed by immunohistochemistry, which has been indicated as a suitable surrogate biomarker. Recent studies have highlighted that p16^{INK4A} overexpression is not a reliable surrogate marker of HPV presence in non-oropharyngeal head and neck sites. Moreover, its use in OPCs should be cautiously advised to validate a positive result of HPV DNA evaluation and should not be used as a solitary diagnostic tool [].

It has been suggested that virus-infected cancer cells communicate with stromal cells through the secretion of cytokines and chemokines, or by releasing tumor exosomes to alter the tumor microenvironment. Previous studies have identified the relationship between HPV infection and T-cell-inflamed phenotype. These findings also supported the improved prognosis of patients with HPV-positive HNSCC that probably resulted from activated immune cell subtypes. Wang J, *et al.* (2019) also verified that HPV-positive status was significantly correlated with lymphocyte infiltration (T-eff cells, NK cells, B cells) and cytolytic activity based on an integrated analysis [].

Immunoscore Assessing HNSCC

The clinical application of the prognostic significance of TILs is to establish an Immunoscore, system which will be a potential algorithm to define antitumor immune responses using quantitative pathology. Immunoscore is based on the quantification of CD3+ and CD8+ TILs in the core and the invasive margin of resected tumors and uses this enumeration of TILs to provide a scale ranging from Immunoscore 0 (when low numbers of both cell types are described in both regions), to Immunoscore 4 (when high numbers are described in both regions). Immunoscore has been applied in colorectal cancer in large cohorts []. In HNSCC, CD8+ T cells infiltrate in the tumor component of the invasive margin and PD-L1 expression in the tumor were predictive for disease recurrence [].

Follow-up of HNSCC Patients

HNSCC patients may develop recurrent or second primary tumors highlighting the importance of regular and lifelong monitoring after treatment. However, repeated visits to the clinic may be inconvenient, time-consuming, and expensive, emphasizing the need to develop an alternative monitoring approach. The convenience of saliva collection and changes in salivary composition in healthy *versus* disease conditions have shown the suitability of saliva as a diagnostic fluid. When applied to a high-risk group like HNSCC survivors, a saliva-based test utilizing a panel of biomarkers for HNSCC could provide a non-invasive, reasonably accurate, and less expensive monitoring method. The initial job in developing such a test is characterizing post-treatment changes in saliva. Interestingly, this is a challenge due to the unavailability of saliva. This xerostomia or salivary hypofunction (decreased salivary flow) is due to the destruction of salivary glands, the most common complication of conventional radiotherapy. The impact is usually long-lasting. The IMRT, a sophisticated method of radiotherapy for HNSCC, spares salivary glands and is associated with preferential recovery of stimulated saliva but unstimulated volumes remain depressed. To maximize the probability of detecting pre- to post-treatment changes, post-IMRT recovery of stimulated saliva is advantageous [].

Determination of the source of OPCs related salivary biomarkers remains a challenge. Exfoliate cancer cells, oral mucosa cells, alterations in the salivary gland secretion patterns could contribute to the saliva biomarker profile. Although the further stratification of biomarker sources remains an important scientific arena, only the focus on an effective screening method using easily obtainable whole saliva will allow wider clinical implementation. While the results are promising and demarcate the power of the salivary transcriptome and proteome markers, further studies with larger prospective cohorts will be needed to allow a population-level clinical application [].

Conclusion

Head and neck squamous cell carcinoma (HNSCC) is paramount, as evidenced by a growing number of patients diagnosed every year, yet the prognosis and survival remain dismal despite multimodality treatment regimes. In the near future, with the advancement in molecular analysis and genomic imprinting, biomarkers hold great promise as effective diagnostic, therapeutic, and prognostic agents for HNSCC, which will be able to yield better patient survival and prognosis. Numerous biomarkers have been identified with a potentially high impact on screening, diagnosis as well as treating HNSCC.

More research and commitment are needed from the scientific community in making the quest for versatile biomarkers come into reality.

CONSENT FOR PUBLICATION

Not applicable.

CONFLICT OF INTEREST

The author declares no conflict of interest, financial or otherwise.

ACKNOWLEDGEMENTS

Declared none.

REFERENCES

[1]   Beynon RA, Lang S, Schimansky S, *et al.* Tobacco smoking and alcohol drinking at diagnosis of head and neck cancer and all-cause mortality: Results from head and neck 5000, a prospective observational cohort of people with head and neck cancer. Int J Cancer 2018; 143(5): 1114-27.[http://dx.doi.org/10.1002/ijc.31416] [PMID: 29607493]

[2]   Sterba KR, Garrett-Mayer E, Carpenter MJ, *et al.* Smoking status and symptom burden in surgical head and neck cancer patients. Laryngoscope 2017; 127(1): 127-33.[http://dx.doi.org/10.1002/lary.26159] [PMID: 27392821]

[3]   Williams MD. Integration of biomarkers including molecular targeted therapies in head and neck cancer. Head Neck Pathol 2010; 4(1): 62-9.[http://dx.doi.org/10.1007/s12105-010-0166-6] [PMID: 20237991]

[4]   Argiris A, Karamouzis MV, Raben D, Ferris RL. Head and neck cancer. Lancet 2008; 371(9625): 1695-709.[http://dx.doi.org/10.1016/S0140-6736(08)60728-X] [PMID: 18486742]

[5]   Khariwala SS, Hatsukami D, Hecht SS. Tobacco carcinogen metabolites and DNA adducts as biomarkers in head and neck cancer: potential screening tools and prognostic indicators. Head Neck 2012; 34(3): 441-7.[http://dx.doi.org/10.1002/hed.21705] [PMID: 21618325]

[6]   Hecht SS. Biochemistry, biology, and carcinogenicity of tobacco-specific N-nitrosamines. Chem Res Toxicol 1998; 11(6): 559-603.[http://dx.doi.org/10.1021/tx980005y] [PMID: 9625726]

[7]   Yuan JM, Koh WP, Murphy SE, *et al.* Urinary levels of tobacco-specific nitrosamine metabolites in relation to lung cancer development in two prospective cohorts of cigarette smokers. Cancer Res 2009; 69(7): 2990-5.[http://dx.doi.org/10.1158/0008-5472.CAN-08-4330] [PMID: 19318550]

[8]   Khariwala SS, Carmella SG, Stepanov I, *et al.* Elevated levels of 1-hydroxypyrene and N′-nitrosonornicotine in smokers with head and neck cancer: A matched control study. Head Neck 2013; 35(8): 1096-100.[http://dx.doi.org/10.1002/hed.23085] [PMID: 22807150]

[9]   Pöschl G, Seitz HK. Alcohol and cancer. Alcohol 2004; 39(3): 155-65.[http://dx.doi.org/10.1093/alcalc/agh057] [PMID: 15082451]

[10]   Dal Maso L, Torelli N, Biancotto E, *et al.* Combined effect of tobacco smoking and alcohol drinking in the risk of head and neck cancers: a re-analysis of case-control studies using bi-dimensional spline models. Eur J Epidemiol 2016; 31(4): 385-93.[http://dx.doi.org/10.1007/s10654-015-0028-3] [PMID: 25855002]

[11]   Price G, Roche M, Crowther R. Profile of head and neck cancers in England: incidence, mortality and survival. Natl Cancer Intelligence Netw 2011. http://www.ncin.org.uk/view?rid=69

[12] NHS Digital [homepage on the internet]National Head and Neck Cancer Audit. DAHNO Tenth Annual Report[internet] 2014. http://digital.nhs.uk/catalogue/PUB18081

[13] Ang KK, Harris J, Wheeler R, *et al*. Human papillomavirus and survival of patients with oropharyngeal cancer. N Engl J Med 2010; 363(1): 24-35.[http://dx.doi.org/10.1056/NEJMoa0912217] [PMID: 20530316]

[14] Dahlstrom KR, Bell D, Hanby D, *et al*. Socioeconomic characteristics of patients with oropharyngeal carcinoma according to tumor HPV status, patient smoking status, and sexual behavior. Oral Oncol 2015; 51(9): 832-8.[http://dx.doi.org/10.1016/j.oraloncology.2015.06.005] [PMID: 26120093]

[15] Leemans CR, Braakhuis BJ, Brakenhoff RH. The molecular biology of head and neck cancer. Nat Rev Cancer 2011; 11(1): 9-22.[http://dx.doi.org/10.1038/nrc2982] [PMID: 21160525]

[16] Maitra R. Viruses and Head and Neck Cancer. Head and Cancer Res 2015; 1(1:3): 1-3.

[17] Chan KC, Hung EC, Woo JK, *et al*. Early detection of nasopharyngeal carcinoma by plasma Epstein-Barr virus DNA analysis in a surveillance program. Cancer 2013; 119(10): 1838-44.[http://dx.doi.org/10.1002/cncr.28001] [PMID: 23436393]

[18] Gupta B, Johnson NW. Emerging and established global life-style risk factors for cancer of the upper aero-digestive tract. Asian Pac J Cancer Prev 2014; 15(15): 5983-91.[http://dx.doi.org/10.7314/APJCP.2014.15.15.5983] [PMID: 25124561]

[19] Sarode SC, Sarode GS, Karmarkar S, Tupkari JV. A new classification for potentially malignant disorders of the oral cavity. Oral Oncol 2011; 47(9): 920-1.[http://dx.doi.org/10.1016/j.oraloncology.2011.06.005] [PMID: 21715215]

[20] Randhawa T, Shameena P, Sudha S, Nair R. Squamous cell carcinoma of tongue in a 19-year-old female. Indian J Cancer 2008; 45(3): 128-30.[http://dx.doi.org/10.4103/0019-509X.44071] [PMID: 19018119]

[21] Orbak R, Bayraktar C, Kavrut F, Gündogdu C. Poor oral hygiene and dental trauma as the precipitating factors of squamous cell carcinoma. Oral Oncology Extra 2005; 41(6): 109-13.[http://dx.doi.org/10.1016/j.ooe.2005.02.006]

[22] Lin WW, Karin M. A cytokine-mediated link between innate immunity, inflammation, and cancer. J Clin Invest 2007; 117(5): 1175-83.[http://dx.doi.org/10.1172/JCI31537] [PMID: 17476347]

[23] Mantovani A, Allavena P, Sica A, Balkwill F. Cancer-related inflammation. Nature 2008; 454(7203): 436-44.[http://dx.doi.org/10.1038/nature07205] [PMID: 18650914]

[24] Culig Z. Cytokine disbalance in common human cancers. Biochimica et Biophysica Acta (BBA)-. Molecular Cell Research 2011; 1813(2): 308-14.

[25] Zhu Z, Zhong S, Shen Z. Targeting the inflammatory pathways to enhance chemotherapy of cancer. Cancer Biol Ther 2011; 12(2): 95-105.[http://dx.doi.org/10.4161/cbt.12.2.15952] [PMID: 21623164]

[26] Loesche WJ, Grossman NS. Periodontal disease as a specific, albeit chronic, infection: diagnosis and treatment. Clin Microbiol Rev 2001; 14(4): 727-52.[http://dx.doi.org/10.1128/CMR.14.4.727-752.2001] [PMID: 11585783]

[27] Armitage GC. Periodontal diagnoses and classification of periodontal diseases. Periodontol 2000 2004; 34(1): 9-21.[http://dx.doi.org/10.1046/j.0906-6713.2002.003421.x] [PMID: 14717852]

[28] Burt B. Research, Science and Therapy Committee of the American Academy of PeriodontologyPosition paper: epidemiology of periodontal diseases. J Periodontol 2005; 76(8): 1406-19.[http://dx.doi.org/10.1902/jop.2005.76.8.1406] [PMID: 16101377]

[29] Scannapieco FA, Ng P, Hovey K, Hausmann E, Hutson A, Wactawski-Wende J. Salivary biomarkers associated with alveolar bone loss. Ann N Y Acad Sci 2007; 1098(1): 496-7.[http://dx.doi.org/10.1196/annals.1384.034] [PMID: 17435158]

[30] Giannobile WV, Beikler T, Kinney JS, Ramseier CA, Morelli T, Wong DT. Saliva as a diagnostic tool for periodontal disease: current state and future directions. Periodontol 2000 2009; 50(1): 52-64.[http://dx.doi.org/10.1111/j.1600-0757.2008.00288.x] [PMID: 19388953]

[31] Scannapieco FA, Wang B, Shiau HJ. Oral bacteria and respiratory infection: effects on respiratory pathogen adhesion and epithelial cell proinflammatory cytokine production. Ann Periodontol 2001; 6(1): 78-86.[http://dx.doi.org/10.1902/annals.2001.6.1.78] [PMID: 11887474]

[32] Genco RJ, Trevisan M, Wu T, Beck JD. Periodontal disease and risk of coronary heart disease. JAMA 2001; 285(1): 40-1.[http://dx.doi.org/10.1001/jama.285.1.40] [PMID: 11150098]

[33] Nichols TC, Fischer TH, Deliargyris EN, Baldwin AS, Jr. Role of nuclear factor-kappa B (NF-kappa B) in inflammation, periodontitis, and atherogenesis. Ann Periodontol 2001; 6(1): 20-9.[http://dx.doi.org/10.1902/annals.2001.6.1.20] [PMID: 11887466]

[34] Shultis WA, Weil EJ, Looker HC, *et al*. Effect of periodontitis on overt nephropathy and end-stage renal

disease in type 2 diabetes. Diabetes Care 2007; 30(2): 306-11.[http://dx.doi.org/10.2337/dc06-1184] [PMID: 17259499]

[35] Mealey BL, Rose LF. Diabetes mellitus and inflammatory periodontal diseases. Curr Opin Endocrinol Diabetes Obes 2008; 15(2): 135-41.[http://dx.doi.org/10.1097/MED.0b013e3282f824b7] [PMID: 18316948]

[36] Haraszthy VI, Zambon JJ, Trevisan M, Zeid M, Genco RJ. Identification of periodontal pathogens in atheromatous plaques. J Periodontol 2000; 71(10): 1554-60.[http://dx.doi.org/10.1902/jop.2000.71.10.1554] [PMID: 11063387]

[37] Dorn BR, Dunn WA, Jr, Progulske-Fox A. Invasion of human coronary artery cells by periodontal pathogens. Infect Immun 1999; 67(11): 5792-8.[http://dx.doi.org/10.1128/IAI.67.11.5792-5798.1999] [PMID: 10531230]

[38] Ruma M, Boggess K, Moss K, et al. Maternal periodontal disease, systemic inflammation, and risk for preeclampsia. Am J Obstet Gynecol 2008; 198(4): 389.e1-5.[http://dx.doi.org/10.1016/j.ajog.2007.12.002] [PMID: 18295179]

[39] Graham S, Dayal H, Rohrer T, et al. Dentition, diet, tobacco, and alcohol in the epidemiology of oral cancer. J Natl Cancer Inst 1977; 59(6): 1611-8.[http://dx.doi.org/10.1093/jnci/59.6.1611] [PMID: 926184]

[40] Zheng TZ, Boyle P, Hu HF, et al. Dentition, oral hygiene, and risk of oral cancer: a case-control study in Beijing, People's Republic of China. Cancer Causes Control 1990; 1(3): 235-41.[http://dx.doi.org/10.1007/BF00117475] [PMID: 2102296]

[41] Winn DM, Blot WJ, McLaughlin JK, et al. Mouthwash use and oral conditions in the risk of oral and pharyngeal cancer. Cancer Res 1991; 51(11): 3044-7.[PMID: 2032242]

[42] Marshall JR, Graham S, Haughey BP, et al. Smoking, alcohol, dentition and diet in the epidemiology of oral cancer. Eur J Cancer B Oral Oncol 1992; 28B(1): 9-15.[http://dx.doi.org/10.1016/0964-1955(92)90005-L] [PMID: 1422474]

[43] Bundgaard T, Wildt J, Frydenberg M, Elbrønd O, Nielsen JE. Case-control study of squamous cell cancer of the oral cavity in Denmark. Cancer Causes Control 1995; 6(1): 57-67.[http://dx.doi.org/10.1007/BF00051681] [PMID: 7718736]

[44] Velly AM, Franco EL, Schlecht N, et al. Relationship between dental factors and risk of upper aerodigestive tract cancer. Oral Oncol 1998; 34(4): 284-91.[http://dx.doi.org/10.1016/S1368-8375(98)80009-2] [PMID: 9813724]

[45] Moreno-López LA, Esparza-Gómez GC, González-Navarro A, Cerero-Lapiedra R, González-Hernández MJ, Domínguez-Rojas V. Risk of oral cancer associated with tobacco smoking, alcohol consumption and oral hygiene: a case-control study in Madrid, Spain. Oral Oncol 2000; 36(2): 170-4.[http://dx.doi.org/10.1016/S1368-8375(99)00084-6] [PMID: 10745168]

[46] Talamini R, Vaccarella S, Barbone F, et al. Oral hygiene, dentition, sexual habits and risk of oral cancer. Br J Cancer 2000; 83(9): 1238-42.[http://dx.doi.org/10.1054/bjoc.2000.1398] [PMID: 11027440]

[47] Balaram P, Sridhar H, Rajkumar T, et al. Oral cancer in southern India: the influence of smoking, drinking, paan-chewing and oral hygiene. Int J Cancer 2002; 98(3): 440-5.[http://dx.doi.org/10.1002/ijc.10200] [PMID: 11920597]

[48] Lissowska J, Pilarska A, Pilarski P, et al. Smoking, alcohol, diet, dentition and sexual practices in the epidemiology of oral cancer in Poland. Eur J Cancer Prev 2003; 12(1): 25-33.[http://dx.doi.org/10.1097/00008469-200302000-00005] [PMID: 12548107]

[49] Rosenquist K, Wennerberg J, Schildt EB, Bladström A, Göran Hansson B, Andersson G. Oral status, oral infections and some lifestyle factors as risk factors for oral and oropharyngeal squamous cell carcinoma. A population-based case-control study in southern Sweden. Acta Otolaryngol 2005; 125(12): 1327-36.[http://dx.doi.org/10.1080/00016480510012273] [PMID: 16303683]

[50] Guha N, Boffetta P, Wünsch Filho V, et al. Oral health and risk of squamous cell carcinoma of the head and neck and esophagus: results of two multicentric case-control studies. Am J Epidemiol 2007; 166(10): 1159-73.[http://dx.doi.org/10.1093/aje/kwm193] [PMID: 17761691]

[51] Tezal M, Grossi SG, Genco RJ. Is periodontitis associated with oral neoplasms? J Periodontol 2005; 76(3): 406-10.[http://dx.doi.org/10.1902/jop.2005.76.3.406] [PMID: 15857075]

[52] Tezal M, Sullivan MA, Reid ME, et al. Chronic periodontitis and the risk of tongue cancer. Arch Otolaryngol Head Neck Surg 2007; 133(5): 450-4.[http://dx.doi.org/10.1001/archotol.133.5.450] [PMID: 17515503]

[53] Tezal M, Sullivan MA, Hyland A, et al. Chronic periodontitis and the incidence of head and neck squamous cell carcinoma. Cancer Epidemiol Biomarkers Prev 2009; 18(9): 2406-12.[http://dx.doi.org/10.1158/1055-9965.EPI-09-0334] [PMID: 19745222]

[54] Jayaprakash V, Rigual NR, Moysich KB, et al. Chemoprevention of head and neck cancer with aspirin: a

case-control study. Arch Otolaryngol Head Neck Surg 2006; 132(11): 1231-6.[http://dx.doi.org/10.1001/archotol.132.11.1231] [PMID: 17116820]

[55] Lax AJ, Thomas W. How bacteria could cause cancer: one step at a time. Trends Microbiol 2002; 10(6): 293-9.[http://dx.doi.org/10.1016/S0966-842X(02)02360-0] [PMID: 12088666]

[56] Karin M, Lawrence T, Nizet V. Innate immunity gone awry: linking microbial infections to chronic inflammation and cancer. Cell 2006; 124(4): 823-35.[http://dx.doi.org/10.1016/j.cell.2006.02.016] [PMID: 16497591]

[57] Huycke MM, Gaskins HR. Commensal bacteria, redox stress, and colorectal cancer: mechanisms and models. Exp Biol Med (Maywood) 2004; 229(7): 586-97.[http://dx.doi.org/10.1177/153537020422900702] [PMID: 15229352]

[58] Homann N, Tillonen J, Rintamäki H, Salaspuro M, Lindqvist C, Meurman JH. Poor dental status increases acetaldehyde production from ethanol in saliva: a possible link to increased oral cancer risk among heavy drinkers. Oral Oncol 2001; 37(2): 153-8.[http://dx.doi.org/10.1016/S1368-8375(00)00076-2] [PMID: 11167142]

[59] Visapää JP, Götte K, Benesova M, et al. Increased cancer risk in heavy drinkers with the alcohol dehydrogenase 1C*1 allele, possibly due to salivary acetaldehyde. Gut 2004; 53(6): 871-6.[http://dx.doi.org/10.1136/gut.2003.018994] [PMID: 15138216]

[60] Salaspuro MP. Acetaldehyde, microbes, and cancer of the digestive tract. Crit Rev Clin Lab Sci 2003; 40(2): 183-208.[http://dx.doi.org/10.1080/713609333] [PMID: 12755455]

[61] Shapiro KB, Hotchkiss JH, Roe DA. Quantitative relationship between oral nitrate-reducing activity and the endogenous formation of N-nitrosoamino acids in humans. Food Chem Toxicol 1991; 29(11): 751-5.[http://dx.doi.org/10.1016/0278-6915(91)90183-8] [PMID: 1761254]

[62] Mirvish SS. Role of N-nitroso compounds (NOC) and N-nitrosation in etiology of gastric, esophageal, nasopharyngeal and bladder cancer and contribution to cancer of known exposures to NOC. Cancer Lett 1995; 93(1): 17-48.[http://dx.doi.org/10.1016/0304-3835(95)03786-V] [PMID: 7600541]

[63] Rüegg C. Leukocytes, inflammation, and angiogenesis in cancer: fatal attractions. J Leukoc Biol 2006; 80(4): 682-4.[http://dx.doi.org/10.1189/jlb.0606394] [PMID: 16849612]

[64] Asting AG, Carén H, Andersson M, Lönnroth C, Lagerstedt K, Lundholm K. COX-2 gene expression in colon cancer tissue related to regulating factors and promoter methylation status. BMC Cancer 2011; 11(1): 238.[http://dx.doi.org/10.1186/1471-2407-11-238] [PMID: 21668942]

[65] Grivennikov SI, Karin M. Inflammatory cytokines in cancer: tumour necrosis factor and interleukin 6 take the stage. Ann Rheum Dis 2011; 70 (Suppl. 1): i104-8.[http://dx.doi.org/10.1136/ard.2010.140145] [PMID: 21339211]

[66] Tatemichi M, Ogura T, Esumi H. Impact of inducible nitric oxide synthase gene on tumor progression. Eur J Cancer Prev 2009; 18(1): 1-8.[http://dx.doi.org/10.1097/CEJ.0b013e3282f75f29] [PMID: 19077558]

[67] Allen C, Duffy S, Teknos T, et al. Nuclear factor-kappaB-related serum factors as longitudinal biomarkers of response and survival in advanced oropharyngeal carcinoma. Clin Cancer Res 2007; 13(11): 3182-90.[http://dx.doi.org/10.1158/1078-0432.CCR-06-3047] [PMID: 17545521]

[68] Greten FR, Eckmann L, Greten TF, et al. IKKbeta links inflammation and tumorigenesis in a mouse model of colitis-associated cancer. Cell 2004; 118(3): 285-96.[http://dx.doi.org/10.1016/j.cell.2004.07.013] [PMID: 15294155]

[69] Wang D, Wang H, Shi Q, et al. Prostaglandin E(2) promotes colorectal adenoma growth via transactivation of the nuclear peroxisome proliferator-activated receptor δ. Cancer Cell 2004; 6(3): 285-95.[http://dx.doi.org/10.1016/j.ccr.2004.08.011] [PMID: 15380519]

[70] Stetler-Stevenson WG. The tumor microenvironment: regulation by MMP-independent effects of tissue inhibitor of metalloproteinases-2. Cancer Metastasis Rev 2008; 27(1): 57-66.[http://dx.doi.org/10.1007/s10555-007-9105-8] [PMID: 18058195]

[71] Leaner VD, Donninger H, Birrer MJ. Transcription factors as targets for cancer therapy: AP-1 a potential therapeutic target. Curr Cancer Ther Rev 2007; 3(1): 1-6.[http://dx.doi.org/10.2174/157339407780126665]

[72] Sparmann A, Bar-Sagi D. Ras-induced interleukin-8 expression plays a critical role in tumor growth and angiogenesis. Cancer Cell 2004; 6(5): 447-58.[http://dx.doi.org/10.1016/j.ccr.2004.09.028] [PMID: 15542429]

[73] Dauer DJ, Ferraro B, Song L, et al. Stat3 regulates genes common to both wound healing and cancer. Oncogene 2005; 24(21): 3397-408.[http://dx.doi.org/10.1038/sj.onc.1208469] [PMID: 15735721]

[74] Cassatella MA, Huber V, Calzetti F, et al. Interferon-activated neutrophils store a TNF-related apoptosis-inducing ligand (TRAIL/Apo-2 ligand) intracellular pool that is readily mobilizable following exposure to

proinflammatory mediators. J Leukoc Biol 2006; 79(1): 123-32.[http://dx.doi.org/10.1189/jlb.0805431] [PMID: 16244105]

[75] Williams DA. Inflammatory cytokines and mucosal injury. J Natl Cancer Inst Monogr 2001; 2001(29): 26-30.[http://dx.doi.org/10.1093/oxfordjournals.jncimonographs.a003435] [PMID: 11694562]

[76] Chuang SC, Jenab M, Heck JE, et al. Diet and the risk of head and neck cancer: a pooled analysis in the INHANCE consortium. Cancer Causes Control 2012; 23(1): 69-88.[http://dx.doi.org/10.1007/s10552-011-9857-x] [PMID: 22037906]

[77] Bloching M, Reich W, Schubert J, Grummt T, Sandner A. The influence of oral hygiene on salivary quality in the Ames Test, as a marker for genotoxic effects. Oral Oncol 2007; 43(9): 933-9.[http://dx.doi.org/10.1016/j.oraloncology.2006.11.006] [PMID: 17257882]

[78] Negri E, Boffetta P, Berthiller J, et al. Family history of cancer: pooled analysis in the International Head and Neck Cancer Epidemiology Consortium. Int J Cancer 2009; 124(2): 394-401.[http://dx.doi.org/10.1002/ijc.23848] [PMID: 18814262]

[79] Gaudet MM, Olshan AF, Chuang SC, et al. Body mass index and risk of head and neck cancer in a pooled analysis of case-control studies in the International Head and Neck Cancer Epidemiology (INHANCE) Consortium. Int J Epidemiol 2010; 39(4): 1091-102.[http://dx.doi.org/10.1093/ije/dyp380] [PMID: 20123951]

[80] Balkwill F, Mantovani A. Inflammation and cancer: back to Virchow? Lancet 2001; 357(9255): 539-45.[http://dx.doi.org/10.1016/S0140-6736(00)04046-0] [PMID: 11229684]

[81] Bekes EM, Schweighofer B, Kupriyanova TA, et al. Tumor-recruited neutrophils and neutrophil TIMP-free MMP-9 regulate coordinately the levels of tumor angiogenesis and efficiency of malignant cell intravasation. Am J Pathol 2011; 179(3): 1455-70.[http://dx.doi.org/10.1016/j.ajpath.2011.05.031] [PMID: 21741942]

[82] Wang F, Arun P, Friedman J, Chen Z, Van Waes C. Current and potential inflammation targeted therapies in head and neck cancer. Curr Opin Pharmacol 2009; 9(4): 389-95.[http://dx.doi.org/10.1016/j.coph.2009.06.005] [PMID: 19570715]

[83] Panagiotakos DB, Dimakopoulou K, Katsouyanni K, et al. AIRGENE Study GroupMediterranean diet and inflammatory response in myocardial infarction survivors. Int J Epidemiol 2009; 38(3): 856-66.[http://dx.doi.org/10.1093/ije/dyp142] [PMID: 19244256]

[84] Esposito K, Marfella R, Ciotola M, et al. Effect of a mediterranean-style diet on endothelial dysfunction and markers of vascular inflammation in the metabolic syndrome: a randomized trial. JAMA 2004; 292(12): 1440-6.[http://dx.doi.org/10.1001/jama.292.12.1440] [PMID: 15383514]

[85] Chrysohoou C, Panagiotakos DB, Pitsavos C, Das UN, Stefanadis C. Adherence to the Mediterranean diet attenuates inflammation and coagulation process in healthy adults: The ATTICA Study. J Am Coll Cardiol 2004; 44(1): 152-8.[http://dx.doi.org/10.1016/j.jacc.2004.03.039] [PMID: 15234425]

[86] Hanahan D, Weinberg RA. Hallmarks of cancer: the next generation. Cell 2011; 144(5): 646-74.

[87] Galvão-Moreira LV, da Cruz MC. Oral microbiome, periodontitis and risk of head and neck cancer. Oral Oncol 2016; 53: 17-9.[http://dx.doi.org/10.1016/j.oraloncology.2015.11.013] [PMID: 26684542]

[88] Brieger J, Jacob R, Riazimand HS, et al. Chromosomal aberrations in premalignant and malignant squamous epithelium. Cancer Genet Cytogenet 2003; 144(2): 148-55.[http://dx.doi.org/10.1016/S0165-4608(02)00936-6] [PMID: 12850378]

[89] Zuo C, Zhang H, Spencer HJ, et al. Increased microsatellite instability and epigenetic inactivation of the hMLH1 gene in head and neck squamous cell carcinoma. Otolaryngol Head Neck Surg 2009; 141(4): 484-90.[http://dx.doi.org/10.1016/j.otohns.2009.07.007] [PMID: 19786217]

[90] Mao L, Lee JS, Fan YH, et al. Frequent microsatellite alterations at chromosomes 9p21 and 3p14 in oral premalignant lesions and their value in cancer risk assessment. Nat Med 1996; 2(6): 682-5.[http://dx.doi.org/10.1038/nm0696-682] [PMID: 8640560]

[91] Rosin MP, Cheng X, Poh C, et al. Use of allelic loss to predict malignant risk for low-grade oral epithelial dysplasia. Clin Cancer Res 2000; 6(2): 357-62.[PMID: 10690511]

[92] Visapää JP, Götte K, Benesova M, et al. Increased cancer risk in heavy drinkers with the alcohol dehydrogenase 1C*1 allele, possibly due to salivary acetaldehyde. Gut 2004; 53(6): 871-6.[http://dx.doi.org/10.1136/gut.2003.018994] [PMID: 15138216]

[93] Salaspuro MP. Acetaldehyde, microbes, and cancer of the digestive tract. Crit Rev Clin Lab Sci 2003; 40(2): 183-208.[http://dx.doi.org/10.1080/713609333] [PMID: 12755455]

[94] Shapiro KB, Hotchkiss JH, Roe DA. Quantitative relationship between oral nitrate-reducing activity and the endogenous formation of N-nitrosoamino acids in humans. Food Chem Toxicol 1991; 29(11): 751-5.[http://dx.doi.org/10.1016/0278-6915(91)90183-8] [PMID: 1761254]

[95] Mirvish SS. Role of N-nitroso compounds (NOC) and N-nitrosation in etiology of gastric, esophageal, nasopharyngeal and bladder cancer and contribution to cancer of known exposures to NOC. Cancer Lett 1995; 93(1): 17-48.[http://dx.doi.org/10.1016/0304-3835(95)03786-V] [PMID: 7600541]

[96] Rüegg C. Leukocytes, inflammation, and angiogenesis in cancer: fatal attractions. J Leukoc Biol 2006; 80(4): 682-4.[http://dx.doi.org/10.1189/jlb.0606394] [PMID: 16849612]

[97] Asting AG, Carén H, Andersson M, Lönnroth C, Lagerstedt K, Lundholm K. COX-2 gene expression in colon cancer tissue related to regulating factors and promoter methylation status. BMC Cancer 2011; 11(1): 238.[http://dx.doi.org/10.1186/1471-2407-11-238] [PMID: 21668942]

[98] Grivennikov SI, Karin M. Inflammatory cytokines in cancer: tumour necrosis factor and interleukin 6 take the stage. Ann Rheum Dis 2011; 70 (Suppl. 1): i104-8.[http://dx.doi.org/10.1136/ard.2010.140145] [PMID: 21339211]

[99] Tatemichi M, Ogura T, Esumi H. Impact of inducible nitric oxide synthase gene on tumor progression. Eur J Cancer Prev 2009; 18(1): 1-8.[http://dx.doi.org/10.1097/CEJ.0b013e3282f75f29] [PMID: 19077558]

[100 Allen C, Duffy S, Teknos T, et al. Nuclear factor-kappaB-related serum factors as longitudinal biomarkers of
] response and survival in advanced oropharyngeal carcinoma. Clin Cancer Res 2007; 13(11): 3182-90.[http://dx.doi.org/10.1158/1078-0432.CCR-06-3047] [PMID: 17545521]

[101 Greten FR, Eckmann L, Greten TF, et al. IKKbeta links inflammation and tumorigenesis in a mouse model of
] colitis-associated cancer. Cell 2004; 118(3): 285-96.[http://dx.doi.org/10.1016/j.cell.2004.07.013] [PMID: 15294155]

[102 Wang D, Wang H, Shi Q, et al. Prostaglandin E(2) promotes colorectal adenoma growth via transactivation
] of the nuclear peroxisome proliferator-activated receptor δ. Cancer Cell 2004; 6(3): 285-95.[http://dx.doi.org/10.1016/j.ccr.2004.08.011] [PMID: 15380519]

[103 Stetler-Stevenson WG. The tumor microenvironment: regulation by MMP-independent effects of tissue
] inhibitor of metalloproteinases-2. Cancer Metastasis Rev 2008; 27(1): 57-66.[http://dx.doi.org/10.1007/s10555-007-9105-8] [PMID: 18058195]

[104 Leaner VD, Donninger H, Birrer MJ. Transcription factors as targets for cancer therapy: AP-1 a potential
] therapeutic target. Curr Cancer Ther Rev 2007; 3(1): 1-6.[http://dx.doi.org/10.2174/157339407780126665]

[105 Sparmann A, Bar-Sagi D. Ras-induced interleukin-8 expression plays a critical role in tumor growth and
] angiogenesis. Cancer Cell 2004; 6(5): 447-58.[http://dx.doi.org/10.1016/j.ccr.2004.09.028] [PMID: 15542429]

[106 Dauer DJ, Ferraro B, Song L, et al. Stat3 regulates genes common to both wound healing and cancer.
] Oncogene 2005; 24(21): 3397-408.[http://dx.doi.org/10.1038/sj.onc.1208469] [PMID: 15735721]

[107 Dauer DJ, Ferraro B, Song L, et al. Stat3 regulates genes common to both wound healing and cancer.
] Oncogene 2005; 24(21): 3397-408.[http://dx.doi.org/10.1038/sj.onc.1208469] [PMID: 15735721]

[108 Williams DA. Inflammatory cytokines and mucosal injury. J Natl Cancer Inst Monogr 2001; 2001(29): 26-
] 30.[http://dx.doi.org/10.1093/oxfordjournals.jncimonographs.a003435] [PMID: 11694562]

[109 Pöllänen MT, Salonen JI, Uitto VJ. Structure and function of the tooth-epithelial interface in health and
] disease. Periodontol 2000 2003; 31(1): 12-31.[http://dx.doi.org/10.1034/j.1600-0757.2003.03102.x] [PMID: 12656993]

[110 Kinzler KW, Vogelstein B. Lessons from hereditary colorectal cancer. Cell 1996; 87(2): 159-
] 70.[http://dx.doi.org/10.1016/S0092-8674(00)81333-1] [PMID: 8861899]

[111 Califano J, van der Riet P, Westra W, et al. Genetic progression model for head and neck cancer:
] implications for field cancerization. Cancer Res 1996; 56(11): 2488-92.[PMID: 8653682]

[112 Ha PK, Benoit NE, Yochem R, et al. A transcriptional progression model for head and neck cancer. Clin
] Cancer Res 2003; 9(8): 3058-64.[PMID: 12912957]

[113 Park BJ, Chiosea SI, Grandis JR. Molecular changes in the multistage pathogenesis of head and neck cancer.
] Cancer Biomark 2010; 9(1-6): 325-39.

[114 Weber RG, Scheer M, Born IA, et al. Recurrent chromosomal imbalances detected in biopsy material from
] oral premalignant and malignant lesions by combined tissue microdissection, universal DNA amplification, and comparative genomic hybridization. Am J Pathol 1998; 153(1): 295-303.[http://dx.doi.org/10.1016/S0002-9440(10)65571-X] [PMID: 9665491]

[115 Brieger J, Jacob R, Riazimand HS, et al. Chromosomal aberrations in premalignant and malignant squamous
] epithelium. Cancer Genet Cytogenet 2003; 144(2): 148-55.[http://dx.doi.org/10.1016/S0165-4608(02)00936-6] [PMID: 12850378]

[116 Zuo C, Zhang H, Spencer HJ, et al. Increased microsatellite instability and epigenetic inactivation of the

] hMLH1 gene in head and neck squamous cell carcinoma. Otolaryngol Head Neck Surg 2009; 141(4): 484-90.[http://dx.doi.org/10.1016/j.otohns.2009.07.007] [PMID: 19786217]

[117 Mao L, Lee JS, Fan YH, *et al.* Frequent microsatellite alterations at chromosomes 9p21 and 3p14 in oral
] premalignant lesions and their value in cancer risk assessment. Nat Med 1996; 2(6): 682-5.[http://dx.doi.org/10.1038/nm0696-682] [PMID: 8640560]

[118 Rosin MP, Cheng X, Poh C, *et al.* Use of allelic loss to predict malignant risk for low-grade oral epithelial
] dysplasia. Clin Cancer Res 2000; 6(2): 357-62.[PMID: 10690511]

[119 Zhang L, Rosin MP. Loss of heterozygosity: a potential tool in management of oral premalignant lesions?
] Journal of Oral Pathology & Medicine: Review article 2001; 30(9): 513-20.[http://dx.doi.org/10.1034/j.1600-0714.2001.300901.x]

[120 Shin DM, Charuruks N, Lippman SM, *et al.* p53 protein accumulation and genomic instability in head and
] neck multistep tumorigenesis. Cancer Epidemiol Biomarkers Prev 2001; 10(6): 603-9.[PMID: 11401909]

[121 Soni S, Kaur J, Kumar A, *et al.* Alterations of rb pathway components are frequent events in patients with
] oral epithelial dysplasia and predict clinical outcome in patients with squamous cell carcinoma. Oncology
2005; 68(4-6): 314-25.[http://dx.doi.org/10.1159/000086970] [PMID: 16020958]

[122 Yarbrough WG. The ARF-p16 gene locus in carcinogenesis and therapy of head and neck squamous cell
] carcinoma. Laryngoscope 2002; 112(12): 2114-28.[http://dx.doi.org/10.1097/00005537-200212000-00002]
[PMID: 12461329]

[123 Ha PK, Tong BC, Westra WH, *et al.* Mitochondrial C-tract alteration in premalignant lesions of the head and
] neck: a marker for progression and clonal proliferation. Clin Cancer Res 2002; 8(7): 2260-5.[PMID: 12114429]

[124 Rubin Grandis J, Tweardy DJ, Melhem MF. Asynchronous modulation of transforming growth factor alpha
] and epidermal growth factor receptor protein expression in progression of premalignant lesions to head and
neck squamous cell carcinoma. Clin Cancer Res 1998; 4(1): 13-20.[PMID: 9516947]

[125 Grandis JR, Drenning SD, Zeng Q, *et al.* Constitutive activation of Stat3 signaling abrogates apoptosis in
] squamous cell carcinogenesis *in vivo.* Proc Natl Acad Sci USA 2000; 97(8): 4227-32.[http://dx.doi.org/10.1073/pnas.97.8.4227] [PMID: 10760290]

[126 Srinivasan M, Jewell SD. Evaluation of TGF-α and EGFR expression in oral leukoplakia and oral submucous
] fibrosis by quantitative immunohistochemistry. Oncology 2001; 61(4): 284-92.[http://dx.doi.org/10.1159/000055335] [PMID: 11721175]

[127 Gollin SM. Chromosomal alterations in squamous cell carcinomas of the head and neck: window to the
] biology of disease. Head Neck 2001; 23(3): 238-53.[http://dx.doi.org/10.1002/1097-0347(200103)23:3<238::AID-HED1025>3.0.CO;2-H] [PMID: 11428 456]

[128 Patmore HS, Ashman JN, Stafford ND, *et al.* Genetic analysis of head and neck squamous cell carcinoma
] using comparative genomic hybridisation identifies specific aberrations associated with laryngeal origin.
Cancer Lett 2007; 258(1): 55-62.[http://dx.doi.org/10.1016/j.canlet.2007.08.014] [PMID: 17920192]

[129 Nordkvist A, Gustafsson H, Juberg-Ode M, Stenman G. Recurrent rearrangements of 11q14-22 in
] mucoepidermoid carcinoma. Cancer Genet Cytogenet 1994; 74(2): 77-83.[http://dx.doi.org/10.1016/0165-4608(94)90001-9] [PMID: 8019965]

[130 Tonon G, Modi S, Wu L, *et al.* t(11;19)(q21;p13) translocation in mucoepidermoid carcinoma creates a novel
] fusion product that disrupts a Notch signaling pathway. Nat Genet 2003; 33(2): 208-13.[http://dx.doi.org/10.1038/ng1083] [PMID: 12539049]

[131 Tirado Y, Williams MD, Hanna EY, Kaye FJ, Batsakis JG, El-Naggar AK. CRTC1/MAML2 fusion
] transcript in high grade mucoepidermoid carcinomas of salivary and thyroid glands and Warthin's tumors:
implications for histogenesis and biologic behavior. Genes Chromosomes Cancer 2007; 46(7): 708-15.[http://dx.doi.org/10.1002/gcc.20458] [PMID: 17437281]

[132 Jin YT, Kayser S, Kemp BL, *et al.* The prognostic significance of the biomarkers p21WAF1/CIP1, p53, and
] bcl-2 in laryngeal squamous cell carcinoma. Cancer 1998; 82(11): 2159-65.[http://dx.doi.org/10.1002/(SICI)1097-0142(19980601)82:11<2159::AID-CNCR10>3.0.CO;2-T] [PMID: 9610695]

[133 Narayana A, Vaughan AT, Gunaratne S, Kathuria S, Walter SA, Reddy SP. Is p53 an independent prognostic
] factor in patients with laryngeal carcinoma? Cancer 1998; 82(2): 286-91.[http://dx.doi.org/10.1002/(SICI)1097-0142(19980115)82:2<286::AID-CNCR7>3.0.CO;2-P] [PMID: 9445184]

[134 Erber R, Conradt C, Homann N, *et al.* TP53 DNA contact mutations are selectively associated with allelic
] loss and have a strong clinical impact in head and neck cancer. Oncogene 1998; 16(13): 1671-

59

9.[http://dx.doi.org/10.1038/sj.onc.1201690] [PMID: 9582015]

[135] Mineta H, Borg A, Dictor M, Wahlberg P, Akervall J, Wennerberg J. p53 mutation, but not p53 overexpression, correlates with survival in head and neck squamous cell carcinoma. Br J Cancer 1998; 78(8): 1084-90.[http://dx.doi.org/10.1038/bjc.1998.632] [PMID: 9792155]

[136] Nagai MA, Miracca EC, Yamamoto L, et al. TP53 genetic alterations in head-and-neck carcinomas from Brazil. Int J Cancer 1998; 76(1): 13-8.[http://dx.doi.org/10.1002/(SICI)1097-0215(19980330)76:1<13::AID-IJC3>3.0.CO;2-0] [PMID: 9533755]

[137] Hegde PU, Brenski AC, Caldarelli DD, et al. Tumor angiogenesis and p53 mutations: prognosis in head and neck cancer. Arch Otolaryngol Head Neck Surg 1998; 124(1): 80-5.[http://dx.doi.org/10.1001/archotol.124.1.80] [PMID: 9440785]

[138] Shin DM, Mao L, Papadimitrakopoulou VM, et al. Biochemopreventive therapy for patients with premalignant lesions of the head and neck and p53 gene expression. J Natl Cancer Inst 2000; 92(1): 69-73.[http://dx.doi.org/10.1093/jnci/92.1.69] [PMID: 10620636]

[139] Clayman GL, el-Naggar AK, Lippman SM, et al. Adenovirus-mediated p53 gene transfer in patients with advanced recurrent head and neck squamous cell carcinoma. J Clin Oncol 1998; 16(6): 2221-32.[http://dx.doi.org/10.1200/JCO.1998.16.6.2221] [PMID: 9626224]

[140] Lee BJ, Wang SG, Choi JS, Lee JC, Goh EK, Kim MG. The prognostic value of telomerase expression in peripheral blood mononuclear cells of head and neck cancer patients. Am J Clin Oncol 2006; 29(2): 163-7.[http://dx.doi.org/10.1097/01.coc.0000207372.64733.b0] [PMID: 16601436]

[141] Thurnher D, Knerer B, Formanek M, Kornfehl J. Non-radioactive semiquantitative testing for the expression levels of telomerase activity in head and neck squamous cell carcinomas may be indicative for biological tumour behaviour. Acta Otolaryngol 1998; 118(3): 423-7.[http://dx.doi.org/10.1080/00016489850183557] [PMID: 9655221]

[142] Gillison ML, Shah KV. Human papillomavirus-associated head and neck squamous cell carcinoma: mounting evidence for an etiologic role for human papillomavirus in a subset of head and neck cancers. Curr Opin Oncol 2001; 13(3): 183-8.[http://dx.doi.org/10.1097/00001622-200105000-00009] [PMID: 11307062]

[143] Herbst RS, Arquette M, Shin DM, et al. Phase II multicenter study of the epidermal growth factor receptor antibody cetuximab and cisplatin for recurrent and refractory squamous cell carcinoma of the head and neck. J Clin Oncol 2005; 23(24): 5578-87.[http://dx.doi.org/10.1200/JCO.2005.07.120] [PMID: 16009949]

[144] Baselga J, Trigo JM, Bourhis J, et al. Phase II multicenter study of the antiepidermal growth factor receptor monoclonal antibody cetuximab in combination with platinum-based chemotherapy in patients with platinum-refractory metastatic and/or recurrent squamous cell carcinoma of the head and neck. J Clin Oncol 2005; 23(24): 5568-77.[http://dx.doi.org/10.1200/JCO.2005.07.119] [PMID: 16009950]

[145] Burtness B, Goldwasser MA, Flood W, Mattar B, Forastiere AA. Eastern Cooperative Oncology GroupPhase III randomized trial of cisplatin plus placebo compared with cisplatin plus cetuximab in metastatic/recurrent head and neck cancer: an Eastern Cooperative Oncology Group study. J Clin Oncol 2005; 23(34): 8646-54.[http://dx.doi.org/10.1200/JCO.2005.02.4646] [PMID: 16314626]

[146] Cohen EE, Kane MA, List MA, et al. Phase II trial of gefitinib 250 mg daily in patients with recurrent and/or metastatic squamous cell carcinoma of the head and neck. Clin Cancer Res 2005; 11(23): 8418-24.[http://dx.doi.org/10.1158/1078-0432.CCR-05-1247] [PMID: 16322304]

[147] Soulieres D, Senzer NN, Vokes EE, Hidalgo M, Agarwala SS, Siu LL. Multicenter phase II study of erlotinib, an oral epidermal growth factor receptor tyrosine kinase inhibitor, in patients with recurrent or metastatic squamous cell cancer of the head and neck. J Clin Oncol 2004; 22(1): 77-85.[http://dx.doi.org/10.1200/JCO.2004.06.075] [PMID: 14701768]

[148] Caponigro F, Milano A, Basile M, Ionna F, Iaffaioli RV. Recent advances in head and neck cancer therapy: the role of new cytotoxic and molecular-targeted agents. Curr Opin Oncol 2006; 18(3): 247-52.[http://dx.doi.org/10.1097/01.cco.0000219253.53091.fb] [PMID: 16552236]

[149] Sumitani K, Kamijo R, Toyoshima T, et al. Specific inhibition of cyclooxygenase-2 results in inhibition of proliferation of oral cancer cell lines via suppression of prostaglandin E2 production. J Oral Pathol Med 2001; 30(1): 41-7.[http://dx.doi.org/10.1034/j.1600-0714.2001.300107.x] [PMID: 11140899]

[150] Zweifel BS, Davis TW, Ornberg RL, Masferrer JL. Direct evidence for a role of cyclooxygenase 2-derived prostaglandin E2 in human head and neck xenograft tumors. Cancer Res 2002; 62(22): 6706-11.[PMID: 12438270]

[151] Kubicek GJ, Machtay M, Axelrod RA. Phase I trial of bortezomib (VELCADE), cisplatin and radiotherapy for advanced head and neck cancer. J Clin Oncol 2008; 26(15_suppl): 6028.

[152] Caponigro F, Formato R, Caraglia M, Normanno N, Iaffaioli RV. Monoclonal antibodies targeting epidermal

] growth factor receptor and vascular endothelial growth factor with a focus on head and neck tumors. Curr Opin Oncol 2005; 17(3): 212-7.[http://dx.doi.org/10.1097/01.cco.0000159623.68506.cf] [PMID: 15818163]

[153 Vokes EE, Cohen EE, Mauer AM. A phase I study of erlotinib and bevacizumab for recurrent or metastatic
] squamous cell carcinoma of the head and neck (HNC). Journal of Clinical Oncology 2005; 23(16_suppl): 5504.

[154 Seiwert TY, Davis DW, Yan D. pKDR/KDR ratio predicts response in a phase I/II pharmacodynamic study
] of erlotinib and bevacizumab for recurrent or metastatic head and neck cancer (HNC). J Clin Oncol 2007; 25(18_suppl): 6021.

[155 Hoa M, Davis SL, Ames SJ, Spanjaard RA. Amplification of wild-type K-ras promotes growth of head and
] neck squamous cell carcinoma. Cancer Res 2002; 62(24): 7154-6.[PMID: 12499248]

[156 Tanaka N, Odajima T, Ogi K, Ikeda T, Satoh M. Expression of E-cadherin, α-catenin, and β-catenin in the
] process of lymph node metastasis in oral squamous cell carcinoma. Br J Cancer 2003; 89(3): 557-63.[http://dx.doi.org/10.1038/sj.bjc.6601124] [PMID: 12888830]

[157 Shintani S, Li C, Mihara M, Nakashiro K, Hamakawa H. Gefitinib ('Iressa'), an epidermal growth factor
] receptor tyrosine kinase inhibitor, mediates the inhibition of lymph node metastasis in oral cancer cells. Cancer Lett 2003; 201(2): 149-55.[http://dx.doi.org/10.1016/S0304-3835(03)00464-6] [PMID: 14607328]

[158 Kawata R, Shimada T, Maruyama S, Hisa Y, Takenaka H, Murakami Y. Enhanced production of matrix
] metalloproteinase-2 in human head and neck carcinomas is correlated with lymph node metastasis. Acta Otolaryngol 2002; 122(1): 101-6.[http://dx.doi.org/10.1080/00016480252775823] [PMID: 11876588]

[159 Howell GM, Grandis JR. Molecular mediators of metastasis in head and neck squamous cell carcinoma. Head
] Neck 2005; 27(8): 710-7.[http://dx.doi.org/10.1002/hed.20222] [PMID: 15952195]

[160 Saad MA, Kuo SZ, Rahimy E, et al. Alcohol-dysregulated miR-30a and miR-934 in head and neck squamous
] cell carcinoma. Mol Cancer 2015; 14: 181.[http://dx.doi.org/10.1186/s12943-015-0452-8] [PMID: 26472042]

[161 Franzmann EJ, Reategui EP, Pedroso F, et al. Soluble CD44 is a potential marker for the early detection of
] head and neck cancer. Cancer Epidemiol Biomarkers Prev 2007; 16(7): 1348-55.[http://dx.doi.org/10.1158/1055-9965.EPI-06-0011] [PMID: 17627000]

[162 Batsakis JG. Surgical excision margins: a pathologist's perspective. Adv Anat Pathol 1999; 6(3): 140-
] 8.[http://dx.doi.org/10.1097/00125480-199905000-00002] [PMID: 10342011]

[163 Rosas SL, Koch W, da Costa Carvalho MG, et al. Promoter hypermethylation patterns of p16, O6-
] methylguanine-DNA-methyltransferase, and death-associated protein kinase in tumors and saliva of head and neck cancer patients. Cancer Res 2001; 61(3): 939-42.[PMID: 11221887]

[164 Goldenberg D, Harden S, Masayesva BG, et al. Intraoperative molecular margin analysis in head and neck
] cancer. Arch Otolaryngol Head Neck Surg 2004; 130(1): 39-44.[http://dx.doi.org/10.1001/archotol.130.1.39] [PMID: 14732766]

[165 Belbin TJ, Singh B, Barber I, et al. Molecular classification of head and neck squamous cell carcinoma using
] cDNA microarrays. Cancer Res 2002; 62(4): 1184-90.[PMID: 11861402]

[166 Gomes CC, Gomez RS. MicroRNA and oral cancer: future perspectives. Oral Oncol 2008; 44(10): 910-
] 4.[http://dx.doi.org/10.1016/j.oraloncology.2008.01.002] [PMID: 18620891]

[167 Bouquot JE, Gorlin RJ. Leukoplakia, lichen planus, and other oral keratoses in 23,616 white Americans over
] the age of 35 years. Oral Surg Oral Med Oral Pathol 1986; 61(4): 373-81.[http://dx.doi.org/10.1016/0030-4220(86)90422-6] [PMID: 3458148]

[168 Bouquot JE, Whitaker SB. Oral leukoplakia--rationale for diagnosis and prognosis of its clinical subtypes or
] "phases". Quintessence Int 1994; 25(2): 133-40.[PMID: 8183979]

[169 Silverman S, Jr, Gorsky M, Lozada F. Oral leukoplakia and malignant transformation. A follow-up study of
] 257 patients. Cancer 1984; 53(3): 563-8.[http://dx.doi.org/10.1002/1097-0142(19840201)53:3<563::AID-CNCR2820530332>3.0.CO;2-F] [PMID: 6537892]

[170 Lumerman H, Freedman P, Kerpel S. Oral epithelial dysplasia and the development of invasive squamous
] cell carcinoma. Oral Surg Oral Med Oral Pathol Oral Radiol Endod 1995; 79(3): 321-9.[http://dx.doi.org/10.1016/S1079-2104(05)80226-4] [PMID: 7621010]

[171 Gupta PC, Murti PR, Bhonsle RB, Mehta FS, Pindborg JJ. Effect of cessation of tobacco use on the incidence
] of oral mucosal lesions in a 10-yr follow-up study of 12,212 users. Oral Dis 1995; 1(1): 54-8.[http://dx.doi.org/10.1111/j.1601-0825.1995.tb00158.x] [PMID: 7553382]

[172 Sudbø J, Kildal W, Risberg B, Koppang HS, Danielsen HE, Reith A. DNA content as a prognostic marker in
] patients with oral leukoplakia. N Engl J Med 2001; 344(17): 1270-8.[http://dx.doi.org/10.1056/NEJM200104263441702] [PMID: 11320386]

[173] Pindborg JJ, Reichart PA, Smith CJ, Waal I, Van Der. World Health Organization international histological classification of tumours. Histological typing of cancer and precancer of the oral mucosa 1997.

[174] Tabor MP, Braakhuis BJ, van der Wal JE. Comparative molecular and histological grading of epithelial dysplasia of the oral cavity and the oropharynx. J Pathol Soc Great Britain and Ireland 2003; 199(3): 354-60.[http://dx.doi.org/10.1002/path.1285]

[175] Fischer DJ, Epstein JB, Morton TH, Jr, Schwartz SM. Interobserver reliability in the histopathologic diagnosis of oral pre-malignant and malignant lesions. J Oral Pathol Med 2004; 33(2): 65-70.[http://dx.doi.org/10.1111/j.1600-0714.2004.0037n.x] [PMID: 14720191]

[176] Kujan O, Khattab A, Oliver RJ, Roberts SA, Thakker N, Sloan P. Why oral histopathology suffers inter-observer variability on grading oral epithelial dysplasia: an attempt to understand the sources of variation. Oral Oncol 2007; 43(3): 224-31.[http://dx.doi.org/10.1016/j.oraloncology.2006.03.009] [PMID: 16931119]

[177] Abbey LM, Kaugars GE, Gunsolley JC, et al. The effect of clinical information on the histopathologic diagnosis of oral epithelial dysplasia. Oral Surg Oral Med Oral Pathol Oral Radiol Endod 1998; 85(1): 74-7.[http://dx.doi.org/10.1016/S1079-2104(98)90401-2] [PMID: 9474618]

[178] Kujan O, Oliver RJ, Khattab A, Roberts SA, Thakker N, Sloan P. Evaluation of a new binary system of grading oral epithelial dysplasia for prediction of malignant transformation. Oral Oncol 2006; 42(10): 987-93.[http://dx.doi.org/10.1016/j.oraloncology.2005.12.014] [PMID: 16731030]

[179] Silverman S, Jr, Gorsky M, Lozada-Nur F. A prospective follow-up study of 570 patients with oral lichen planus: persistence, remission, and malignant association. Oral Surg Oral Med Oral Pathol 1985; 60(1): 30-4.[http://dx.doi.org/10.1016/0030-4220(85)90210-5] [PMID: 3862010]

[180] van der Meij EH, Mast H, van der Waal I. The possible premalignant character of oral lichen planus and oral lichenoid lesions: a prospective five-year follow-up study of 192 patients. Oral Oncol 2007; 43(8): 742-8.[http://dx.doi.org/10.1016/j.oraloncology.2006.09.006] [PMID: 17112770]

[181] Kern SE. Why your new cancer biomarker may never work: recurrent patterns and remarkable diversity in biomarker failures. Cancer Res 2012; 72(23): 6097-101.[http://dx.doi.org/10.1158/0008-5472.CAN-12-3232] [PMID: 23172309]

[182] Moons KG, Altman DG, Reitsma JB, Collins GS. Transparent reporting of a multivariate prediction model for individual prognosis or development initiativeNew guideline for the reporting of studies developing, validating, or updating a multivariable clinical prediction model: the TRIPOD statement. Adv Anat Pathol 2015; 22(5): 303-5.[http://dx.doi.org/10.1097/PAP.0000000000000072] [PMID: 26262512]

[183] Hanahan D, Weinberg RA. Hallmarks of cancer: the next generation. Cell 2011; 144(5): 646-74.

[184] Economopoulou P, Agelaki S, Perisanidis C, Giotakis EI, Psyrri A. The promise of immunotherapy in head and neck squamous cell carcinoma. Ann Oncol 2016; 27(9): 1675-85.[http://dx.doi.org/10.1093/annonc/mdw226] [PMID: 27380958]

[185] Galon J, Costes A, Sanchez-Cabo F, et al. Type, density, and location of immune cells within human colorectal tumors predict clinical outcome. Science 2006; 313(5795): 1960-4.[http://dx.doi.org/10.1126/science.1129139] [PMID: 17008531]

[186] Huang Y, Ma C, Zhang Q, et al. CD4+ and CD8+ T cells have opposing roles in breast cancer progression and outcome. Oncotarget 2015; 6(19): 17462-78.[http://dx.doi.org/10.18632/oncotarget.3958] [PMID: 25968569]

[187] Donnem T, Hald SM, Paulsen EE, et al. Stromal CD8+ T-cell density—a promising supplement to TNM staging in non–small cell lung cancer. Clin Cancer Res 2015; 21(11): 2635-43.[http://dx.doi.org/10.1158/1078-0432.CCR-14-1905] [PMID: 25680376]

[188] Shang B, Liu Y, Jiang SJ, Liu Y. Prognostic value of tumor-infiltrating FoxP3+ regulatory T cells in cancers: a systematic review and meta-analysis. Sci Rep 2015; 5: 15179.[http://dx.doi.org/10.1038/srep15179] [PMID: 26462617]

[189] Krupar R, Robold K, Gaag D, et al. Immunologic and metabolic characteristics of HPV-negative and HPV-positive head and neck squamous cell carcinomas are strikingly different. Virchows Arch 2014; 465(3): 299-312.[http://dx.doi.org/10.1007/s00428-014-1630-6] [PMID: 25027580]

[190] Näsman A, Romanitan M, Nordfors C, et al. Tumor infiltrating CD8+ and Foxp3+ lymphocytes correlate to clinical outcome and human papillomavirus (HPV) status in tonsillar cancer. PLoS One 2012; 7(6): e38711.[http://dx.doi.org/10.1371/journal.pone.0038711] [PMID: 22701698]

[191] Partlová S, Bouček J, Kloudová K, et al. Distinct patterns of intratumoral immune cell infiltrates in patients with HPV-associated compared to non-virally induced head and neck squamous cell carcinoma. OncoImmunology 2015; 4(1): e965570.[http://dx.doi.org/10.4161/21624011.2014.965570] [PMID:

25949860]

[192 Ward MJ, Thirdborough SM, Mellows T, *et al.* Tumour-infiltrating lymphocytes predict for outcome in
] HPV-positive oropharyngeal cancer. Br J Cancer 2014; 110(2): 489-
500.[http://dx.doi.org/10.1038/bjc.2013.639] [PMID: 24169344]

[193 Ou D, Adam J, Garberis I, *et al.* Clinical relevance of tumor infiltrating lymphocytes, PD-L1 expression and
] correlation with HPV/p16 in head and neck cancer treated with bio- or chemo-radiotherapy.
OncoImmunology 2017; 6(9): e1341030.[http://dx.doi.org/10.1080/2162402X.2017.1341030] [PMID:
28932643]

[194 Vassilakopoulou M, Avgeris M, Velcheti V, *et al.* Evaluation of PD-L1 expression and associated tumor-
] infiltrating lymphocytes in laryngeal squamous cell carcinoma. Clin Cancer Res 2016; 22(3): 704-
13.[http://dx.doi.org/10.1158/1078-0432.CCR-15-1543] [PMID: 26408403]

[195 Uppaluri R, Dunn GP, Lewis JS, Jr. Focus on TILs: prognostic significance of tumor infiltrating lymphocytes
] in head and neck cancers. Cancer Immun 2008; 8(1): 16.[PMID: 19053167]

[196 Balermpas P, Michel Y, Wagenblast J, *et al.* Tumour-infiltrating lymphocytes predict response to definitive
] chemoradiotherapy in head and neck cancer. Br J Cancer 2014; 110(2): 501-
9.[http://dx.doi.org/10.1038/bjc.2013.640] [PMID: 24129245]

[197 Balermpas P, Rödel F, Rödel C, *et al.* CD8+ tumour-infiltrating lymphocytes in relation to HPV status and
] clinical outcome in patients with head and neck cancer after postoperative chemoradiotherapy: A multicentre
study of the German cancer consortium radiation oncology group (DKTK-ROG). Int J Cancer 2016; 138(1):
171-81.[http://dx.doi.org/10.1002/ijc.29683] [PMID: 26178914]

[198 Oguejiofor K, Hall J, Slater C, *et al.* Stromal infiltration of CD8 T cells is associated with improved clinical
] outcome in HPV-positive oropharyngeal squamous carcinoma. Br J Cancer 2015; 113(6): 886-
93.[http://dx.doi.org/10.1038/bjc.2015.277] [PMID: 26313665]

[199 Mandal R, Şenbabaoğlu Y, Desrichard A, *et al.* The head and neck cancer immune landscape and its
] immunotherapeutic implications. JCI Insight 2016; 1(17):
e89829.[http://dx.doi.org/10.1172/jci.insight.89829] [PMID: 27777979]

[200 Badoual C, Hans S, Rodriguez J, *et al.* Prognostic value of tumor-infiltrating CD4+ T-cell subpopulations in
] head and neck cancers. Clin Cancer Res 2006; 12(2): 465-72.[http://dx.doi.org/10.1158/1078-0432.CCR-05-
1886] [PMID: 16428488]

[201 Erdman SE, Rao VP, Olipitz W, *et al.* Unifying roles for regulatory T cells and inflammation in cancer. Int J
] Cancer 2010; 126(7): 1651-65.[http://dx.doi.org/10.1002/ijc.24923] [PMID: 19795459]

[202 Matta A, Ralhan R. Overview of current and future biologically based targeted therapies in head and neck
] squamous cell carcinoma. Head Neck Oncol 2009; 1: 6.[http://dx.doi.org/10.1186/1758-3284-1-6] [PMID:
19284526]

[203 Liang C, Marsit CJ, McClean MD. Biomarkers of HPV in head and neck squamous cell carcinoma. Cancer
] Res 2012; 72(19): 5004-13.[http://dx.doi.org/10.1158/0008-5472.CAN-11-3277]

[204 Smith EM, Rubenstein LM, Ritchie JM. Does pretreatment seropositivity to human papillomavirus have
] prognostic significance for head and neck cancers? Cancer Epidemiol Biomarkers Prev 2008; 17(8): 2087-
96.[http://dx.doi.org/10.1158/1055-9965.EPI-08-0054]

[205 Bishop JA, Ma XJ, Wang H. Detection of transcriptionally active high-risk HPV in patients with head and
] neck squamous cell carcinoma as visualized by a novel E6/E7 mRNA in situ hybridization method. Am J
Surg Pathol 2012; 36(12): 1874-82.

[206 Principe S, Dikova V, Bagán J. Salivary Cytokines in patients with Head and Neck Cancer (HNC) treated
] with Radiotherapy. J Clin Exp Dent 2019; 11(11): e1072-7.[http://dx.doi.org/10.4317/jced.56318] [PMID:
31700580]

[207 Russo N, Bellile E, Murdoch-Kinch CA, *et al.* Cytokines in saliva increase in head and neck cancer patients
] after treatment. Oral Surg Oral Med Oral Pathol Oral Radiol 2016; 122(4): 483-
90.[http://dx.doi.org/10.1016/j.oooo.2016.05.020] [PMID: 27554375]

[208 Boscolo-Rizzo P, Del Mistro A, Bussu F, *et al.* New insights into human papillomavirus-associated head and
] neck squamous cell carcinoma. Acta Otorhinolaryngol Ital 2013; 33(2): 77-87.[PMID: 23853396]

[209 Wang J, Sun H, Zeng Q, *et al.* HPV-positive status associated with inflamed immune microenvironment and
] improved response to anti-PD-1 therapy in head and neck squamous cell carcinoma. Sci Rep 2019; 9(1):
13404.[http://dx.doi.org/10.1038/s41598-019-49771-0] [PMID: 31527697]

[210 Pagès F, Kirilovsky A, Mlecnik B, *et al. In situ* cytotoxic and memory T cells predict outcome in patients
] with early-stage colorectal cancer. J Clin Oncol 2009; 27(35): 5944-
51.[http://dx.doi.org/10.1200/JCO.2008.19.6147] [PMID: 19858404]

63

[211 Galon J, Fox BA, Bifulco CB, *et al.* Immunoscore and Immunoprofiling in cancer: an update from the
]   melanoma and immunotherapy bridge 2015. J Transl Med 2016; 14: 273.[http://dx.doi.org/10.1186/s12967-
      016-1029-z] [PMID: 27650038]

[212 Brinkmann O, Kastratovic DA, Dimitrijevic MV, *et al.* Oral squamous cell carcinoma detection by salivary
]   biomarkers   in   a   Serbian   population.   Oral   Oncol   2011;   47(1):   51-
      5.[http://dx.doi.org/10.1016/j.oraloncology.2010.10.009] [PMID: 21109482]

Targeting Inflammation: Window for Therapeutic Strategy in Head and Neck Malignancy

Norhafiza Mat Lazim*

Department of Otorhinolaryngology-Head and Neck Surgery, School of Medical Sciences, Universiti Sains Malaysia, Health Campus 16150, Kubang Kerian, Kelantan, Malaysia

Abstract

Inflammation is a hallmark of cancer. Inflammation is closely linked to head and neck malignancy and other solid tumors. Arrays of inflammation cascades and markers have been identified and proven to play significant roles in carcinogenesis. Many substances and molecules are secreted in response to the inflammation and its ecosystem and can be effectively measured and quantified at various stages of the carcinogenesis process. A spectrum of available inflammatory biomarkers can be a potentially effective therapeutic approach in the management armamentarium of head and neck malignancy. However, the cost, practicality, and availability are some of the major obstacles that need to be counteracted in order to progress in this challenging oncologic arena. Together with the continuous commitment from scientists, clinicians, laboratory personnel, and other related health staff, with the combination of technology updates, this new treatment approach and strategy are coming to reality. This chapter will discuss selected inflammatory biomarkers of significance critical for the armamentarium management of head and neck malignancy. Hopefully, this will escalate the treatment response of head and neck cancer patients. Hence, this ensures the patient's survival with the best quality of life.

Keywords: Carcinogenesis, Chemoradiation, Cytokines, Growth factors, Head and neck malignancy, Inflammation markers, Macrophages, Metastases, Neck nodes, Prognosis, Quality of life, Residual diseases, Survival.

* **Corresponding author Norhafiza Mat Lazim:** Department of Otorhinolaryngology-Head and Neck Surgery, School of Medical Sciences, Universiti Sains Malaysia, Health Campus 16150, Kubang Kerian, Kelantan, Malaysia; Tel:+60199442664; Fax: +6097676424; E-mail: norhafiza@usm.my

INTRODUCTION

Nowadays, head and neck malignancy is showing great progress in its management due to the advancement and refinement of the technology, instrumentation, and operation theatre set up. Head and neck squamous cell carcinoma (HNSCC) continues to be a challenge as the incidence is on the rise and its involvement with vital facial and head anatomic complexes that respons-

ible for breathing, speech, eating, hearing, and vision. Late presentation is a common feature of HNSCC patients, and this may be attributed to ignorance, poverty, poor access to health services, and patients consulting traditional healers and usage of traditional medicines [1]. Clinical presentation will depend on the regional anatomic involvement. Computed tomography is the mainstay for assessing and staging the head and neck malignancy whereas magnetic resonance imaging is the preferred tool for evaluating cartilage, bone, perineural, and perivascular invasion. Furthermore, in selected cases, a combination of fine-needle aspiration and neck ultrasonography increases the accuracy of cervical lymph node staging [2]. The prognosis of selected groups of HNSCC remains dismal despite extensive multimodality treatment incorporating surgery and chemoradiation.

With a median overall survival of less than 1 year, patients with chronic or metastatic HNSCC have a poor prognosis. This population includes patients whose disease has recurred locally or who, after initial treatment for localized disease, have developed distant metastases. A fair number of head and neck cancer patients present with loco-regional advanced disease or distant metastases at first presentation. The rate of second primary tumors after a diagnosis of HNC is about 3-7% per year [3]. A small number of patients with a limited recurrent disease can still be treated with curative intent, but the vast majority are treated with systemic therapy for palliative care [4]. Early-stage diseases are mainly treated with surgery and most patients experience a good quality of life with a regular follow-up scheme. A selected patient who presented with recurrent disease, locally or regionally, may be offered salvage surgery or chemoradiation.

For instance, conventionally, the normal treatment of NPC requires chemoradiation and surgery, in the majority of cases. Radiation therapy alone is known to be the main approach to NPC treatment, especially for early-stage disease. The concurrent chemoradiation has been a standard practice for stage III-IV diseases. Surgery mainly involves neck dissection in recurrent cases, in the patient who had exhausted chemoradiation and present with neck nodes that is not amenable to radiation. Surgery can also be performed in case of the patient had a small and limited recurrent tumor at the nasopharynx that can be addressed *via* transnasal nasopharyngectomy. Critically, deciding the best possible treatment method for a specific patient will depend on multiple factors such as tumor factors, patient's comorbidity, expertise and equipment availability, and committed rehabilitation team.

At the time, as more treatment choices become available, it is rational to postulate that the results for HNSCC patients could be optimized with an acceptable succession of treatment regimens. This translates to better prognosis and survival for this subset of patients. One of the most effective instruments for providing full benefit to the patients is to increase the number of therapy lines and choices and refine the order in which these therapies should be delivered. Therefore, to produce a maximally efficient and tolerable multi-line continuum of care, it is important to incorporate as many potentially effective therapies as possible into the treatment model of head and neck malignancy [3]. In addition, only a minority of patients with HNSCC benefit from immunotherapy in clinical practice, and the need to discover novel biomarkers to improve treatment strategies is becoming increasingly important. Immunotherapy is based on host immune system functional restoration to counteract different strategies of tumor evasion. Immunotherapeutic approaches generally comprised of tumor-specific antibodies, cancer vaccines, cytokines, adoptive T-cell transfer, and immune-modulating agents [5]. Immune checkpoint inhibitor and EGFR inhibitor is a strong example of immune-targeted therapy [6, 7]. EGFR inhibitor overexpression is seen in most head and neck cancer and is associated with poor prognosis [8, 9].

Presently, many ongoing trials focusing on discovering new biomarkers that can be used in managing head and neck malignancy are in progress. For instance, a study assessing the outcomes of using a combination of antiepileptic plus cisplatin and cetuximab that might escalate treatment outcomes with minimal complications [10]. There are other scientific studies that look at other combinations of therapy in order to escalate the treatment outcomes of head and neck malignancy [11]. This effort needs full support from the government and non-governmental bodies in terms of financial assistance and mutual collaborative work and programs. This will have a great impact on the discovery of potent new therapeutic markers or agents for

HNSCC. These new agents can be made available locally at a fair cost and accessible to all disadvantaged HNSCC patients.

With regards to the management of HNSCC, primary tumor management is essential in order to reduce the progression of the tumor and later appearance of distant metastases. However, the side effects of radiotherapy cannot be overlooked, as it can cause second primaries and many significant related toxicities that can impair the patient's quality of life. Multiple new techniques of radiation have been investigated in head and neck cancer patients in order to improve survival rates whilst minimizing the morbidities associated with radiation toxicity. Such regimes include hyperfractionated radiotherapy with the intention to reduce malignant cell repopulations by shortening the treatment interval time [10].

Critically, *via* modifying the tumor microenvironment, radiotherapy can also induce distant metastases. This may be partly attributed to the radioresistance that can be modulated *via* for instance microRNAs regulation [12]. MicroRNAs and their associated factors are responsible for controlling the intracellular pathways involved in DNA damage, repair, apoptosis, angiogenesis, and cell proliferation. For instance, in NPC, the microRNAs are upregulated and are reported to be responsible for the radiation resistance [13, 14]. Other inflammatory markers and gene aberrations have also been documented to involve in producing the radioresistance effects of radiation.

In addition, some studies have also shown that accelerated tumor cell growth and proliferation may occur about 3 to 4 weeks after radiation exposure, which can have significant clinical sequelae. If we can identify this critical stage of cell proliferation and inflammatory cascades that are involved in carcinogenesis, metastasis, and response to treatment, we might be able to identify and develop potential therapeutic targets that address this critical point of cell biology. These potential targets can modulate the important markers, proteins, cytokines, and peptides in the inflammation ecosystem and can be applied to produce the desired effects with minimal side effects. Thus, the molecular mechanisms of radiation resistance in head and neck cancer, for instance in NPC treatment, need to be thoroughly understood [15].

Chemotherapy also carries its own risk of complications and benefits. Multiple factors are involved in producing the desired chemotherapeutic effects and the unwanted side effects, and this largely involves the inflammatory markers and the immune-mediated mechanisms. Targeting the inflammatory-immune markers as a potential therapeutic target for NPC and other head and neck malignancy will allow the transformation of head and neck cancer management to another level. The finesse treatment approaches will produce highly efficacious therapeutic agents and avoid all unwanted complications that have significantly impaired head and neck cancer patient's quality of life.

INFLAMMATION IN HEAD AND NECK MALIGNANCY

As in the previous chapter, several critical elements of inflammation concerning head and neck malignancy have been highlighted and discussed. This pertaining to the risk factors, assessment tools as well as treatment for head and neck cancer. In terms of the treatment paradigm of head and neck malignancy, currently, available therapy such as chemoradiation, targeted therapy, and immunotherapy are based on the critical elements of inflammation and their related mechanisms of actions within the inflammation ecosystem. Immunotherapy has been shown to be a highly effective therapeutic agent, especially for selected recurrent and metastatic HNSCC.

The most active immunotherapy field in HNSCC over the last decade has been the production of monoclonal antibodies (mAbs) targeting the tumor antigen (TA) on the cell surface. This targeted therapy focused on the unique tumor characteristic and aimed to improve the therapeutic response while minimizing the toxicity [16]. The bulk of research focused on the epidermal growth factor receptor (EGFR). EGFR is a transmembrane surface receptor that can be activated and modulated by multiple mechanisms. Overexpression of EGFR is linked with poor treatment response and impaired patient's prognosis. Interestingly, tobacco can cause activation and upregulate the EGFR *via* specific mechanisms and is responsible for reduced treatment effectiveness [17].

Cetuximab is the most common EGFR monoclonal antibody (mAb) used in head and neck malignancy management. It is currently, the only FDA-approved EGFR targeting drugs for HNSCC. It is approved for three particular uses, firstly, in combination with radiation for locally aggressive disease, secondly, as a single agent for recurrent or metastatic disease following the failure of platinum-based chemotherapy, and thirdly, in combination with platinum-based chemotherapy plus 5-FU for first-line recurrent or metastatic HNSCC [16]. This existing treatment can be potentially enhanced with a combination of targeted inflammatory markers in the coming years in order to escalate the therapeutic ratio. This will be highly possible with the continuous effort from the scientific community at large. Another important anti-EGFR mAbs that were clinically tested in HNSCC is Panitumumab. This is a fully human IgG2 mAb which is potentially less immunogenic.

At this juncture, immunotherapy is a promising treatment strategy for effective management of head and neck malignancy. The immune landscape of the head and neck cancer microenvironment is heterogeneous. Multiple immune-targeted agents have been used in treating aggressive and locally advanced head and neck malignancies. As aforementioned, the monoclonal antibodies have been showing a good treatment response. Such example of mAbs that was used in malignant tumor management including, as mentioned earlier, cetuximab and trastuzumab. In comparison, Cetuximab is an EGFR receptor antibody, whereas trastuzumab is the anti-human epidermal growth factor receptor 2 (HER2). These two immune-targeted agents mainly act to counteract the proliferation and apoptosis mediated signaling pathways which are regulated by the growth factor transmembrane receptors.

In selected cases, for the same receptors involved, targeting mAbs yields superior clinical outcomes compared to targeting non-immunogenic small molecules of the same receptors. This can be explained by different immune mechanisms and signaling pathways that underlie the pathogenesis of mAB which give varied therapeutic efficacy. The EGFR overexpression in relation to intracellular phosphorylation cascades has a significant prognostication value in head and neck malignancy [18]. Cetuximab, the first molecularly targeted drug approved by the FDA for the treatment of HNSCC in combination with radiation for locally advanced disease [19]. It is a prototype of mAb with dual signaling and immunological mechanisms [20]. It has minimal side effects and its application has been extended to the new emerging HPV positive head and neck cancers [21]. For instance, the efficacy of cetuximab in combination with chemotherapy has been investigated in patients with low-risk oropharyngeal carcinoma [22, 23]. Multiple other factors especially the immune-related inflammatory markers that can be further explored for gaining maximal therapeutic outcomes for these HNSCC patients. The identification of specific immune-mediated inflammatory markers can be further investigated and incorporated into the immuno-targeted therapy armamentarium. Significant advances and refinement have been made in the assessment of the intrinsic and adaptive resistance mechanisms to immunotherapy [24]. Emerging evidence is looking at the Cetuximab resistance in the treatment paradigm of head and neck malignancy. Several mechanisms have been postulated to underlie the cetuximab radioresistance. These include activation of MET/MAPK signaling pathways, EGFR gene mutation that causes persistent activation of EGFR, and reactivation of selected signaling pathways such as tyrosine kinase, Her 2 and 3 [25].

At the other end of the spectrum, HPV-related head and neck malignancy has surged at certain geographic regions globally. Importantly, this subset of head and neck malignancy has a different biological profile in comparison with other HNSCC. However, the reason why HPV-positive head and neck carcinoma patients have a better prognosis than HPV negative patients remains controversial. The inflammatory constituents and their various mechanisms may play exquisite roles in these critical differences. In particular, the improved overall survival of positive HPV patients may rely on multiple immuno-inflammatory factors. The HPV-positive patients mainly involved the tonsillar carcinoma or oropharyngeal carcinoma and the oral cavity carcinoma [26]. The main modality of treatment of this subset of cancer is transoral surgery for early tumors (T1 and T2 tumor) and chemoradiation for late-stage tumor (T3 and T4 tumor). Importantly the HPV oncogenic proteins may influence the outcomes of the treatment approach. The positive factors that are related to patients with HPV positive tumors include younger age at diagnosis, higher performance status, lower smoking and alcohol-related morbidities, decreased risk of secondary primary tumors, and can tolerate a more aggressive treatment plan. Younger patients may have significant inflammatory responses that able to modify the effect of treatment. In addition, the beneficial outcome of HPV-positive HNSCC could be due to improved sensitivity to chemoradiation. Numerous proteins, peptides, and cytokines in the signaling pathways modulate the cell proliferation, the extent of DNA damage and repair, thus allowing the apoptotic response of cancer cells to chemoradiation [27]. The chemotherapy regime is continuously being investigated in terms of dosing, frequency, and interval of infusion in order to improve treatment outcomes and lessen the toxicity [28].

The ability to prevent immune destruction, in particular by T-lymphocytes and B-lymphocytes, macrophages and natural killer cells, is a proven hallmark of the multistep evolution of cancer. The complex process of initiation, activation, and progression leads to carcinogenesis with the resultant malignant tissue formation. Immunosuppression is frequently viewed as a failure of immunosurveillance, but this does not completely describe the dynamic interplay between cancer and immunity. Treatment of head and neck cancer with immune checkpoint blockade is potentially efficacious. The immune landscape of head and neck cancer serves as a promising frontier for research in immunotherapy [29]. This ultimately will enhance the therapeutic approach of head and neck malignancy.

Immunosurveillance is just part of a wider, complex mechanism known as cancer immunosurveillance. This cancer surveillance consists of three phases of tumor removal, balance, and escape from clinically overt disease. The immune system is thus capable of preventing and encouraging the development and growth of neoplastic tissue [9]. Immunomodulation and inflammation may act synergistically in producing numerous effects in carcinogenesis. This interaction also has significant value in therapeutic immunotherapy and can be exploited and enhanced to yield potent newer therapeutic markers.

Immunotherapy is based on the functional restoration of the immune system of the host. Its role is to help combat various techniques for tumor evasion. Interestingly certain malignant tumors are immunogenic than other tumors. This may be associated with tumor-associated antigens that drive immune activation activations, which may include the oncogenic HPV viral antigens [30]. Broadly speaking, immunotherapeutic methods may include tumor-specific antibodies, cancer vaccinations, cytokines, T-cell adoption, and immunomodulating agents [5]. Multiple immune cells, peptides, humoral factors, and cytokines influence and regulate the tumor microenvironment. The balance between these factors can either modulate the cells and tissue towards malignant changes or can be used as a target to treat cancer. Specifically, cancer immunotherapy is based on the functional restoration of certain signal cascades of the host immune system. It has been applied in clinical practice in the majority of solid human malignancy with the aim to effectively kills cancer cells and preserves viable normal cells. Cancer immunotherapy serves as an interesting research avenue to expand and facilitate the discovery of novel therapeutic agents.

The signal cascades help to counteract various strategies for tumor evasion. These include immunosuppressive microenvironment growth, cellular immune escape through regulatory T-cells or myeloid-derived suppressor cells a reduced antigen processing and presentation, and increased tumor-permissive cytokine profiles [29]. For instance, cancer-associated fibroblast (CAFs) play important roles in shaping the immunosuppressive microenvironment of the tumor in oral cavity cancers by inducing pro-tumoral TAM phenotypes [31]. CAFs also mediated autophagy reactions in oral cancers that are responsible for tumor progression. By controlling secreted factors involved in the autophagy, this CAF mediated autophagy can be controlled and allows blockage of the malignant cell proliferation [32, 33]. In the coming years, many of these modified therapeutic strategies to reverse this CAF-mediated immunosuppression should be considered.

These critical elements play dominant roles in the inflammation ecosystem and may be applied to the current understanding of radioresistance of head and neck cancers to chemoradiation as well as to the targeted therapy. Early immunosuppression identification in HNSCC patients resulted in clinical trials of available immunostimulatory strategies. The immunomodulation approach involves critical molecules, including interleukin (IL)-2 and interferon (IFN)-2a. The interleukin is an important protein that regulates many functions and signaling pathways in the process of carcinogenesis. This again will escalate possible effective treatment strategies for HNSCC. Tumor stromal cells, including immune system cells, modulate the development and progression of cancer. Regulatory T (Treg) cells that express transcription factors are often found at elevated levels of tumor lesions and are essential for the prevention of autoimmunity and maintenance of immune homeostasis [34]. Multiple cytokines and interleukins secreted in response to CAFs such as interleukin 6 play a significant role in head and neck cancer progression [35]. With numerous researches coming in the future, more molecules and markers can be identified.

TARGETTING INFLAMMATION AND REDUCE THE RISK FACTORS OF HEAD AND NECK MALIGNANCY

Roles of inflammation in carcinogenesis of head and neck malignancy has been extensively discussed in previous chapters. The risk factors serve as a target for screening and prevention programs for HNSCC, and this can be implemented at very early in the disease process. The chemoradiation as an integral treatment of the majority of recurrent and metastatic HNSCC carries several limitations inclusive of its significant related toxicities. The radiation-induced DNA damage not only occurs in the cancerous tissues but also within surrounding normal tissues. Of note, after radiation, cell death is proportionate to the dosage of radiation delivered. Critically, the percentage of apoptotic cells is also increased gradually in a dose-dependent manner. The adjacent tissues also exposed to radiation and are at risk of collateral damage. The evidence of damage induced by radiations which mainly involves the chromosomal double strands breakage can be visualized on immunofluorescence. They will appear as speckles of fluorescent foci [36]. The inflammatory markers can be identified and tagged in combination with immunofluorescence in order to further delineate the effects of radiation as well as chemotherapy on both the malignant and healthy tissues.

As described above, the function of the epidermal growth factor receptor in the development and progression of squamous cell carcinoma of the head and neck has been extensively studied. It is a promising biomarker that can be further assessed. It has multiple roles at various molecular levels including protein expression, polymorphism, genes activation, polymorphism, mutation, and EGFR ligand expression [37]. EGFR is a transmembrane glycoprotein member of the tyrosine kinase growth factor family that controls cell growth, apoptotic signaling, angiogenesis, cell proliferation, and metastases [18]. Several studies investigated the potential roles of EGFR as a prognostic indicator in head and neck cancer that was treated with surgery and radiation. The study by Lin *et al*. reported that overexpression of EGFR in laryngeal cancer is associated with the invasion and metastasis potential of the malignant laryngeal cells. Thus, by inhibiting the EGFR expression, the risk of malignant transformation and progression can be blocked.

Imperatively, this receptor is overexpressed in up to 90% of HNSCC and has been associated with reduced survival [38-40]. Multiple studies reported on the potential roles of EGFR in monitoring response, predict survival, reducing the morbidity related effects, and improved prognosis. Accumulating evidence has contributed to the evaluation of EGFR pathways and their signaling cascades and the potential agents that can be combined with the current therapeutic approach in the armamentarium management of head and neck malignancy [11]. Cetuximab, Trastuzumab, Panitumumab, Olipamuzumab are examples of EGFR receptor antibodies that have been extensively studied. Cetuximab is a chimeric monoclonal IgG1 subclass antibody binds to the EGFR extracellular domain with a higher affinity [11]. Apart from the growth factor receptors, another interesting group biomarker in the immune-mediated inflammatory ecosystem that is of promising high values is the immune checkpoint inhibitors.

In reality, immunotherapy was revolutionized by the development of immune checkpoint inhibitors. The immune checkpoint inhibitors (ICIs) have transformed the treatment landscape of head and neck malignancy and other human solid malignancies. Immune checkpoint proteins are physiologically responsible for regulating immune tolerance and preventing excessive immune injury. Tumor-induced immune evasion, partially mediated by T cell-suppressive immune checkpoints, is one of the major causes of HNSCC recurrence and metastasis [41]. In recent years, immune checkpoint inhibitors (ICIs) targeting cytotoxic T lymphocyte-associated antigen 4 (CTLA-4) and the programmed cell death protein 1 (PD-1 / PD-L1) pathway have been widely administered and have shown promise in a range of malignancies [41].

In multiple tumor forms, anti-programmed cell death therapy is successful and can offer remarkable clinical advantages with minimal toxicity. Several studies are looking at the potential biomarkers that can predict the tumor response to the ICIs and also the possible adverse reactions [42-44]. By modifying the identified adverse events that are highly linked to ICIs application, a novel effective marker can be developed that can escalate the therapeutic response with minimal or negligible side effects. Since HNSCC 's immune environment is very complex, new immune control point inhibitor applications need to be led by a more detailed understanding [44]. With future research, this brand-new targeted therapy in combination with the inflammatory marker can open up the availability of treatment choices for combatting HNSCC that will transform the whole landscapes of head and neck cancer management.

The head and neck cancer microenvironment is unique. It is characterized by the presence of inflammatory cells, immunosuppressive cytokines, secretory proteins, growth factors receptors, and many more. The cytokines group itself is a major constituent of the tumor microenvironment ecosystem. This family of proteins includes interferons, interleukins, chemokines, tumor necrosis factors, *etc.* Importantly these cytokines regulate cell growth and signaling and modulate cell migration and proliferation. The availability of systemic therapies that able to balance and reverse the immunosuppressive effects of these cytokines holds as a potentially viable therapeutic target. The inflammatory cytokines such as VEGF, IL6, and HGF are found in higher levels in head and neck cancer patients. Numerous studies highlight that these biomarkers are strongly related to disease progression and relapse [45].

ROLE OF INFLAMMATION IN THE APPLICATION OF INVESTIGATION TOOLS OF HEAD AND NECK MALIGNANCY

In the future, some of the inflammatory markers can be combined with imaging like PET scans in order to delineate the active malignant cells. This approach can be highly efficient for detecting recurrent and metastatic diseases very early during the disease process. With the advancement in nanotechnology and artificial intelligence, the assessment of HNSCC will escalate in order to bring out the best possible treatment outcomes. Consequently, head and neck cancer patient's management can be improved, and better survival and prognosis can be attained.

The inflammatory mediators and their response are significant. In addition to playing a critical role in tumor development, such as mediating angiogenesis, inflammatory responses have been shown to play a role in other aspects of cancer progression, such as tissue invasion and metastases. For instance, the application of circulating tumor cells in liquid biopsy can be used in assessing the tumor response by mapping with MRI quantitative imaging [46]. CTCs may present during the diagnosis and circulate in the systemic circulation during the treatment phase. A study by Liu *et al.* investigating the CTCs in hypopharyngeal carcinoma can be used to monitor response to chemoradiation and as a marker for determining progression-free survival and overall survival [47]. Emerging evidence showed numerous technical refinements and molecular characterization of the CTS that can be used as a diagnostic tool of head and neck carcinoma. This will allow the expansion of CTCs clinical applications for personalized treatment approach [48]. A system has been developed based on a microfluidic-based immune capture system, a CytoSorter that can be used to differentiate the malignant locally advanced head and neck cancer from benign disease and for monitoring treatment response and prediction of local recurrence [49].

Angiogenesis itself enhances the vascular invasion of migratory cells. It plays critical steps in malignant cell progression and metastases. The majority of head and neck cancers express angiogenesis factors such as VEGF. Critically, VEGF is associated with patient prognosis [50]. High expression of VEGF is associated with more advanced disease and resistance to traditional cytotoxic agents [51]. Matrix metalloproteases and their antagonists are essential for angiogenesis and the remodeling of the extracellular matrix. Primarily the VEGF influences immune suppression through numerous ways include:

1. Induce programmed death ligand 1 expression
2. Bind to VEGF receptor 1 on myeloid-derived cells
3. Decrease T cell extravasation and adhesions through the vessel wall
4. Increase T reg differentiation [51]

Anti-angiogenesis agents are capable of modulating tumor microenvironment and enhance tumor chemoradiation sensitivity. Several anti-angiogenic agents are in the phase of clinical trials includes bevacizumab, sorafenib, sunitinib, and several larger trials are still underway [52]. The angiogenesis labeled with nanoprobe for instance, can be produced and used as a sophisticated tool to detect malignant mass initiation as well as delivering therapeutic agents simultaneously. This double sword strategy will greatly enhance the management strategy for head and neck malignancy. Other inflammatory markers also possess similar roles and can be modulated to produce a potent agent.

For example, in creating an immunosuppressive tumor environment, stromal cells such as tumor-associated macrophages (TAM) and fibroblasts have a critical function. TAM has both functions as immunostimulatory and immunosup-pressive. TAM activate malignant cell proliferation by stimulating specific signaling pathways. Thus, by knowing the detailed characterization of TAM, it can be regulated and can be used to suppress cancer metastases [53]. The role of PD-L1 and, in particular, PD-L2 in stromal cell tumor permissive function in HPV-positive and HPV-negative HNSCC has not yet been fully understood [54]. The immunomodulators and effectors can be potentially tagged in HPV positive and HPV negative patients in elucidating the consistent markers that can be used for detection as well as monitor the therapeutic response of these patients. Some genetic alterations have been identified in HPV positive oropharyngeal carcinoma with the possibility of application in risk stratifications [55].

EXPLOITING INFLAMMATION FOR THERAPEUTIC AND MANAGEMENT OF HEAD AND NECK MALIGNANCY

At present, there are a number of significant markers that have been studied in the treatment of head and neck cancers in order to gain better treatment response whilst minimizing the treatment-related side effects. Specific inflammatory biomarkers that have gained scientific interest include cytokines, growth factors, angiogenesis factors, microRNAs, circulating tumor cells, and tumor associated macrophages. The roles of these biomarkers in predicting treatment response is critical. Such markers that have been thoroughly examined in head and neck malignancy as prognostic factors include Ki67 proliferative index, hypoxia-inducible factors, apoptotic markers, COX, and other biological tumor markers [40].

Given the substantial toxicity and minimal clinical effectiveness of conventional platinum-based chemotherapy, there is an urgent need for innovative therapeutic methods that can extend the existing HNSCC treatment regime. Numerous significant markers that have been mentioned earlier are of great promise to be used in the future management of head and neck cancer. As such, novel immune markers class can be identified and tailored for developing immune-targeting therapeutic strategies for different subgroups of head and neck malignancy [56]. A novel therapeutic choice has been provided for the development of immune checkpoint inhibitors that may also be useful for recurrent patients. Among the immune checkpoint inhibitors, the PD-1 / PD-L1 and CTLA-4 have shown promising therapeutic results [57]. Clinical studies have already shown that, when used to treat HNSCC patients, anti-PD-1 / PD-L1 therapy provides antitumor activity and it has a reasonable safety profile [44]. As the incidence of HPV driven HNSCC is on the rise, the magnitude of these new therapeutic agents in the management armamentarium of HNSCC is monumental. The development of the HPV vaccine in combination with immune checkpoint inhibitors is in phase II clinical trial with a positive response [58]. A multiplexed panel of serum biomarkers may present a promising new approach for the early detection of head and neck cancer. an expanded panel comprised of multiple cytokines, chemokines, growth factors, and other tumor markers, which individually may show some promising correlation with disease status, might provide higher diagnostic power if used in combination. Thus, we evaluated a novel multianalyte Lab-MAP profiling technology that allows simultaneous measurement of multiple serum biomarkers [59].

In HNSCC patients, current immuno-oncology therapies will show considerable effectiveness and induce long-term remission. In selected cases, despite multimodality treatment regimes, the issues of radioresistance impair the desired treatment outcomes. Given that the majority of squamous cell carcinomas of the head and neck (HNSCC) are characterized by aggressive local invasion and poor prognosis overall, the radioresistance added to the complexity of the treatment regime and expected outcomes. Both the disease and its treatment resulted in substantial patient morbidities in addition to increasing mortality rates. Indeed, treatments for HNSCC patients often affect an individual's most personal attributes, including facial appearance and the ability to eat and talk [60]. Hence in coming years with the expansion of immune-targeted therapy, nanotechnology, and artificial intelligence, it might be possible that the treatment will be non-surgery orientated. The patients can safely consume the tablets or having injections as a potential treatment of their tumors, replacing the surgery and avoiding the dreadful complications from the surgery. This is a highly promising avenue for global advancement in drug therapeutics.

For example, the most commonly studied salivary proteins in salivary gland malignancy are EGF, interleukin 6 and 8, and other NFaB-derived components such as TNFa or interleukin 1β, interleukin 4 and 10, and VEGF [61]. These inflammatory markers have critical immunomodulation effects that can be used to develop agents or sensors that able to detect these biomarkers and predict the treatment response, prognosis and risk of tumor recurrence. Saliva screening in the form of liquid biopsy is a non-invasive approach. This can be developed based on the presence and changes of the mentioned biomarkers may be used to show the local effects of ionizing radiation on the cancer tissue. Of note, salivary cytokines have promising features to be used as biomarkers for upper aerodiges-

tive tract cancer screening, as it is easy to perform, does not require many instruments and can be performed in the outpatient clinic setting.

In oral cavity cancer, studies have also shown that certain pro-inflammatory cytokines, such as TNF-alpha, IL-1alpha, IL-6, IL-8, granulocyte-macrophage colony-stimulating factor (GM-CSF), and VEGF, are found to be significantly elevated in the tumor microenvironment [61]. Epstain *et al.* found that in the first weeks of RT treatment, saliva volume and total EGF production decreased dramatically and continued to decrease during the therapy. The content of inflammatory-related immune markers can be utilized to monitor response to radiations or risk of radiation-related toxicity.

The response to radiotherapy can vary greatly among individuals. Biomarkers of radiosensitivity, whether intrinsic or from hypoxia, would move radiation oncology from precision medicine to precise, personalized medicine. Identifying hypoxic mediated biomarkers can serve as critical modifiers to enhance the radiation effects of malignant cells killing log. EGFR amplification status, in combination with gene expression profiling, may serve as a predictive biomarker for personalized interventional strategies of combined treatment like cetuximab and fractionated radiotherapy. Koi *et al.* studying *in vivo* and *ex vivo* the effect of fractionated irradiation and EGFR inhibition and revealed that the local tumor control and tumor growth were correlated with potential biomarkers. These include the EGFR gene amplification and radioresponse-associated gene expression profiles [62]. The combination of intratumoral EGFR-AS, cetuximab, and intensity-modulated radiation was well tolerated and associated with promising local control in selected head and neck cancer patients [63].

Many salivary cytokines can be affected by radiation or chemoradiation therapy and, therefore, salivary cytokine analysis may be a useful biomarker for predicting the outcome of radiotherapy in HNC [64]. The hematological inflammatory markers such as the neutrophil-to-lymphocyte ratio (NLR), the C-reactive protein (CRP), albumin ratio (CAR), and the platelet-to-lymphocyte ratio (PLR) have been investigated in predicting the treatment side-effects [65]. The CRP can serve as a dual prognostic predictor in solid tumors. Acute-phase proteins may also be useful to identify patients at risk of developing severe immune-mediated toxicity after anticancer immunotherapy. Recent studies also suggest that biomarker profiles as well as alternative inflammatory mediators should be further developed to optimize the predictive utility in cancer patients [66].

MARKERS OF PROMISE FOR EFFECTIVE FOLLOW UP REGIMES

The majority of aforementioned markers are potential to be used during follow up

head and neck cancer patients at the outpatient clinic setting. The characteristics of such markers include:

1. Easy to detect
2. A low false negative value
3. Stable through post-treatment period.
4. Does not influence by other medications
5. Present in higher concentration

Importantly, the availability of noninvasive and effective methods of detection is vital. These can be in the form of blood collection tools, needles for tissue collection, or salivary collection devices. These will ensure a good, safe, and ease of practice at the follow-up clinics. The assisting health personnel and nurses should also be exposed and well versed with the tool storage, specimen collection, and transportation of specimens to the related laboratories.

Recently, with the substantial rise of HPV-positive oropharyngeal cancers, the collection of blood, tissue, or saliva of affected patients *via* sophisticated gadgets and devices will allow a better treatment strategy for this subset of patients. Early diagnosis can be made, and tailored personalized treatment can be instituted. With the development of biomarkers as discussed previously, the treatment-related complications can also be minimized. There are various HPV biomarkers, which include HPV DNA, and serological markers like HPV 16 L1 antibodies, capsid protein viruses, or oncoprotein expressions [66]. The combined HPV DNA status assessment and overexpression of p16INK4a may serve as an accurate surrogate marker for biologically active HPV infection during follow-up schemes [67].

Although one of the hallmarks of cancer is evading anti-cancer immunity, immunotherapy, also harnesses the immune system's power to destroy cancer cells. Despite the recent 'Immunotherapy tsunami in oncology' and numerous studies of immunotherapy treatment resulting in almost miracle cures in cases of extremely refractory cancers, these therapies are for selected patient's group only [60]. Now with the advent of biomolecular markers and gene profiling, the immune-targeted therapies can be expanded to the majority of head and neck cancer patients.

Currently, clinical methods such as biopsy, vital tissue staining, and exfoliative cytology are used only by small groups of patients and have significant limitations. In the setting of oral cancers, the development of devices such as the Oral Fluid Nano Sensor Test (OFNASET) platform would make diagnostic technology for saliva simple to use and can be effectively applied during outpatient clinic review [45]. Compared with other physiological fluids (*i.e.*, blood, urine, *etc.*), bioinformatic analysis of RNA-Seq data showed a special property of saliva because it contains significant quantities of bacterial RNA-Seq reads [69]. As aforementioned, Epidermal growth factor receptor (EGFR) protein, as well as mRNA are reported to be overexpressed in 40% to 90% of head and neck squamous cell carcinomas (HNSCC), which is correlated to increased tumor growth and metastasis, poor prognosis, and resistance to chemotherapy and radiotherapy [69]. Cetuximab is a chimeric human-murine immunoglobulin monoclonal antibody that can bind to EGFR with similar affinity to its natural ligands (EGF and TGFα) and prevent activation of downstream signaling pathways. EGFR protein expression is detected in >90% of all SCCHN tumors. In addition, high levels of EGFR protein expression and increased *EGFR* gene copy numbers are associated with decreased survival, resistance to radiotherapy, locoregional treatment failure, and increased rates of distant metastases [5].

In phase II and III clinical trials for the treatment of SCCHN, multiple novel agents targeting the ErbB / HER receptor family are being tested (Table 1).

Table 1 **Example of immune targeted therapy in head and neck cancer.**

S. No.	Drugs/Agent	Action Target	Method of Administration
1.	Panitumumab	Fully human anti-EGFR mAb	Intravenous (IV)
2.	Nimotuzumab	Humanized anti- EGFR mAb	Intravenous (IV)
3.	Zalutumumab	Fully human anti- EGFR mAb	Per Oral (PO)
4.	Gefitinib	Reversible, small- molecule EGFR-TKI	Per Oral (PO)
5.	Erlotinib	Reversible, small- molecule EGFR TKI	Per Oral (PO)
6.	Lapatinib	Reversibl, small- molecule EGFR/ErbB2 TKI	Per Oral (PO)
7.	Afatinib	Irreversible, small- molecule ErbB family inhibitor	Per Oral (PO)
8.	PF- 00299804	Irreversible, small- molecule pan-HE-TKI	Per Oral (PO)

(Modified from Agulnik M. New approaches to EGFR inhibition for locally advanced or metastatic squamous cell carcinoma of the head and neck (SCCHN). Med Oncol. 2012;29(4): 2481–2491).

FUTURE PROSPECT OF APPLICATION OF INFLAMMATORY MARKERS IN HEAD AND NECK MALIGNANCY TREATMENT

The emergence of myriad's effective biomarkers for head and neck malignancy is vital in order to improve treatment outcomes of HNSCC patients. At present, we have seen big data and experience exponential growth in the technology that will ultimately assist in the discovery of new promising markers and ensure the existing markers able to be applied at the local hospitals and other community health settings. A multidisciplinary team comprised of committed scientists, clinicians, laboratory personnel, postgraduate students, paramedics, and other related health individuals is crucial for continuing work in progress in the arena of oncology and medicine. Giving the current momentum in scientific research and the need for optimum patient treatment, the discovery of versatile biomarkers that easy to use, widely available, inexpensive, cost-effective is highly possible. Subsequently, this will improve the patient's management, prognosis, and quality of life.

Immunotherapy studies for patients with HPV-positive and HPV-negative subtypes are underway. Treatment strategies aim to take advantage of special viral-specific tumor antigens, the oncogenic protein E6 and E7, and the EBV DNA and proteins of the patient with oropharyngeal cancer [70]. Improved immunotherapy and de-escalation of chemoradiation combination hold a great promise for future targeted therapy for head and neck malignancy.

Adoptive T-cell transfer, which utilizes *in vitro* genetically modified autologous tumor-infiltrating T-lymphocytes has demonstrated compelling activity, is another immunotherapeutic HPV-related method [70]. Different combination methods representing a feasible treatment choice are currently being studied, such as in a phase III study in NPC in which randomized EBV-positive NPC patients undergo either a cytotoxic doublet, gemcitabine plus carboplatin, or the same regimen followed by autologous EBV-specific T-lymphocyte reinfusion [70]. This is an example of the potential expansion of immune-targeted therapies in the coming years.

Ipilimumab, the first anti-CTLA-4 antibody, was rapidly introduced into clinical trials and approved in 2011 by the US FDA for the treatment of metastatic melanoma [27]. The nivolumab, pembrolizumab, and durvalumab are currently being investigated, with the EXTREME regimen selected as the comparator arm in several recently opened phase 3 trials EXTREME regimen in the CheckMate 651 trial [4, 71]. Salivary exRNA has specific properties and a wide variety of applications and can be further assessed, for instance, the transcript levels, differential gene expression, alternative splicing, functional analysis, gene fusion detections [68]. Microarray technology has also been used to investigate the biological roles of novel genes, for instance, in NPC at various metastatic and clinical levels. According to the comparison of global patterns of gene expression in NPC cell lines of high and low tumorigenic and metastatic diseases, revealed a cohort of genes involved in the cell cycle, apoptosis, metastases, chemokines, and immunomodulation that potentially mediate their differential metastatic characteristics [72].

As the technology continues to evolve, many more advanced techniques, facility and expertise will be made available in the near future. More studies can focus on each of the inflammatory markers in great depth, and with the scientific community engagement and commitment, it will transform the therapeutic management of head and neck cancer to a better level. Of note, these new therapeutic agents should be made available locally at low cost, so that it will benefit the disadvantaged head and neck cancer patients, who mostly come a from the low socioeconomic background.

CONCLUSION

Treating head and neck malignancy is challenging. Despite the spectrum of multimodality treatment approach available, the prognosis of head and neck malignancy patients remains suboptimal, especially those who present with late-stage disease. This is mainly due to the low socioeconomic status of the patient, scarcity of well-equipped treatment facilities, and many other limiting logistic and human factors. The discovery of effective therapeutic agents and biomarkers can ultimately improve patient prognosis, hence survival. In addition, with the usage of a new therapy, the comorbidities from conventional chemoradiation can be reduced. This is the major limiting factor for maintaining a patient's quality of life during treatment and post-treatment of head and neck cancer patients. The new markers can be made widely available with less cost to facilitate an efficient management practice for all patients across the head and neck surgical oncology centers and hospitals globally.

CONSENT FOR PUBLICATION

Not applicable.

CONFLICT OF INTEREST

The author confirmed that the chapter's contents have no conflict of interest.

ACKNOWLEDGEMENTS

Declared none.

REFERENCES

[1]   Gilyoma JM, Rambau PF, Masalu N, Kayange NM, Chalya PL. Head and neck cancers: a clinico-pathological profile and management challenges in a resource-limited setting. BMC Res Notes 2015; 8: 772.[http://dx.doi.org/10.1186/s13104-015-1773-9] [PMID: 26654449]

[2]   Sanderson RJ, Ironside JA. Squamous cell carcinomas of the head and neck. BMJ 2002; 325(7368): 822-7.[http://dx.doi.org/10.1136/bmj.325.7368.822] [PMID: 12376446]

[3]   Guidi A, Codecà C, Ferrari D. Chemotherapy and immunotherapy for recurrent and metastatic head and neck cancer: a systematic review. Med Oncol 2018; 35(3): 37.[http://dx.doi.org/10.1007/s12032-018-1096-5] [PMID: 29441454]

[4]   Argiris A, Harrington KJ, Tahara M, *et al.* Evidence-based treatment options in recurrent and/or metastatic squamous cell carcinoma of the head and neck. Front Oncol 2017; 7: 72.[http://dx.doi.org/10.3389/fonc.2017.00072] [PMID: 28536670]

[5]   Szturz P, Vermorken JB. Immunotherapy in head and neck cancer: aiming at EXTREME precision. BMC Med 2017; 15(1): 110.[http://dx.doi.org/10.1186/s12916-017-0879-4] [PMID: 28571578]

[6]   Saada-Bouzid E, Peyrade F, Guigay J. Immunotherapy in recurrent and or metastatic squamous cell carcinoma of the head and neck. Curr Opin Oncol 2019; 31(3): 146-51.[http://dx.doi.org/10.1097/CCO.0000000000000522] [PMID: 30893146]

[7]   Saba NF, Chen ZG, Haigentz M, *et al.* Targeting the egfr and immune pathways in squamous cell carcinoma of the head and neck (scchn): forging a new alliance. Mol Cancer Ther 2019; 18(11): 1909-15.[http://dx.doi.org/10.1158/1535-7163.MCT-19-0214] [PMID: 31676542]

[8]   Agarwal V, Subash A, Nayar RC, Rao V. Is EGFR really a therapeutic target in head and neck cancers? J Surg Oncol 2019; 119(6): 685-6.[http://dx.doi.org/10.1002/jso.25387] [PMID: 30701564]

[9]   Nair S, Trummell HQ, Rajbhandari R, *et al.* Novel EGFR ectodomain mutations associated with ligand-independent activation and cetuximab resistance in head and neck cancer. PLoS One 2020; 15(2): e0229077.[http://dx.doi.org/10.1371/journal.pone.0229077] [PMID: 32069320]

[10]   Iannelli F, Zotti AI, Roca MS, *et al.* Valproic acid synergizes with cisplatin and cetuximab *in vitro* and *in vivo* in head and neck cancer by targeting the mechanisms of resistance. Front Cell Dev Biol 2020; 8: 732.[http://dx.doi.org/10.3389/fcell.2020.00732] [PMID: 33015030]

[11]   Taberna M, Oliva M, Mesía R. Cetuximab-containing combinations in locally advanced and recurrent or metastatic head and neck squamous cell carcinoma. Front Oncol 2019; 9: 383.[http://dx.doi.org/10.3389/fonc.2019.00383] [PMID: 31165040]

[12]   Ahmad P, Sana J, Slavik M, Slampa P, Smilek P, Slaby O. MicroRNAs involvement in radioresistance of head and neck cancer. Dis Markers 2017; 2017: 8245345.[http://dx.doi.org/10.1155/2017/8245345] [PMID: 28325958]

[13]   Huang W, Liu J, Hu S, *et al.* miR-181a upregulation promotes radioresistance of nasopharyngeal carcinoma by targeting RKIP. OncoTargets Ther 2019; 12: 10873-84.[http://dx.doi.org/10.2147/OTT.S228800] [PMID: 31849491]

[14]   Huang W, Shi G, Yong Z, *et al.* Downregulation of RKIP promotes radioresistance of nasopharyngeal carcinoma by activating NRF2/NQO1 axis *via* downregulating miR-450b-5p. Cell Death Dis 2020; 11(7): 504.[http://dx.doi.org/10.1038/s41419-020-2695-6] [PMID: 32632129]

[15]   Li MY, Liu JQ, Chen DP, *et al.* Radiotherapy induces cell cycle arrest and cell apoptosis in nasopharyngeal carcinoma *via* the ATM and Smad pathways. Cancer Biol Ther 2017; 18(9): 681-93.[http://dx.doi.org/10.1080/15384047.2017.1360442] [PMID: 28799829]

[16]   Wen Y, Grandis JR. Emerging drugs for head and neck cancer. Expert Opin Emerg Drugs 2015; 20(2): 313-29.[http://dx.doi.org/10.1517/14728214.2015.1031653] [PMID: 25826749]

[17]   Byeon HK, Ku M, Yang J. Beyond EGFR inhibition: multilateral combat strategies to stop the progression of head and neck cancer. Exp Mol Med 2019; 51(1): 1-14.[http://dx.doi.org/10.1038/s12276-018-0202-2] [PMID: 30700700]

[18]   Rong C, Muller MF, Xiang F, *et al.* Adaptive ERK signalling activation in response to therapy and in silico prognostic evaluation of EGFR-MAPK in HNSCC. Br J Cancer 2020; 123(2): 288-97.[http://dx.doi.org/10.1038/s41416-020-0892-9] [PMID: 32424150]

[19]   Concu R, Cordeiro MNDS. Cetuximab and the head and neck squamous cell cancer. Curr Top Med Chem 2018; 18(3): 192-8.[http://dx.doi.org/10.2174/1568026618666180112162412] [PMID: 29332581]

[20]   Gildener-Leapman N, Ferris RL, Bauman JE. Promising systemic immunotherapies in head and neck squamous cell carcinoma. Oral Oncol 2013; 49(12): 1089-96.[http://dx.doi.org/10.1016/j.oraloncology.2013.09.009] [PMID: 24126223]

[21]   Gillison ML, Trotti AM, Harris J, *et al.* Radiotherapy plus cetuximab or cisplatin in human papillomavirus-positive oropharyngeal cancer (NRG Oncology RTOG 1016): a randomised, multicentre, non-inferiority trial. Lancet 2019; 393(10166): 40-50. [published correction appears in Lancet. 2020 Mar 7;395(10226):784].[http://dx.doi.org/10.1016/S0140-6736(18)32779-X] [PMID: 30449625]

[22]   Mehanna H, Robinson M, Hartley A, *et al.* De-escalate hpv trial groupRadiotherapy plus cisplatin or cetuximab in low-risk human papillomavirus-positive oropharyngeal cancer (De-ESCALaTE HPV): an open-label randomised controlled phase 3 trial. Lancet 2019; 393(10166): 51-60.[http://dx.doi.org/10.1016/S0140-6736(18)32752-1] [PMID: 30449623]

[23]   Jones DA, Mistry P, Dalby M. Concurrent cisplatin or cetuximab with radiotherapy for HPV-positive

84

oropharyngeal cancer: Medical resource use, costs, and quality-adjusted survival from the De-ESCALaTE HPV trial. Eur J Cancer 2020; 124: 178-85.

[24] Heath BR, Michmerhuizen NL, Donnelly CR, *et al.* Head and neck cancer immunotherapy beyond the checkpoint blockade. J Dent Res 2019; 98(10): 1073-80.[http://dx.doi.org/10.1177/0022034519864112] [PMID: 31340724]

[25] Novoplansky O, Fury M, Prasad M, *et al.* MET activation confers resistance to cetuximab, and prevents HER2 and HER3 upregulation in head and neck cancer. Int J Cancer 2019; 145(3): 748-62.[http://dx.doi.org/10.1002/ijc.32170] [PMID: 30694565]

[26] Solomon B, Young RJ, Rischin D. Head and neck squamous cell carcinoma: Genomics and emerging biomarkers for immunomodulatory cancer treatments. Semin Cancer Biol 2018; 52(Pt 2): 228-40.[http://dx.doi.org/10.1016/j.semcancer.2018.01.008] [PMID: 29355614]

[27] Boscolo-Rizzo P, Del Mistro A, Bussu F, *et al.* New insights into human papillomavirus-associated head and neck squamous cell carcinoma. Acta Otorhinolaryngol 2013; 33(2): 77-87.[PMID: 23853396]

[28] Szturz P, Wouters K, Kiyota N, *et al.* Weekly low-dose *versus* three-weekly high-dose cisplatin for concurrent chemoradiation in locoregionally advanced non-nasopharyngeal head and neck cancer: a systematic review and meta-analysis of aggregate data. Oncologist 2017; 22(9): 1056-66.[http://dx.doi.org/10.1634/theoncologist.2017-0015] [PMID: 28533474]

[29] Mandal R, Şenbabaoğlu Y, Desrichard A, *et al.* The head and neck cancer immune landscape and its immunotherapeutic implications. JCI Insight 2016; 1(17): e89829.[http://dx.doi.org/10.1172/jci.insight.89829] [PMID: 27777979]

[30] Faden DL, Ding F, Lin Y, *et al.* APOBEC mutagenesis is tightly linked to the immune landscape and immunotherapy biomarkers in head and neck squamous cell carcinoma. Oral Oncol 2019; 96: 140-7.[http://dx.doi.org/10.1016/j.oraloncology.2019.07.020] [PMID: 31422205]

[31] Takahashi H, Sakakura K, Kudo T, *et al.* Cancer-associated fibroblasts promote an immunosuppressive microenvironment through the induction and accumulation of protumoral macrophages. Oncotarget 2017; 8(5): 8633-47.[http://dx.doi.org/10.18632/oncotarget.14374] [PMID: 28052009]

[32] New J, Arnold L, Ananth M, *et al.* Secretory autophagy in cancer-associated fibroblasts promotes head and neck cancer progression and offers a novel therapeutic target. Cancer Res 2017; 77(23): 6679-91.[http://dx.doi.org/10.1158/0008-5472.CAN-17-1077] [PMID: 28972076]

[33] Irani S, Barati I, Badiei M. Periodontitis and oral cancer - current concepts of the etiopathogenesis. Oncol Rev 2020; 14(1): 465.[http://dx.doi.org/10.4081/oncol.2020.465] [PMID: 32231765]

[34] Huang YH, Chang CY, Kuo YZ, *et al.* Cancer-associated fibroblast-derived interleukin-1β activates protumor C-C motif chemokine ligand 22 signaling in head and neck cancer. Cancer Sci 2019; 110(9): 2783-93.[http://dx.doi.org/10.1111/cas.14135] [PMID: 31325403]

[35] Qin X, Yan M, Wang X, *et al.* Cancer-associated fibroblast-derived il-6 promotes head and neck cancer progression *via* the osteopontin-nf-kappa b signaling pathway. Theranostics 2018; 8(4): 921-40.[http://dx.doi.org/10.7150/thno.22182] [PMID: 29463991]

[36] Bossi P, Resteghini C, Paielli N, Licitra L, Pilotti S, Perrone F. Prognostic and predictive value of EGFR in head and neck squamous cell carcinoma. Oncotarget 2016; 7(45): 74362-79.[http://dx.doi.org/10.18632/oncotarget.11413] [PMID: 27556186]

[37] Alterio D, Marvaso G, Maffini F, *et al.* Role of EGFR as prognostic factor in head and neck cancer patients treated with surgery and postoperative radiotherapy: proposal of a new approach behind the EGFR overexpression. Med Oncol 2017; 34(6): 107.[http://dx.doi.org/10.1007/s12032-017-0965-7] [PMID: 28452036]

[38] Stegeman H, Kaanders JH, van der Kogel AJ, *et al.* Predictive value of hypoxia, proliferation and tyrosine kinase receptors for EGFR-inhibition and radiotherapy sensitivity in head and neck cancer models. Radiother Oncol 2013; 106(3): 383-9.[http://dx.doi.org/10.1016/j.radonc.2013.02.001] [PMID: 23453541]

[39] Wang H, Mustafa A, Liu S, *et al.* Immune checkpoint inhibitor toxicity in head and neck cancer: from identification to management. Front Pharmacol 2019; 10: 1254.[http://dx.doi.org/10.3389/fphar.2019.01254] [PMID: 31708780]

[40] Yao L, Jia G, Lu L, Bao Y, Ma W. Factors affecting tumor responders and predictive biomarkers of toxicities in cancer patients treated with immune checkpoint inhibitors. Int Immunopharmacol 2020; 85: 106628.[http://dx.doi.org/10.1016/j.intimp.2020.106628] [PMID: 32474388]

[41] Nakamura Y. Biomarkers for immune checkpoint inhibitor-mediated tumor response and adverse events. Front Med (Lausanne) 2019; 6: 119.[http://dx.doi.org/10.3389/fmed.2019.00119] [PMID: 31192215]

[42] Fan Y, Geng Y, Shen L, Zhang Z. Advances on immune-related adverse events associated with immune

checkpoint inhibitors. Front Med 2020. [published online ahead of print, 2020 Aug 10].[http://dx.doi.org/10.1007/s11684-019-0735-3] [PMID: 32779094]

[43] Zhou X, Yao Z, Yang H, Liang N, Zhang X, Zhang F. Are immune-related adverse events associated with the efficacy of immune checkpoint inhibitors in patients with cancer? A systematic review and meta-analysis. BMC Med 2020; 18(1): 87.[http://dx.doi.org/10.1186/s12916-020-01549-2] [PMID: 32306958]

[44] Wang J, Sun H, Zeng Q, et al. HPV-positive status associated with inflamed immune microenvironment and improved response to anti-PD-1 therapy in head and neck squamous cell carcinoma. Sci Rep 2019; 9(1): 13404.[http://dx.doi.org/10.1038/s41598-019-49771-0] [PMID: 31527697]

[45] Kaczor-Urbanowicz KE, Kim Y, Li F, et al. Novel approaches for bioinformatic analysis of salivary RNA sequencing data for development. Bioinformatics 2018; 34(1): 1-8.[http://dx.doi.org/10.1093/bioinformatics/btx504] [PMID: 28961734]

[46] Ng SP, Bahig H, Wang J, et al. Predicting treatment response based on dual assessment of magnetic resonance imaging kinetics and circulating tumor cells in patients with head and neck cancer (PREDICT-HN): matching 'liquid biopsy' and quantitative tumor modeling. BMC Cancer 2018; 18(1): 903.[http://dx.doi.org/10.1186/s12885-018-4808-5] [PMID: 30231854]

[47] Liu K, Chen N, Wei J, Ma L, Yang S, Zhang X. Clinical significance of circulating tumor cells in patients with locally advanced head and neck squamous cell carcinoma. Oncol Rep 2020; 43(5): 1525-35.[http://dx.doi.org/10.3892/or.2020.7536] [PMID: 32323844]

[48] Tinhofer I, Staudte S. Circulating tumor cells as biomarkers in head and neck cancer: recent advances and future outlook. Expert Rev Mol Diagn 2018; 18(10): 897-906.[http://dx.doi.org/10.1080/14737159.2018.1522251] [PMID: 30199647]

[49] Zheng W, Zhang Y, Guo L, et al. Evaluation of therapeutic efficacy with CytoSorter® circulating tumor cell-capture system in patients with locally advanced head and neck squamous cell carcinoma. Cancer Manag Res 2019; 11: 5857-69.[http://dx.doi.org/10.2147/CMAR.S208409] [PMID: 31303792]

[50] Vassilakopoulou M, Psyrri A, Argiris A. Targeting angiogenesis in head and neck cancer. Oral Oncol 2015; 51(5): 409-15.[http://dx.doi.org/10.1016/j.oraloncology.2015.01.006] [PMID: 25680863]

[51] Micaily I, Johnson J, Argiris A. An update on angiogenesis targeting in head and neck squamous cell carcinoma. Cancers Head Neck 2020; 5: 5.[http://dx.doi.org/10.1186/s41199-020-00051-9] [PMID: 32280512]

[52] Seiwert TY, Cohen EE. Targeting angiogenesis in head and neck cancer. Semin Oncol 2008; 35(3): 274-85.[http://dx.doi.org/10.1053/j.seminoncol.2008.03.005] [PMID: 18544442]

[53] Gao L, Zhang W, Zhong WQ, et al. Tumor associated macrophages induce epithelial to mesenchymal transition via the EGFR/ERK1/2 pathway in head and neck squamous cell carcinoma. Oncol Rep 2018; 40(5): 2558-72.[http://dx.doi.org/10.3892/or.2018.6657] [PMID: 30132555]

[54] Baruah P, Bullenkamp J, Wilson POG, Lee M, Kaski JC, Dumitriu IE. TLR9 mediated tumor-stroma interactions in human papilloma virus (HPV)-positive head and neck squamous cell carcinoma up-regulate PD-L1 and PD-L2. Front Immunol 2019; 10: 1644.[http://dx.doi.org/10.3389/fimmu.2019.01644] [PMID: 31379843]

[55] Dogan S, Xu B, Middha S, et al. Identification of prognostic molecular biomarkers in 157 HPV-positive and HPV-negative squamous cell carcinomas of the oropharynx. Int J Cancer 2019; 145(11): 3152-62.[http://dx.doi.org/10.1002/ijc.32412] [PMID: 31093971]

[56] Chen YP, Wang YQ, Lv JW, et al. Identification and validation of novel microenvironment-based immune molecular subgroups of head and neck squamous cell carcinoma: implications for immunotherapy. Ann Oncol 2019; 30(1): 68-75.[http://dx.doi.org/10.1093/annonc/mdy470] [PMID: 30407504]

[57] Darvin P, Toor SM, Sasidharan Nair V, Elkord E. Immune checkpoint inhibitors: recent progress and potential biomarkers. Exp Mol Med 2018; 50(12): 1-11.[http://dx.doi.org/10.1038/s12276-018-0191-1] [PMID: 30546008]

[58] Massarelli E, William W, Johnson F, et al. Combining immune checkpoint blockade and tumor-specific vaccine for patients with incurable human papillomavirus 16-related cancer: a phase 2 clinical trial. JAMA Oncol 2019; 5(1): 67-73.[http://dx.doi.org/10.1001/jamaoncol.2018.4051] [PMID: 30267032]

[59] Linkov F, Lisovich A, Yurkovetsky Z, et al. Early detection of head and neck cancer: development of a novel screening tool using multiplexed immunobead-based biomarker profiling. Cancer Epidemiol Biomarkers Prev 2007; 16(1): 102-7.[http://dx.doi.org/10.1158/1055-9965.EPI-06-0602] [PMID: 17220337]

[60] Gameiro SF, Ghasemi F, Barrett JW. Treatment-naïve HPV+ head and neck cancers display a T-cell-inflamed phenotype distinct from their HPV- counterparts that has implications for immunotherapy. Oncoimmunology 2018; 7(10): e1498439.

[61] Principe S, Dikova V, Bagán J. Salivary cytokines in patients with head and neck cancer (HNC) treated with radiotherapy. J Clin Exp Dent 2019; 11(11): e1072-7.[http://dx.doi.org/10.4317/jced.56318] [PMID: 31700580]

[62] Koi L, Löck S, Linge A, et al. EGFR-amplification plus gene expression profiling predicts response to combined radiotherapy with EGFR-inhibition: A preclinical trial in 10 HNSCC-tumour-xenograft models. Radiother Oncol 2017; 124(3): 496-503.[http://dx.doi.org/10.1016/j.radonc.2017.07.009] [PMID: 28807520]

[63] Bauman JE, Duvvuri U, Thomas S, et al. Phase 1 study of EGFR-antisense DNA, cetuximab, and radiotherapy in head and neck cancer with preclinical correlatives Cancer 2018; 124(19): 3881-9.[http://dx.doi.org/10.1002/cncr.31651] [PMID: 30291796]

[64] Liang C, Marsit CJ, McClean MD, et al. Biomarkers of HPV in head and neck squamous cell carcinoma. Cancer Res 2012; 72(19): 5004-13.[http://dx.doi.org/10.1158/0008-5472.CAN-11-3277] [PMID: 22991304]

[65] Mikoshiba T, Ozawa H, Saito S, et al. Usefulness of hematological inflammatory markers in predicting severe side-effects from induction chemotherapy in head and neck cancer patients. Anticancer Res 2019; 39(6): 3059-65.[http://dx.doi.org/10.21873/anticanres.13440] [PMID: 31177149]

[66] Aldalwg MAH, Brestovac B. Human papillomavirus associated cancers of the head and neck: an australian perspective. Head Neck Pathol 2017; 11(3): 377-84.[http://dx.doi.org/10.1007/s12105-017-0780-7] [PMID: 28176136]

[67] Brinkmann O, Kastratovic DA, Dimitrijevic MV, et al. Oral squamous cell carcinoma detection by salivary biomarkers in a Serbian population. Oral Oncol 2011; 47(1): 51-5.[http://dx.doi.org/10.1016/j.oraloncology.2010.10.009] [PMID: 21109482]

[68] Ju H, Hu Z, Lu Y, et al. TLR4 activation leads to anti-EGFR therapy resistance in head and neck squamous cell carcinoma. Am J Cancer Res 2020; 10(2): 454-72.[PMID: 32195020]

[69] Agulnik M. New approaches to EGFR inhibition for locally advanced or metastatic squamous cell carcinoma of the head and neck (SCCHN). Med Oncol 2012; 29(4): 2481-91.[http://dx.doi.org/10.1007/s12032-012-0159-2] [PMID: 22252310]

[70] Canning M, Guo G, Yu M, et al. Heterogeneity of the head and neck squamous cell carcinoma immune landscape and its impact on immunotherapy. Front Cell Dev Biol 2019; 7: 52.[http://dx.doi.org/10.3389/fcell.2019.00052] [PMID: 31024913]

[71] Hargadon KM, Johnson CE, Williams CJ. Immune checkpoint blockade therapy for cancer: An overview of FDA-approved immune checkpoint inhibitors. Int Immunopharmacol 2018; 62: 29-39.[http://dx.doi.org/10.1016/j.intimp.2018.06.001] [PMID: 29990692]

[72] Janvilisri T. Omics-based identification of biomarkers for nasopharyngeal carcinoma. Dis Markers 2015; 2015: 762128.[http://dx.doi.org/10.1155/2015/762128] [PMID: 25999660]

www.ingramcontent.com/pod-product-compliance
Lightning Source LLC
Chambersburg PA
CBHW050806220326
41598CB00006B/135